car·bi·vore

\\ˈkär-bə-ˌvȯr\\

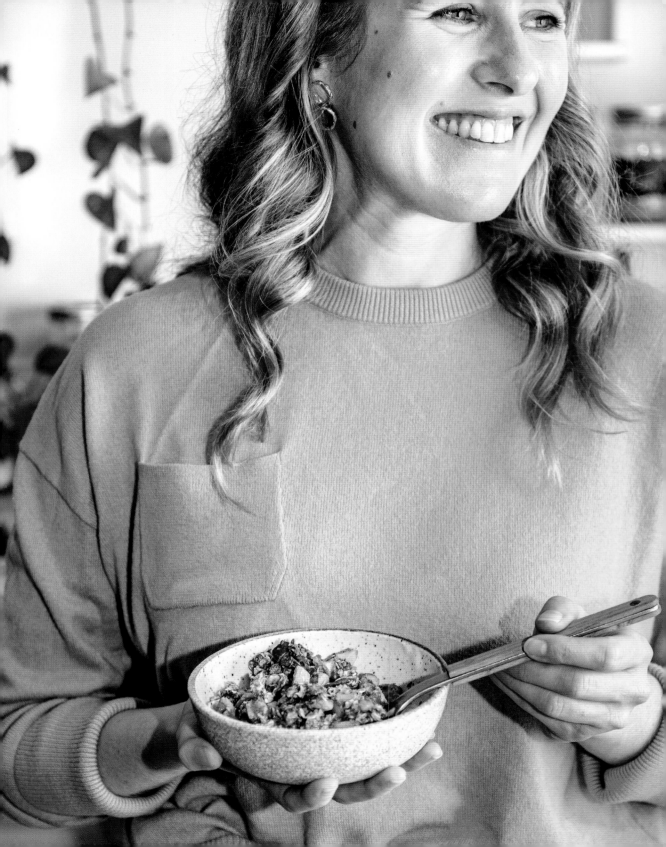

car·bi·vore

\\'kär-bə-,vȯr\\

**130 Healthy Recipes to Stop Fearing
Carbs and Embrace the Comfort
Foods You Love**

PHOEBE LAPINE

Go

hachette
BOOKS

Hachette Go, an imprint of Hachette Books
Hachette Book Group
1290 Avenue of the Americas
New York, NY 10104
HachetteGo.com
Facebook.com/HachetteGo
Instagram.com/HachetteGo

First Edition: March 2024

Hachette Books is a division of Hachette Book Group, Inc. The Hachette Go and Hachette Books name and logos are trademarks of Hachette Book Group, Inc.

The Hachette Speakers Bureau provides a wide range of authors for speaking events. To find out more, go to hachettespeakersbureau.com or email HachetteSpeakers@hbgusa.com.

Hachette Go books may be purchased in bulk for business, educational, or promotional use. For information, please contact your local bookseller or Hachette Book Group Special Markets Department at special.markets@hbgusa.com.

The publisher is not responsible for websites (or their content) that are not owned by the publisher.

Print book interior design by Sheryl Kober

Library of Congress Control Number: 2023011653

ISBNs: 9780306830907 (paper over board); 9780306830914 (ebook)

Printed in China

APS

10 9 8 7 6 5 4 3 2 1

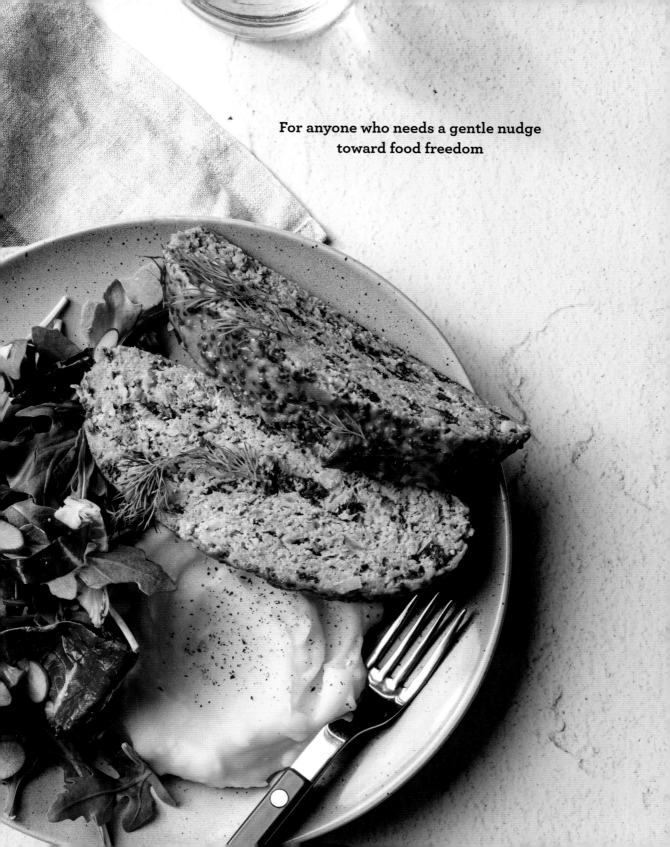

For anyone who needs a gentle nudge
toward food freedom

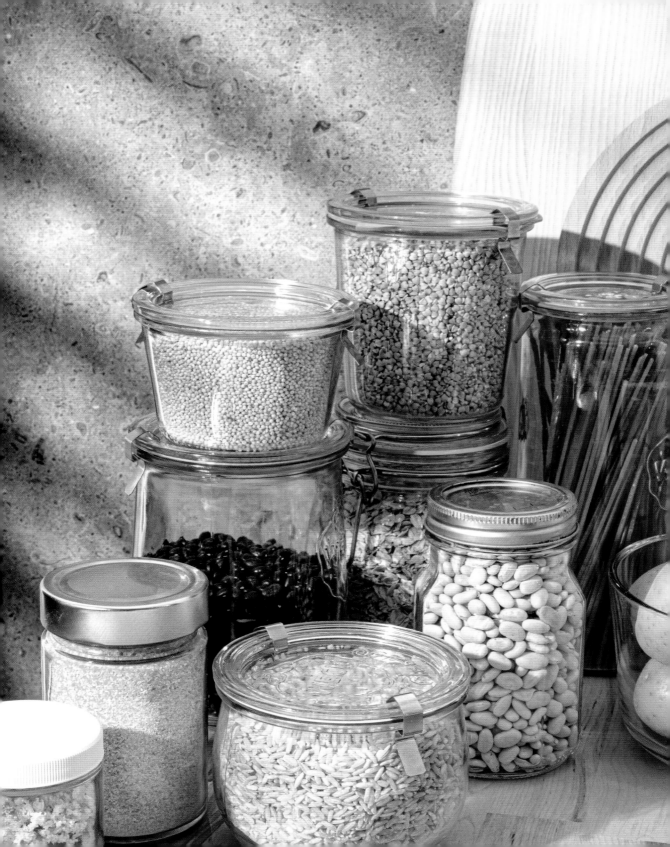

Contents

Introduction **ix**

PART ONE:
TO CARB OR NOT TO CARB
A Carbivore List of Essential Terms **2**

Anatomy of a Carb (& What Happens When It Enters Your Body) **4**

CHAPTER ONE: This Is Your Body on Carbs **7**

CHAPTER TWO: How to Have Your Cake & Eat It Too **19**

CHAPTER THREE: Cooking Like a Carbivore **39**

PART TWO:
THE RECIPES
Carb Companions: Sauces, Condiments, Toppings & Starters **57**

Oats **87**

Rice **115**

Whole Grains from Around the World **141**

Noodles **171**

Spuds **203**

Loaves & Crusts **235**

Corn **267**

Legumes **297**

Recipe Index by Type **326**

Acknowledgments **329**

Resources **330**

Notes **332**

Index **333**

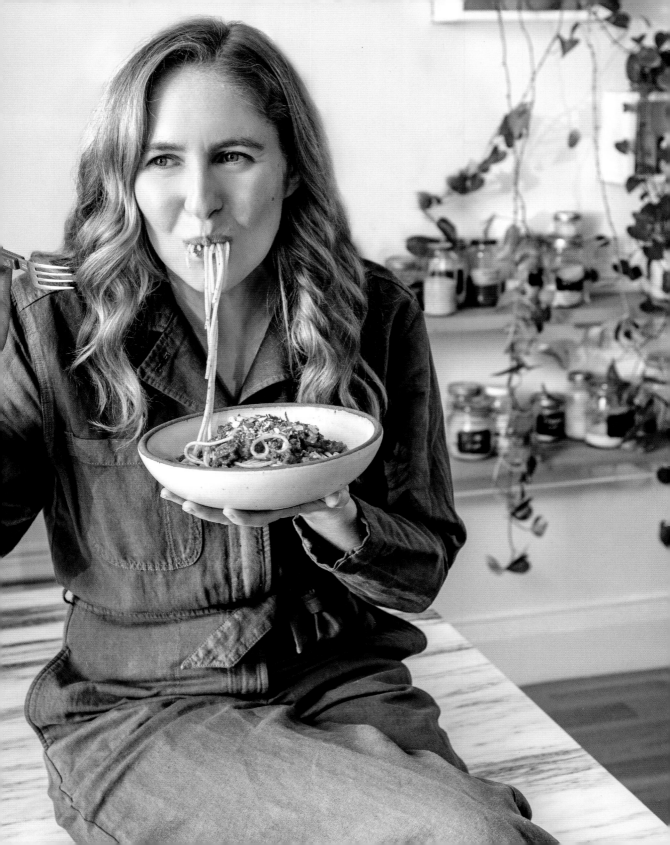

Introduction

If you asked me to describe my desert island meal, it would be something along the lines of what the author David Sedaris answered to a similar interview question: I'd like pasta, served on a plate made entirely of pasta, with shaved pasta on top. I might even add a set of french fry flatware to eat it with and a napkin knit from tiny strands of ramen with which to dab my salivating mouth.

Though I've never actually eaten this fantasy meal, it is safe to say that carbs and I have had a torrid love affair over the years. Sometimes my attraction is healthy, sometimes it's not. In the moment, that pile of spaghetti can make me feel so warm, comforted, and taken care of. But friends (and medical professionals) warn that it's a one-sided entanglement with toxic long-term consequences. One day, at the end of our honeymoon, carbs will leave me at the bottom of Health Mountain and I'll have no choice but to walk back up it again all alone.

I've found myself in this exact position once before. When I was twenty-two, I was diagnosed with the autoimmune disease Hashimoto's thyroiditis. During the years that followed, I transformed from a vibrant, albeit naïve, young professional who ran four miles a day into a thin-haired, sluggish insomniac who could barely make it up the subway steps. Having just left my corporate job to pursue a career in food, I was terrified of the idea that a change in diet was the key to getting back on my feet. But at the urging of an integrative doctor, I finally agreed to go gluten-free for a short period to see the effect.

This was my first time eliminating a food group, and I experienced both the promise and the pain. It became clear that I had been completely subsisting on wheat—muffins for breakfast, sandwiches for lunch, pasta or pizza for dinner. Once my mind got through the first few stages of grief, I opened my eyes to the transformation my body was experiencing. All my symptoms—the fatigue, skin rashes, weight fluctuations, gut problems—were dialed down to a much more manageable volume. So, I stayed off gluten and never looked back.

Except that wasn't the end to my carb confusion.

I kept getting conflicting advice from doctors. Some said it was dangerous for women to be super low carb; others said I hadn't gone far enough—strict approaches like the autoimmune paleo plan were the only way to get thyroid antibodies under control. The same pushing of ultra-low-carb approaches came up again as I dealt with my next health hurdle: SIBO, small intestinal bacterial overgrowth. Some said you couldn't heal the gut without taking out all grains; others said that removing them would be detrimental to the long-term health of my microbiome.

Meanwhile, disaffected former keto-philes kept knocking on my virtual door. These were people who had also experienced the highs and lows of a restrictive diet and, ultimately, found themselves belly-up by the side of the road as the wagon full of cheese and meat sticks sped away. Like many of my readers, they had come to my website, *Feed Me Phoebe*, to find healthy comfort food and a saner way of eating. And to weed out the barrage of conflicting diet information on the internet that ranges from doomsday scientific scare tactics to wishy-washy lore from so-and-so's energy-healer aunt.

My philosophy of "healthy hedonism" has long been my guiding light in and out of the kitchen. I learned the hard way through my elimination diets, autoimmune struggles, and bouts of obsession that **if you're stressing about what you're eating all the time, no amount of kale can make you healthy**. Rather, we all have to find that sweet spot where the things that nourish our body can be offset by the practices (or foods) that feed our spirit. And for some of us, french fries speak to our soul.

Yet, we also know what carbs can do to our blood sugar, and how constant instability can affect every corner of our health. The science has been clear: metabolic issues are the cornerstone of so many modern chronic illnesses, including diabetes, fatty liver disease, polycystic ovary syndrome (PCOS)—potentially Alzheimer's, autoimmune disease, and depression, too.

We also know that the lies we were told in the '90s about fat was misguided. It was the carbs all along.

So, how do we marry these two truths? How do we have a healthier relationship with carbs, embrace being an omnivore, and not ignore the writing on the wall? How do we face this uphill battle with a food industry and production system that seem to be stacked against us? How do we have our cake (or french fries) and eat it too—without the fatigue, insomnia, breakouts, depression, and chronic illness?

That is the goal of this book: to reteach you how macronutrients work in tandem, and how to adjust your habits so they do so in harmony. Common-sense lifestyle changes don't sell books as well as rule-based fad diets, but they are often the backbone of what we need to do to be healthy, be it balancing blood sugar, supporting hormones, or fighting inflammation.

And you can do all these things, believe it or not, while still eating carbs.

•　•　•

Carbivore is a culinary and dietary road map for making a carb-inclusive diet part of a healthy lifestyle and nutritious meal.

The first half of this book, Part One, will up your knowledge base and allow you to strategize how to incorporate carbs into your life. Part Two is dedicated to the recipes that will make it even more delicious.

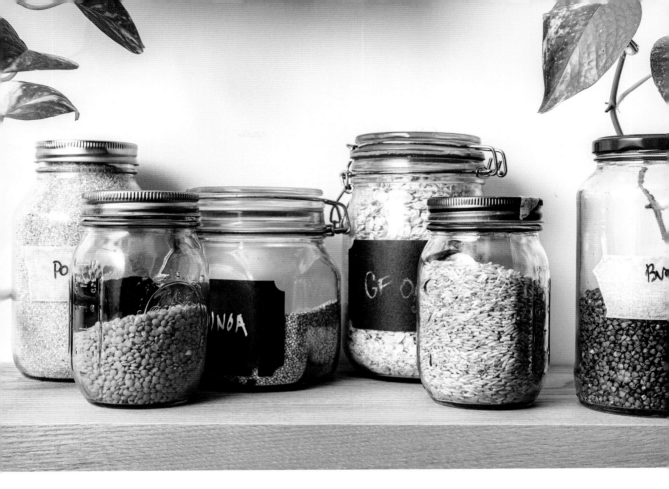

In Chapter 1, we will look at how the body uses and metabolizes carbohydrates, balancing ancient wisdom with existing data on how diet affects gut health, hormone production, and the development or prevention of modern diseases. A hundred years ago, your great-grandparents got more than 50 percent of their nutrients from carbs, and yet the chronic conditions we grapple with today were rare. The rise in global diabetes and other chronic illnesses has become widespread only since the debut of MTV. We will take a deep dive into how our food system has changed since the 1980s, and how the barrage of added sugar has fundamentally changed our collective eating habits.

With this foundation, in Chapter 2, I'll show you how to harness carbs to work better for your body—and not just by changing what's on your plate, but also by improving your stress levels and your sleep. You'll learn about the role of fiber and other "carb companions" to balance blood sugar. By the end of this chapter, you will have a better idea of how to choose your own carb adventure.

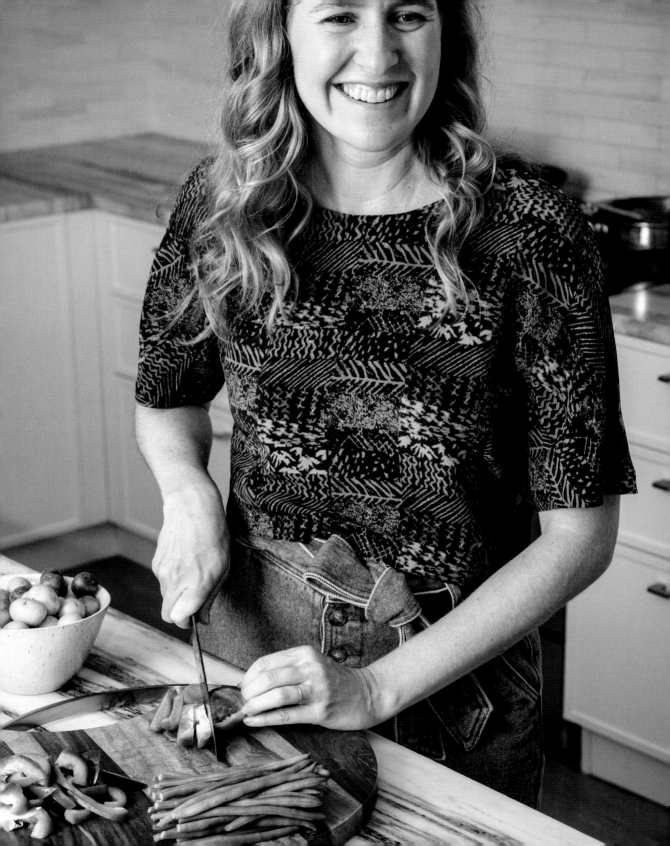

I'll get you prepared to enter your kitchen in Chapter 3 with advice on how to rethink your grocery list with your blood sugar in mind. You'll also learn about the concept of "slow carbs": sprouting grains, sourdough fermentation, and activating resistant starches—ancient practices that have a big impact on metabolism. And I will shine a spotlight on the carb all-stars of this book, teaching you about their origin stories and nutrition content.

Part Two is your carb cookbook with 130+ recipes organized by type of carb: Oats, Rice, Whole Grains from Around the World, Noodles, Spuds, Loaves & Crusts, Corn, and Legumes. The recipes borrow wisdom from the Mediterranean diet and marry them with anti-inflammatory culinary philosophies from across the globe. Every dish is gluten-free because that is my way of eating, but you can easily be a Carbivore and still enjoy wheat. Each recipe has modification advice and labels for a variety of diets, including low-FODMAP. The goal is not to preach one specific approach to food, but to showcase the many ways carbs can be incorporated into a healthy lifestyle, whatever that means to you.

If writing my book on gut health, *SIBO Made Simple*, taught me anything, it's that **what you eat is so much less important than *how* you eat it**. When you eliminate whole food groups—be it fat or carbs or animal protein—fundamentally, you shift the balance on your plate toward something else that might not be good for you in high quantities (animal protein, cheese, sugar, etc.). And more important, it moves you further away from the ultimate goal: a balanced meal.

Striking that balance often isn't possible without acknowledging the elephant in the room: PLEASURE. There is a way to find joy in a pasta dinner and prevent that meal from causing so much chaos in the body. (Not serving it on a plate also made entirely of pasta is a start.) We are coming of age in a post–diet culture where we recognize that whole food groups, like carbs, don't need to be demonized. That food is a product of love and something to be savored. That black-and-white thinking is worse for us than black-and-white cookies.

Carbivore, like a good sourdough starter, will help bake those lessons into a long, healthy life.

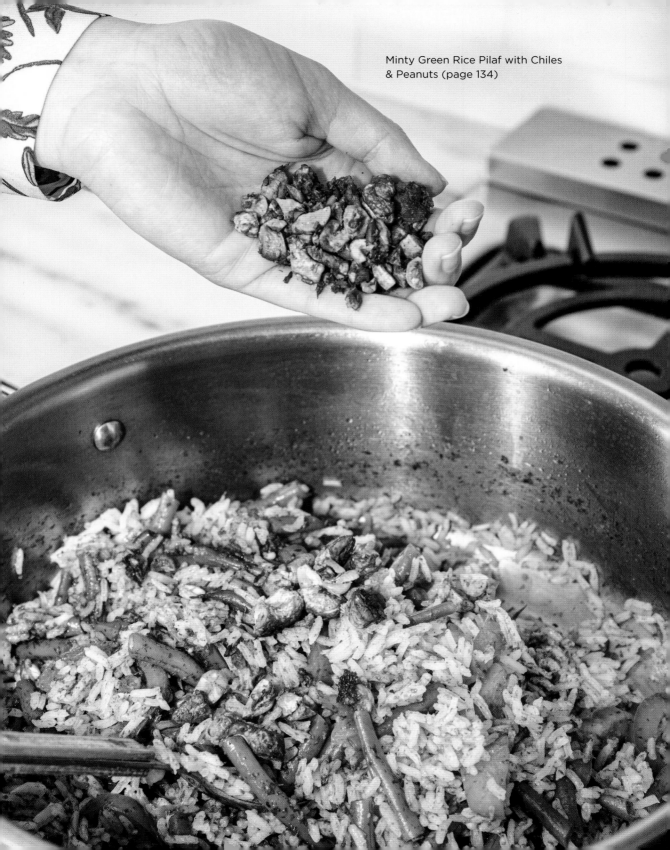

Minty Green Rice Pilaf with Chiles & Peanuts (page 134)

PART ONE

TO CARB OR NOT TO CARB

A Carbivore List of Essential Terms

I'm putting this little glossary up front so we can all get on the same page. Consider it a bare-bones cheat sheet for the most referenced bodily processes, conditions, and building blocks discussed in this book, along with definitions for made-up words like . . . *Carbivore*. Flip back here if you ever feel confused or need a refresher.

BLOOD SUGAR—Another way of saying the amount of glucose in your bloodstream at any given moment.

CARB COMPANION—A whole food with fat, fiber, or protein added to a meal to slow the carbs' roll to your bloodstream.

CARBOHYDRATES—The parent company for all sugars and compounds they create, including starches and fiber.

FASTING GLUCOSE—Your standing blood sugar after fasting for an eight-hour period, usually overnight.

CARB—Colloquial term referring to plants that contain higher ratios of starches or sugars, compared to fiber, and the foods they create. For example, wheat, rice, oats and the pancakes, pastas, and breads they form.

CARBIVORE—Someone who embraces carbs as part of a balanced diet without letting them cause chaos in the body.

CONTINUOUS GLUCOSE MONITOR (CGM)—A small device that attaches to your body and automatically tracks blood glucose levels (blood sugar) throughout the day and night.

FODMAP—An acronym for certain subcategories of carbohydrates (disaccharide, fructose, etc.) that can be digested poorly in the body in high quantities. The low-FODMAP diet is a common therapeutic tool for irritable bowel syndrome (IBS) sufferers.

GLUCOSE SPIKES—When too much sugar (glucose) enters the bloodstream at once (usually after eating) before insulin can be released to bring down those levels and store excess energy as fat.

GLYCEMIC INDEX—A value assigned to foods based on their relationship to our blood glucose levels. Foods low on the GI scale enter the bloodstream slowly. Foods deemed high on the scale cause glucose spikes. The relevance of these values is debatable (see page 25).

HANGER—The cross between hunger and anger, usually as a result of a low-level hypoglycemic event when our mood becomes overly dysregulated and unhinged after a period of not eating.

HIGH FRUCTOSE CORN SYRUP—A cheap alternative sweetener that has twice the sweetness of table sugar due to its higher concentration of fructose versus glucose.

HYPOGLYCEMIA—A common glucose-regulation condition during which blood sugar dips too low after a meal, often as a result of too much insulin being released into the body, that causes us to feel shaky, hungry, and moody.

INSULIN—A hormone produced in the pancreas that controls the amount of glucose in your bloodstream at any given moment. To reduce those glucose levels, insulin's presence tells the liver to store sugar for later.

METABOLISM—The body's process of converting food into energy. Our carbohydrate metabolism involves the formation, breakdown, and conversion of carbohydrates into usable glucose.

MICROBIOME—The community of microorganisms (bacteria and fungi) that inhabits our body, primarily in the large intestine.

RESISTANT STARCH—A type of starch that acts like fiber in that it does not get absorbed by the body and, instead, passes to the large intestine to feed your gut bacteria.

SIBO—An acronym that stands for "small intestinal bacterial overgrowth," an acute condition where normal populations of bacteria begin to colonize too far up the digestive canal, often leading to IBS symptoms.

SLOW CARB—A carb-based meal that hits your bloodstream at a slower pace, allowing you to enjoy your favorite comfort foods without intense glucose spikes.

SUGARS—The group that includes monosaccharides, like glucose and fructose, and their combined form, sucrose (a disaccharide). "Table sugar" refers solely to sucrose.

Anatomy of a Carb
(& What Happens When It Enters Your Body)

Before we dive into the fun stuff, we have to cover some biology basics. Though carbs have become synonymous in everyday conversation with bread, pasta, and cupcakes, the actual macronutrient, *carbohydrate*, is a building block for most of life on earth. You may fancy yourself on a "low-carb diet," but if you were to truly eliminate all carbohydrates, you would also eliminate vegetables and fruits—and exponentially increase your risk of mortality.

Carbohydrates are sugar molecules that your body breaks down into glucose. This is the main source of energy for your body's cells, tissues, and organs. Here's a brief description of how glucose comes together in various clusters—glucose, fructose, sucrose, starch, and fiber—to form the foods we eat.

GLUCOSE

Glucose is the fuel by which all plants are powered. It is a self-made, self-contained energy source in its simplest form. To make it, plants harness solar power to turn carbon dioxide and water into glucose. Just like our wallets would be weighed down if we kept all our usable cash in pennies, **plants combine glucose molecules to save space.** Being industrious, adaptable, and organized living things, instead of jumbling all those tiny particles together in a pile, plants have their own equivalent of Container Store organizers to take that heap and neatly store it under the bed for another season.

FRUCTOSE

If there was one marketing slogan for fructose, it would be *double the pleasure, double the fun.* Like glucose, fructose is a simple sugar, but it has twice the sweetness. Plants use this compound in their fruit as a survival measure. The addictive quality allows theirs seeds to proliferate through the animals that consume, digest, and excrete them. **Fructose is what sets fruits apart from vegetables.** We may seek it out for the sake of pleasure. However, it is not necessary to fuel our cells. A portion of fructose gets converted into glucose in our gut, but the rest is excess.

SUCROSE

One of the aforementioned storage mechanisms for glucose and fructose is sucrose, which is a disaccharide made up of half of each compound. It is like a zip file compression tool for your energy. The resulting molecule is smaller than the sum of its parts. **Sucrose is also what we have come to know as table sugar**—sweeter than pure glucose, but not as sweet as fructose on its own.

STARCH

Long chains of glucose form a "complex carbohydrate" called starch, which is often stored for later in a plant's roots and seeds. Many of the foods we think of as traditional "carbs" are root vegetables, like potatoes and yams, and seed-like grains (from legumes to rice to quinoa), and this is all thanks to their starch content. When we digest starch, enzymes in our saliva and small intestine break it back down into glucose—usable energy. Without the presence of fat, fiber, and protein—as is the case with refined flours—starch can quickly and easily be converted into simple sugars.

FIBER

Another type of complex glucose is fiber. It is found most commonly in leaves, branches, and trunks, which is why, if you're looking for the most fiber-rich vegetable, you can turn toward varieties that have thick stems or stringy, woody leaves, like artichoke, asparagus, or celery. But fiber can be found in all plant matter. Where there are plants in their natural, whole state, there is always fiber. **The percentage of fiber versus starch or sugar is what factors in when we talk about a plant's cost/ benefit.** Fruit has a high ratio of sugar compared to fiber, whereas green vegetables are mostly fiber with a little starch. What we think of as "carbs"—many of the recipe categories in this book—are plants with higher degrees of starch than fiber.

The reason fiber is so important for our overall health, and especially blood sugar, is that although it is made from glucose, **once fiber has formed, it can't be broken down again into energy**. Instead, fiber passes through our digestive tract until it reaches the large intestine, where it becomes fuel for the body's network of hard-working settlers: the beneficial bacteria that make up our microbiome.

These organisms outnumber our own cells three to one and assist in many of our body's essential functions. Needless to say, keeping them happy and well fed fuels our body by extension. Because of this impact, **fiber is one of the most consequential parts of our diet** for aiding digestion, moderating the immune system, and preventing chronic illness—all things a healthy microbiome has been intimately linked to.

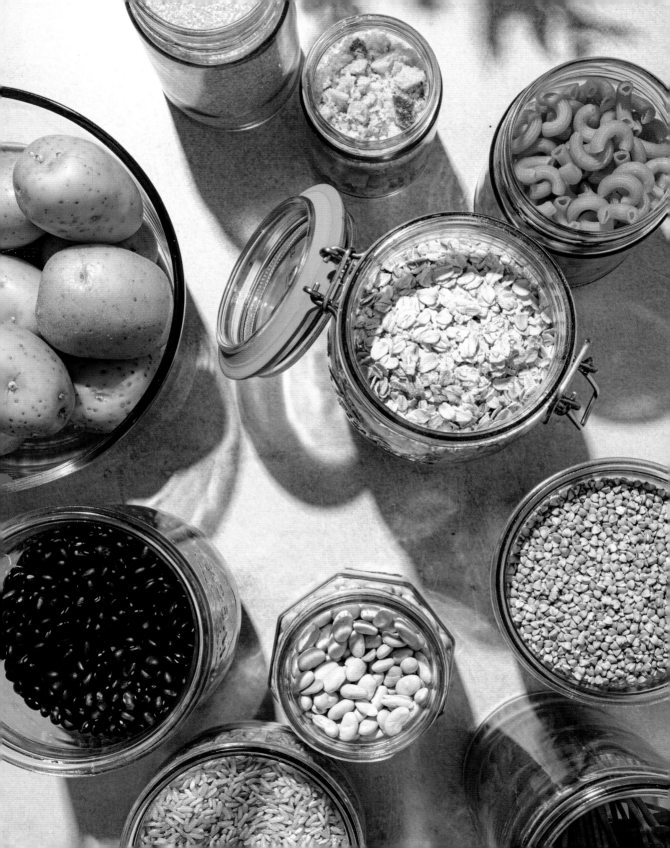

CHAPTER 1

This Is Your Body on Carbs

In many ways, I was a typical '90s kid.

I started my day with a bowl of Honey Nut Cheerios cereal or a Chewy granola bar and ended it with a few low-fat SnackWells cookies from the cupboard. When I reached high school and became more concerned with how I was fitting into my Mavi jeans, I swapped out the whole milk in my syrupy Starbucks caramel macchiato for soy and didn't think twice when I ended up face planting into my math homework by mid-afternoon.

What we know now—thanks to overwhelming scientific evidence—is that the fat-free, high-carb movement that began three decades ago created an epidemic we're still digging our way out of, emotionally and physically. When fat was demonized and removed from packaged food—from our cookies, our milk, our cheese—in came more carbs.

As insulin resistance, weight gain, mental health issues, and chronic illness took hold, the conversation turned to calories. We counted them painstakingly. Soon, chain restaurants were forced to print them on menus. So, we ordered fizzy soda that, despite the 35 grams of sugar, had only 125 calories. And we were taught that a ten-piece order of McDonald's chicken McNuggets had half the calories of a nutrient-dense lentil salad from Le Pain Quotidien.

When diabetes rates continued soaring and autoimmune disease became the leading cause of death in young women, we were told to move more. A calorie in, a calorie out. The problem wasn't the system we lived within, it was simply willpower. And yet, we wondered how we could eat less, when we were already so hungry all the time!

Perhaps we were too distracted by our own (supposed) personal shortcomings that we didn't sense something wasn't adding up. Big food kept chugging, taking us along for the ride. And it took us years to look under the hood and see all the malfunctions.

So why, you ask, am I writing a book promoting carbs when this is the destruction left in their wake?

Because it's not the carbs' fault. Well, not totally.

SUGAR HIDE & SEEK: A MODERN GAME WITH NO WINNERS

Sugar has been used for centuries, not just as a treat, but also as a preservative. By stabilizing the water content in fruits and vegetables, sugar helps prevent or slow the growth of bacteria, mold, and yeast in foods like jam and pickled vegetables. It's the reason whole societies were able to make it through tough winters, and it is still used today in canned foods (think peaches in syrup) for this same purpose.

Similarly, fiber often gets removed to make fresh food last longer on shelves. Whole wheat flour is more likely to spoil than white flour because of the bran. So, slowly, food manufacturers switched to the latter for convenience and longevity.

But stability alone doesn't explain the extreme increase of sugar in packaged foods.

Today, sugar is tucked away on the ingredient labels of **80 percent of products at the supermarket**. This is true regardless of how "high end" your grocery store is, and applies to both commercial brands and those that purport to be gluten-free, healthy, non-GMO, organic, or paleo.

Big food conglomerates have entire science departments dedicated to studying the biology and physiology of our appetites—all for the purpose of learning what combinations of flavors, ingredients, and textures make us eat and buy more food. You might wonder why there is added sugar in sandwich bread, crackers, and peanut butter—savory items that don't need it for any preservative function. It's because the addition of sugar makes a food harder to resist, especially when combined with fat and salt.

Some of us look at the sugar content of ice cream and modify our portions accordingly. But the addition of sugar in foods we don't think of as sweet (along with the elimination of fat, and the stripping away of fiber) drives much of our unconscious consumption—and lack of moderation.

A quality issue, thereby, becomes a quantity issue.

•   •   •

A few generations ago, our ancestors might have been served a few wedges of apple or mango as a snack. And it was savored, knowing additional portions wouldn't be in the cards.

Today, a bag of dried apples or mangoes contains five times that amount of fruit. We eat it in one sitting without thinking twice about the volume of sugar, or even noticing that more sugar has been added in the form of "juice concentrate." It's fruit, right? That's supposed to be the healthy choice.

Unfortunately, the fruit we get our hands on today is so different from what we would find in nature a hundred years ago. It's been domesticated and bred to be sweeter. We eat it by the handful in dried pieces or in small gummies shaped like strawberries. We pack it into smoothies and pouches, and extract its juices to drink with more added sugar.

The result is, we are consuming more sugar, specifically fructose, than ever before. The average American in the early 1900s consumed about forty pounds of added sugar a year. Today, it is more than one hundred pounds.

The American Heart Association recommends that the average woman consume no more than **25 grams (or 6 teaspoons) of added sugar a day; 36 grams or 9 teaspoons for men**. That means my teenage breakfast—a bowl of Honey Nut Cheerios with skim milk—put me at almost the halfway mark for my daily quota. With a sweetened latte added to the mix (33 grams of sugar!), I had been blowing my sugar load (by a lot!) before the day even began.

Like many of you, I had no way of knowing at the time that my erratic energy levels, raging acne, disrupted sleep, insatiable hunger, and unpleasant mood swings could be a result of my diet. My parents certainly didn't think my (occasional) bitchiness was a side effect of anything other than being a teenager!

Knowledge is power to some extent. But when it comes to sugar, it doesn't always make a difference. Despite an iron will in other corners of life, there are few people who can open a bag of candy and eat just one piece. The same goes for a bag of dried mango. Some of us keep eating—not because we don't know better or have no will power, but because it's addictive. **The problem with sugar is that if it's hiding, you will unknowingly seek more.**

ONCE YOU POP, YOU CAN'T STOP

We are hardwired to want sugar.

It's part of our brain's natural survival instinct to make extremely effective, quick energy light up all our pleasure centers. Although other parts of the body (like the intestines) may let you know you've gone overboard after eating a pound of Halloween candy, as far as your brain is concerned, there's no such thing as too much of a good thing. With every hit of dopamine, our brain tells us to get more.

Many researchers have likened the brain on sugar to the brain on hard drugs, like cocaine. One French study found that when given the option, 94 percent of cocaine-addicted rats actually preferred sugar water as their drug of choice.[1] Another study looked at men's brains four hours after a sugary snack and found similar neurological activity to what is seen in drug abusers who need a fix.[2]

Then there is another type of brainwashing: the fact that sugar is, literally, everywhere. There's candy perched at the checkout counter of the gas station, the pharmacy, and even the doctor's office. Seeing these cues can trick your brain into wanting quick energy, even if you aren't hungry.

Although this might sound hopeless, there are elements of this addiction that we can overcome. **Our taste buds are far more adaptable than our brains.** Though our taste buds become increasingly numb to the onslaught of sugar and salt in our everyday meals, they can reset easily once these substances are reduced. The cells on the tongue are constantly turning over and the average lifespan of a taste bud is ten days. That means it takes only a few weeks to deprogram your tongue's love of sugar, even if your brain will never receive the memo.

Though some part of our craving rollercoaster is primal and preprogrammed, our susceptibility to sugar's lure can be decreased, or lit on fire, by many lifestyle factors we'll talk about in Chapter 2—things like your stress levels or sleep. But most important, staying strong in the face of that sugary assault depends on keeping your blood glucose levels steady from the moment you wake up.

ALL ABOARD THE BLOOD SUGAR MOBILE!

Like all animals, we need glucose coursing through our veins to power our entire bodily enterprise. The amount of glucose we need at any given time, though, depends on the amount of activity we're doing. Our blood glucose is generally lowest before the first meal of the day, after fasting overnight. This is called your *fasting glucose*. It is the average needed to keep your organs running on schedule. According to the Centers for Disease Control (CDC), **a fasting blood sugar level of 99 mg/dL or lower is normal**, 100 to 125 mg/dL puts you at risk and is considered prediabetes, and 126 mg/dL or higher indicates you have diabetes.

If you're engaging in an activity that requires more strain on the body—say, a workout or a mad dash to catch the train—more glucose will be brought out of storage and released into the bloodstream to compensate for the additional energy required. This explains why you will sometimes see a blood sugar increase on a continuous glucose monitor after you exercise—especially if you do so on an empty stomach. But the vast majority of the time, blood sugar rises can be tied to a meal.

Just like a car's gas gauge will go up upon refueling, when we eat food, more glucose is introduced to the body. The rate at which that energy hits our bloodstream depends on how complex the carbohydrates that we've eaten are, the efficiency of our digestive organs in breaking them down, and how well our hormones step in as traffic cops to prevent a deluge.

Which brings us back to the subject of added sugar.

The honey in our tea, "fruit juice concentrate" added to dried cranberries, and table sugar sprinkled on oatmeal is all the same thing once it hits your body: some combination of glucose, fructose, or sucrose. Whether the sources are natural or manufactured in a lab, all types of sugar are energy molecules in their simplest form, and on an empty stomach, **can reach your bloodstream within just five minutes of eating them**.

This immediacy might be helpful if you were found lost and starving in the wilderness, but since we know the average American eats one hundred pounds of added sugar a year, most of us rarely experience an energy deficit. Rather, we are dealing with the problems that arise when you have too much of a good thing, all at once.

THE PLIGHT OF MIDDLE MANAGEMENT

The blood sugar rollercoaster will, ultimately, reach its peak about an hour or two after eating. This is when two major digestive workhorses come together to bring down your glucose levels: your liver and your pancreas.

Your liver is the ultimate Cinderella of the digestive system with five hundred chores and not enough hours in the day (or helpful mice interns) to get them all done. Pop science often compares the liver to a sanitation worker. It processes everything—both emotionally and physically—that we put in our body. It does so without bias, treating food the same as supplements, shots of whiskey, and stress. And the work is dirty and thankless.

In addition to sorting through what's coming into the plant, this scrappy organ also produces a vast reservoir of the body's proteins, regulates hormones, and cleans your blood. One reason it is so overworked in modern life is that **your liver is solely responsible for managing the storage of excess sugar**. When there is too much glucose in your bloodstream, your liver will convert it into glycogen—our own space-efficient storage solution—or fat. Excess fructose, on the other hand, will always be stored as fat.

Though it might be more efficient if your liver could make these judgment calls on its own—storing excess energy when you don't need it, and converting it back again when you do—its hands are tied without the green light from another member of middle management: your pancreas.

Your pancreas produces and manages the hormone insulin. In the org chart of your digestive system, the pancreas has fewer direct reports, but its role is so specialized that your liver wouldn't be able to do its primary job without it. **Insulin, when released, lets your liver know it's time to stow away extra glucose.** Like any additional cog in the workflow, it takes time for insulin to enter stage left, and then for your liver to pick up on that cue. Which is why **it often takes more than an hour after a meal for your blood glucose levels to start receding**.

When sugar was hard to come by in the wild, this process worked like a well-oiled machine. The problems arise when middle management becomes overwhelmed, or when communication between coworkers gets lost altogether.

WHAT GOES UP, MUST COME DOWN

The overconsumption of sugar can lead to a crash when it comes to both your energy levels and the organs in charge of managing them.

When a lot of insulin enters your bloodstream, you run the risk of overcorrecting. This will land you on the other side of the valley—with low blood sugar. You may have experienced symptoms of low blood sugar before. Along with hunger comes shakiness, sweating, dizziness, anxiety, and irritability. It's so common in our culture that we've invented our own adjective for this hypoglycemic event: hanger.

Having too much insulin hanging out in the bloodstream on a regular basis means that your liver will be constantly storing glucose for later. It makes losing weight virtually impossible—your body is being programmed to hold on to fat and create more of it. The additional fat converted from fructose can also start to interfere with your organs' abilities to function—it is one of the leading drivers of fatty liver disease.

In many ways, the '90s food movement, which swapped one macronutrient for another, was nothing less than a deal with the devil. **We were promised less fat in the box, but through the equation of our body's storage mechanisms, were all but guaranteed more fat stuffed inside our bodies as a result.**

Needless to say, when insulin levels become dysregulated, your whole metabolism goes with it. If levels are elevated for too long, your pancreas can't keep up its production of insulin and you run the risk of exhausting your reserves entirely, as is the case with diabetes. Your cells can also become resistant, ignoring the insulin cues altogether—what many women with PCOS experience.

Eventually, your blood sugar just keeps rising.

Without any system of checks and balances, too much energy floods your cells. This puts them in a state of oxidative stress and stimulates your body's primary protective measure: inflammation.

CODE RED—ALL SYSTEMS DOWN

Back in 2013, when I was deeply in the weeds of my Hashimoto's diagnosis, one of the issues I struggled with most was perioral dermatitis. This is a wonderfully attractive rash that appears around the nose and mouth. It has few treatment options beyond antibiotics from the dermatologist, and I had tried countless rounds from mine. They worked for a few weeks, and then the small, pixelated bumps would emerge anew and unperturbed. When I cried in her office and asked what could possibly be causing this, my doctor shrugged and said, "We don't know. Something is out of balance and your body is reacting."

In short, what she described was inflammation.

Inflammation is your body's normal response to infection or injury. But if the process goes on for too long or gets out of control, the inflammatory chemicals can interfere with the normal function of your cells and cause tissue damage. Many medical professionals see inflammation as the cornerstone of all major degenerative conditions, including Alzheimer's, heart disease, and some cancers. But because inflammation manifests differently in every person, it can often be difficult for doctors to spot its symptoms.

Without any sort of straightforward treatment plan for my skin, I decided to take on a year of health experiments—which I chronicled in my book *The Wellness Project*. I started by giving my liver a little vacay: no sugar, alcohol, or caffeine for

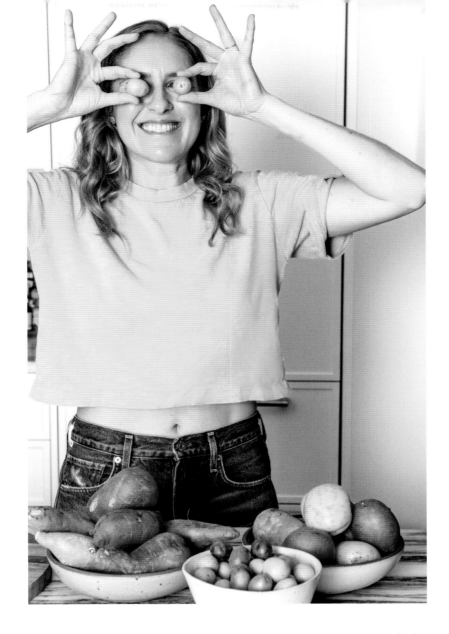

one month. The results of this "vice detox" were astounding. By the end of the thirty days, my face had cleared up entirely. And though I reintegrated sugar into my life in moderation, my perioral dermatitis never came back.

Sugar isn't the only thing to blame, nor is it the only solution to mysterious inflammation—there are other elements of our modern food system and lifestyle that contribute. But we do now know that when one component of our delicately calibrated metabolic system gets out of whack, you play with the hormonal motherboard as a child would a set of elevator buttons.

We often correlate skin issues to hormone imbalances, but the origin of both is often liver overwhelm. When your liver falls down on the job, excess toxins that might have been flushed successfully by way of the bathroom get sent back into circulation, often using the only other escape hatch: your pores.

Because your liver is also in charge of metabolizing estrogen and ushering out any excess, a lagging liver could mean levels become too high. Estrogen dominance can cause skin issues, affect your ability to convert thyroid hormones, and promote yeast overgrowth. And it puts you at higher risk of losing your gallbladder. Riding the sugar rollercoaster can also cause the opposite problem: too much testosterone. As happens to women with PCOS, high insulin levels can result in elevated testosterone levels. This makes it difficult to ovulate and is a leading cause of female infertility.

A lagging liver also affects your whole digestive system. High blood sugar can cause leaky gut syndrome, which, in turn, contributes to food allergies and, potentially, autoimmune issues in the long term. Glucose spikes also slow gut motility, which is one of the biggest drivers of IBS and small intestine bacterial overgrowth (SIBO).

As you can see, dysregulated blood sugar can touch every facet of your health—mood, memory, sleep, skin, and digestion. In the short term, that could mean a weakened immune system, insomnia, headaches, constipation, and acne. Even erectile dysfunction is said to be related to a metabolic issue.

No matter how it manifests for you, **cutting back on sugar could be the key to helping your body break the cycle of inflammation**. Perhaps the most harmful thing that too much insulin can affect is blocking your satiation hormone. This means that the more readily available energy you consume, the hungrier you will become. So, it's no surprise that to the kitchen or corner store we go to grab a granola bar, cookie, bag of dried mango, or sweetened latte, and the cycle begins all over again.

GOING SLOW CARB, NOT LOW CARB

So, are carbs the enemy?

If you've gotten this far, you might think the solution seems obvious: throw this book in the trash and swear off carbs for life.

But here's the thing: A hundred years ago obesity, diabetes, and autoimmune diseases were much rarer, even though the majority of the world's population got half their calories from wheat, rice, or oats. The difference isn't found in *what* people ate, but *how* and *how much*.

Let's take toast, for example. My great-grandparents may have started each day the same way as I might today: with a slice of bread. But, instead of slathering it with jam or jelly—or, gasp, margarine—they were more likely to use full-fat butter. That loaf, if made from white flour, was likely developed from a sourdough starter—a bacterial process that reduces both the gluten and carb content of the loaf. Even more likely, it wasn't made from white flour at all, but from dark, dense whole-grain rye berries. Instead of orange juice, they might have washed down breakfast with a glass of milk, which arrived on their doorstep each morning in a bottle with a slick of cream on top.

On the surface, the comparison seems like a difference of ingredients and taste. But on a molecular level, the stark contrast boils down to macronutrients. Specially carbohydrates' other costars: fat, fiber, and protein.

Just like your digestive organs form an ensemble cast, macronutrients also work synergistically in the body. You need all of them to live. And part of counteracting the worst effects of carbs on blood sugar is to let the rest of the cast get some time in the spotlight alongside them.

As you learned, when you eat or drink pure sugar on an empty stomach, it can hit your bloodstream within five minutes. But if you were to combine that sugar with fat, fiber, or protein—as nature intended—it would be metabolized much more slowly. Depending on the ratio, a Swiss Alps–level spike might be reduced to a mere sloping hill.

When you consume two hundred calories' worth of fresh apple slices, the fiber slows the body's absorption process. Your blood sugar rises more gradually and, without those spikes, your pancreas doesn't have to put in a rush job to release more insulin. Consuming the same number of calories from apple juice, though, which has all the fiber removed, means all that naturally occurring fructose is funneled straight to your liver. Even juice from sweeter vegetables (like beets and carrots) can cause your blood sugar to spike as much as it would if you were drinking a can of soda. There's no fat, fiber, or protein at the party.

You can also see why the concept of calories is meaningless. It is an assigned number for the amount of energy a food contains. The metrics are created by putting food in a box and burning it until there's nothing left—a very different mechanism from how the body actually metabolizes food. Unlike that box, we process nutrients within an open environment. We eat foods together and process them while breathing, sleeping, running, and interacting with the world around us. It's no wonder calories tell us so little about how a food actually affects us.

So, to answer the question: No, all carbs aren't the problem. There are many ways to learn from our ancestors and change the way we enjoy them—going slow carb, versus low carb—which is what the recipes in this book are all about. But the one carb that everyone can seem to agree on as **the supervillain of the century? Sugar.** Sugar provides no additional nutrients that your body needs. It only wreaks havoc.

MEASURING YOUR CARB TOLERANCE

We would all be better off limiting added sugar. But by how much boils down to your individual biology. Just as high insulin levels can throw off your hormonal motherboard, other hormonal imbalances can make you more susceptible to having glucose spikes in the first place.

So, what is a spike, exactly? Studies have shown that when our glucose levels increase by 30 mg/dL or more after a meal, we enter the more perilous part of the rollercoaster for our long-term health. **The biggest issue is variability—steep up and down climbs—not necessarily a numerical threshold.**

The best way to see where you stand is to wear a continuous glucose monitor. This is less intensive than you think: A CGM looks like a small button attached to an area of your body—usually the back of your arm or your stomach. In the center of the patch, a shallow needle is constantly measuring and reporting on the level of glucose in your bloodstream. This small apparatus is commonplace in the lives of some diabetics, but there is much that the average person can learn from it.

Through the company Zoe, I wore my CGM for fourteen days, and even in those two short weeks, the experience was eye-opening. I could see firsthand what would happen when I ate a sweet snack on an empty stomach versus a dessert at the end of a meal. Dishes like mac and cheese that I might have previously deemed "unhealthy" were much better for my blood sugar than a bowl of spaghetti with tomato sauce—and even less disruptive when preceded by a green salad.

Even if I failed to look at the sugar content of my protein bar, I could see the high amount of added sugar just by what it did to my glucose levels first thing in the morning. But when I exercised right afterward, those peaks and valleys disappeared. And after eating a bag of "healthy" candy that claimed to have only three grams of sugar, I could see firsthand what many of us may have already sensed: Packages don't always tell the truth!

Although there were some overarching consistencies—many of which have been validated in larger research studies—I also saw how my blood sugar tolerance was completely individual. I could eat a slice of cake and experience a massive surge, whereas my husband could eat the same portion and be totally fine. One of those blanket truths, however, is that the easiest way to avoid glucose spikes altogether is to reduce carbs—which is, of course, how the keto-mania movement took shape. But it isn't necessary for the average person to be that extreme.

Most people do well eating about half their total calories from carbs. If you suffer from an insulin-related condition—diabetes, PCOS, hypertension, gout, fatty liver disease—you may want to try dialing down your carbs until your metabolism can find its footing again. Others can take a more liberal approach, like the one in this book.

THE PROBLEM WITH CUTTING ALL CARBS

Though keto has become a mainstream diet, the biological process it ignites is a high-level metabolic change—one that's best achieved with supervision.

When you restrict your intake of starch and sugars, your body will look for other ways to convert nutrients into usable energy. During this scenario of extreme deprivation, your liver will step in and begin converting fat and protein into glucose. This is called *nutritional ketosis*, and though it is a process that burns fat for fuel, it shouldn't be viewed as a casual weight-loss tool.

Ketosis is not a state your body should endure for too long. As a diet, it is better suited to short therapeutic phases rather than an ongoing lifestyle. More important, there are people who may not benefit at all from that severe reduction of carbs and the stress of finding fuel from within.

Women's bodies are especially sensitive to changes in diet and energy intake. Though there are many conditions caused by chronically high glucose or insulin levels that affect women in particular, there is also evidence that an extreme low-carb approach isn't the answer either.

Studies have shown that going ultra-low carb can increase our chief stress hormone, cortisol. So, if you're already under a lot of stress, going keto could amplify that hormonal imbalance.[3] For women, cutting carbs overnight and keeping them too low for too long can spur symptoms of adrenal fatigue or HPA axis dysregulation—sleep problems, difficulty getting up in the morning, poor circulation, or thyroid dysfunction. We need carbs to make thyroid hormones and convert them into their active form. Particularly for those of us who already suffer from hypothyroidism or Hashimoto's, a drastic change in carb intake can make our thyroid even more sluggish, leading to more weight gain and fatigue.

Restricting food can also signal to the body that it's time to turn off sex hormones. We are conditioned to know that times of nutrient scarcity are not ideal for incubating another life. This can manifest in changes to the menstrual cycle, causing some women to lose their period or not ovulate. For this reason, most doctors do not recommend ultra-low-carb diets for women trying to conceive.

THE SWEET SPOT

You might find some of this information contradictory, but it just goes to show that the answer to the question "To carb or not to carb?" can swing both ways depending on your individual situation. The most important takeaway is that **extremes in either direction—high carb or low carb—don't benefit the average person**. Either choice can help, or it can hurt.

Whichever camp you fall within, the strategies in Chapter 2 will help you find that sweet spot by teaching you methods of "slow carb" consumption that won't cause as much chaos.

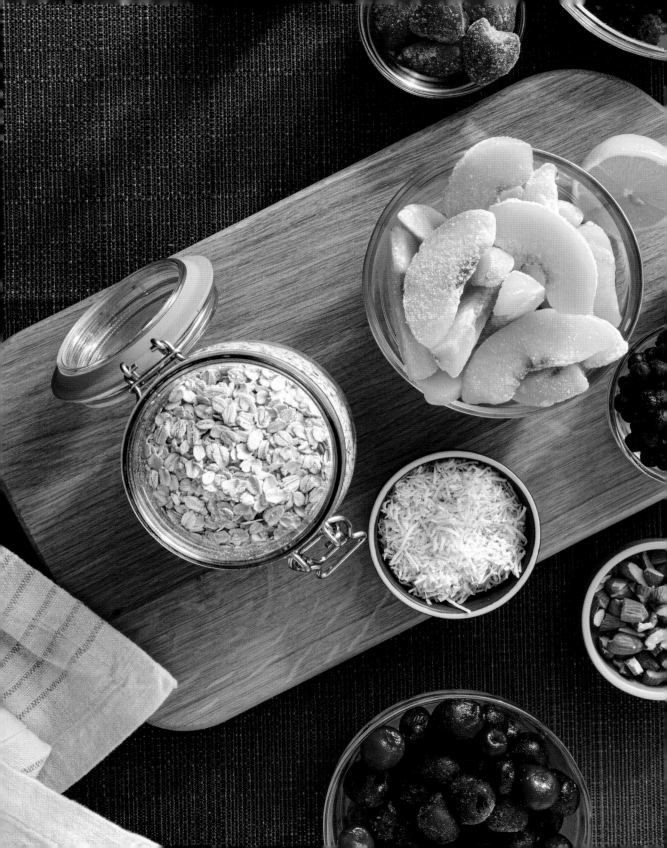

How to Have Your Cake & Eat It Too

I know how hopeless it can seem when the modern food system is stacked against you. But like any of my approaches to healthy hedonism—that sweet spot, where we nourish our body while at the same time feeding our spirit—the key is having a toolkit at your disposal.

There are ways to have your cake and eat it too. And there are healthier recipes for that cake that won't send you into such a tailspin. The array of tips in this chapter can ward off the worst of your blood sugar fluctuations, while still allowing you to include grains and starches as part of a balanced diet. There's even a place for dessert.

You learned why it's important to choose your own carb adventure in Chapter 1. These are the strategies I want you to try on for size, which are broken into three parts: decreasing sugar, rethinking *how* you eat carbs, and changing your lifestyle outside the dining room. **You don't have to do all of them, all at once.** Mix and match to create your own mini Carbivore experiment. Each section has seven tips, so you can easily tackle one a day as a three-week project, or go at your own pace.

The best way to see the impact of each strategy is to test your blood sugar in real time using a continuous glucose monitor or another method. But you can also note how you feel. I created my **Carbivore Symptom & Activity Tracker** (see Resources) to help you monitor how these changes affect all areas of your health.

Remember, you can't make healthier choices until you know what choices are healthy for *you*. Once you know your carb tolerance, you have my permission to pick and choose which Carbivore habits to keep in your arsenal, and which to ignore.

STEP 1: LEARN TO CONSUME SUGAR WITHOUT IT CONSUMING YOU

There is no single tactic that is the be-all and end-all of your blood sugar. That said, if there is one overarching rule to live by, it's that **savory will always be a better choice than sweet**.

We can give ourselves such a huge leg up in the carb department simply by being more vigilant about added sugar. Even if eating white rice, potato, oats, or corn shows the same spike on your glucose monitor as a slice of cake, it is not the complete picture. Studies show that when comparing two foods with the same calories, the one containing fructose will have an overall worse impact on weight gain, mood variation, energy levels, and health.[4] So, on that note, let's start by changing your relationship to sugar.

ADDED SUGAR CHEAT SHEET

Sugar appears on ingredient lists using more than fifty different aliases, from various types of fruit concentrates to compounds like maltodextrin and dextrose that sound like a lab experiment.

Agave nectar/syrup	Diastatic malt	Lactose
Barley malt	Ethyl maltol	Maltodextrin
Beet sugar	Evaporated cane	Maltose
Blackstrap molasses	juice	Malt syrup
Brown rice syrup	Fructose	Maple syrup
Brown sugar	Fruit juice	Molasses
Cane juice crystals	Fruit juice	Muscovado sugar
Cane sugar	concentrate	Panela sugar
Caramel	Galactose	Raw sugar
Carob syrup	Glucose	Refiner's syrup
Castor sugar	Glucose syrup solids	Rice syrup
Coconut sugar	Golden sugar	Sorghum syrup
Confectioners'	Golden syrup	Sucanat
sugar	Grape juice	Sucrose
Corn syrup	concentrate	Sugar (granulated
Corn syrup solids	Grape sugar	or table)
Crystalline fructose	High fructose	Treacle
Date sugar	corn syrup (HFCS)	Turbinado sugar
Demerara sugar	Honey	Yellow sugar
Dextrin	Icing sugar	
Dextrose	Invert sugar	

1. TAKE A FIVE-DAY SUGAR BREAK.

Because of the incredible aftermath of my personal experiment, the first order of business in my 4 Weeks to Wellness program is to take everyone on a brief "vice detox"—eliminating alcohol, caffeine, and **all added sugar** for five days. Whole fruit is allowed, but any packaged foods with sugar on the ingredient list, even a little bit, are out.

For many people, it is the longest five days of their life, but also the most profound. Because sugar is addictive, we can ramp up our consumption without even realizing it. Breaking up with sugar for a period of time helps you find a new equilibrium. Even that short week will begin the process of retraining your taste buds. And more important, it is an opportunity to explore your emotional relationship with sugar. What are you really craving when you want a treat? If you're someone who can't go a day without dessert, why does that make you uncomfortable?

My clients are usually floored by the discoveries from their sugar-free week: acne clearing, sleep regulating, and condiments they didn't think even had sugar—like sriracha—becoming cloyingly sweet. They are also surprised by the withdrawal.

Quitting sugar, like any drug, is not easy and often leads to headaches, crushing fatigue, and irritability. I know that sounds like no fun, but who wants to be married to a substance that can hijack your brain like that? Once you are over the hump, you will have much more steady energy. The quick fix from a candy bar is just a marketing illusion.

Although you may be inspired to keep sugar at bay for longer than five days to enjoy the full benefits of the detox, the goal of this book is moderation. So, eventually reincorporate it intentionally, while keeping the best practices in this chapter in mind.

KEY STRATEGIES TO QUIT SUGAR

- **Eat anything you want as long as it doesn't contain sugar.** This is one of Sarah Wilson's primary tips for starting a sugar detox in her book *I Quit Sugar.* Don't split hairs on other carbs or inflammatory foods. If you want cheese, eat the cheese. Being able to satisfy other cravings will make the sugar omission easier.
- **Allow yourself plenty of time to rest.** Sometimes sugar withdrawal can feel like the flu. Your liver is resetting and your organs might need the extra downtime that sleep brings.
- **Don't let "whole fruit" become a loophole.** Eating a bag of dried mango or making dessert with dates as the sweetener is beside the point. Whole fruit means fruit from the produce aisle. Avoid anything dried or juiced.

2. ELIMINATE MINDLESS SUGAR.

The more we can weed out unnecessary sugar that gives us no conscious pleasure, the more room there is for things that actually feel like treats!

If you aren't the type of person who reads ingredient labels, there could be more added sugar lurking in your pantry than you think. After all, there's added sugar in 80 percent of the grocery store, so it's only natural for that to be reflected as a large percentage of what's in your cupboards. Even "healthy" packaged foods often use sugar as a way to make their products taste like the options from childhood.

Do a deep dive into your fridge and pantry. Use the **Added Sugar Cheat Sheet** (page 20) to help you track down all the potential sources you may not have thought of, like sandwich bread. Although you don't have to throw away all the bad offenders overnight, this exercise will help you identify items that might be good to replace over time.

HOW TO READ AN INGREDIENT LABEL

- Which products should get a second look? There is no perfect answer, as it also depends on how much you love certain brands. But Jessie Inchauspé, author of the fabulous book *Glucose Revolution*, suggests that if an item has more than **five times the amount of sugar than fiber** on the ingredient label, it's not worth it for your blood sugar. This is roughly the ratio in whole fruit, which is how nature intended that we consume fructose: with the added protection of fiber.
- If an ingredient label has more than **three types of sugar listed** or if sugar is one of the **first five ingredients**, put it down. Or don't, but at least know what you're eating.
- **Be more discerning about foods you eat every day**, and particularly the things you consume in the morning, like the milk that goes in your coffee (more on this in the next tip). Remember, this is an exercise to weed out *mindless* sugar. We already know your ice cream has sugar, and that is why you eat it for dessert, not breakfast.

---

3. DON'T CONSUME SUGAR ON AN EMPTY STOMACH.

As you know, sugar can have the biggest impact when fat, fiber, and protein aren't also present. A small bite of fiber-rich food (even a handful of peanuts off the bar!) can slow absorption and limit the negative effects that sweet ingredients have on your blood sugar and hormone levels.

We can define an empty stomach as not having eaten for three hours, which means it is most important to **avoid sweet options for breakfast and as snacks**. Sugar on an empty stomach can impact your blood sugar any time of day, but studies show it has a particularly negative halo effect in the morning.[5] Because you haven't eaten for so long, a bowl of cereal will cause a bigger spike at breakfast than that same bowl would if it were your second or third meal of the day. That glucose dysregulation will make you hungrier again quicker, and also negatively affect your sensitivity to carbs at lunch and dinner. These rules apply regardless of the time of day you have your first meal. So, if you skip breakfast, choose something without sugar for lunch.

Of course, we have been trained, especially in the United States, to embrace sweet things for breakfast, despite their ingredients being almost identical to baked goods we think of as dessert. But don't kid yourself: Muffins are, essentially, breakfast cupcakes. Scones are cookies. And sugar-coated cereal with mini marshmallows is no different than candy.

Eating a high-fiber, low-sugar breakfast will curb your cravings before they start and keep your hormones in check throughout the day. This will also make your need to snack less likely, but if you have to, choose something savory.

10 SAVORY, SLOW CARB BREAKFASTS

1. Seedy "Avocado Toast" Arepas (page 282)

2. Ham & Cheese Dutch Baby with Peas (page 102)

3. Steel Cut Oat Congee with Bok Choy (page 99)

4. Savory Yogurt & Granola Bowls with Avocado & Eggs (page 94)

5. Buckwheat Crepes with Leek Confit, Salmon & Eggs (page 149)

6. Kasha Pilaf with Mushrooms, Bacon & Greens (page 162)

7. Brussels Sprouts & Sweet Potato Hash with Eggs & Leftover Salsa (page 212)

8. Smashed Chickpea Shakshuka with Summer Tomatoes (page 306)

9. Sweet Potato & Cabbage Rosti with Kimchi Aioli (page 231)

10. A big bowl of leftovers from dinner the night before (a personal favorite!)

4. SKIP THE SWEET BEVERAGES (EVEN JUICES AND SMOOTHIES).

Drinking sugar is far worse than eating sugar. You are much more likely to down a bottle of juice or a smoothie in a fraction of the time it would take you to eat a bowl of cereal. This means that those sugars are funneled to your bloodstream that much faster.

Soda isn't the only problem child. Just look at the back of any juice, flavored coffee, energy drink, or coconut water and you'll see there isn't a huge difference in sugar content, and no fiber to slow it down. Even green juices are usually packed with naturally sweet ingredients—apples, pears, or pineapple—to make the greens more palatable. If you can't quit juices, think of them as a supplement, not a meal, and drink them with your lunch for extra nutrients. Better yet, stick with an "all greens" variety that doesn't include fruit, carrots, or beets.

Similarly, kombucha is marketed as a boon to your digestive system. During the fermentation process, bacteria eats the sugar present, leaving little in the final fizzy drink. The problem is, most commercially made kombucha brands add fruit juice *after* the fermentation process, which means it all ends up in the bottle.

Though smoothies begin with whole fruit, we don't get that same safety net when we pulverize the fiber in a high-powered blender (more on this in the next section). It might be better than juicing, which removes the fiber altogether, but not by much.

Any dessert recipe in this book is a better choice than a sweet drink. And just think how much more room in your diet you'd create for them if you just focused on drinking water instead.

---

6 SUGAR-FREE HOMEMADE DRINK IDEAS

1. Hibiscus iced tea

2. "Spa water": add cucumber, lemon, lime, or orange slices to a pitcher of water

3. Fresh ginger or mint tea

4. Sparkling water with lemon or lime juice (homemade Spindrift!)

5. Golden milk latte: add a dash of ground cinnamon, ground turmeric, and ground ginger to unsweetened coconut or almond milk and heat on the stove

6. ACV water: mix 1 tablespoon apple cider vinegar with 8 ounces water—this has a beneficial impact on blood sugar before a meal; add lemon juice and pureed ginger and you've got a kombucha knock-off!

5. TREAT NATURAL SWEETENERS THE SAME AS REGULAR SUGAR.

A lot of "healthy" baking revolves around the idea that switching from table sugar to a natural sweetener, like honey, maple syrup, coconut sugar, or agave is better. But at the end of the day, all sugar is made up of glucose and fructose, in various ratios. The natural options might have slightly better mineral and nutrient profiles, but the substitution isn't necessarily going to mean steadier glucose levels.

The higher the fructose content, the harder a sweetener will be on your body. High fructose corn syrup is among the worst offenders, per its name. One of the other highest? **Agave.** Even though it's marketed as a healthy option, you're better off with table sugar.

This is one reason the glycemic index value assigned to foods is deceiving. It measures only glucose, not fructose. So, agave is considered a low-glycemic option for diabetics, but only because we can't measure its true impact.

My sweeteners of choice, which you'll see in the recipes in this book, are maple syrup and honey. Instead of just adding sweetness, they also lend flavor to a dish. But I try to use them sparingly, and because of their sticky consistency, I can often get away with using less in certain recipes (like granola) without impacting the texture.

6. TREAT ARTIFICIAL SWEETENERS AS WORSE THAN REGULAR SUGAR.

Sugar is addictive, but so is the taste of sugar. There's a tendency to reach for a no-calorie soda as a way to ward off cravings for real food, but in the end, it just makes cravings worse. The perfect storm is Diet Coke. Caffeine stimulates the brain, even if it's exhausted, causing it to overuse energy reserves. With normal soda, some of that energy is supplied in the form of sugar. With artificial aspartame—which is two hundred times sweeter than sucrose—the hunger craving gets doubled: The sweet taste signals to the body that more energy is on the way, but the replenishment never comes. It's a huge rush of promise, followed by no actual nourishment.

Studies have found that artificial sweeteners are actually even more likely to induce glucose intolerance than pure sugar, which may be due partially to the damage they do to your gut microbiome.[6] Sugar alcohols that end in -ol (polyols) are part of the FODMAP acronym and can be irritating to people with IBS. Though these sweeteners are nature based, they are commonly malabsorbed in the gut. If you've noticed your stomach is upset after a sugar-free candy or protein powder, it might be the xylitol or erythritol.[7] Besides killing off healthy bacteria and encouraging leaky gut, the tricky part about these sugar alternatives is that they pull water into your intestines and cause diarrhea, which becomes an even more likely outcome when consumed in tandem with fructose.[8]

Of the sugar-free sweeteners, **stevia and monk fruit are the best options**. But even better would be to wean your taste buds off the sweet stuff and balance your cravings.

7. EMBRACE DESSERT, BUT EAT IT AFTER YOUR MEAL.

Just when you thought your chance with sweets had passed, I go Vanessa Williams on you and save the best for last!

The point of this book is not to deprive you of everything you love. Dessert can still be part of your life as a special-occasion indulgence—I have a few show-stopping tarts and cakes in this book for that very purpose. But per tip #3, save these treats for the end of the meal, when dessert was intended to be eaten, so there's other food in the tank to slow absorption. I'll remind you why this is important in the next section as we talk more about "slow carb" strategies.

STEP 2: REDUCE THE GLUCOSE ROLLERCOASTER BY GOING SLOW CARB

If you've gotten your relationship with sugar under control, you're already ahead of the game. Your glucose spikes should be calmer now. But starch-based carbs like bread, pasta, and rice can also send your blood sugar into a tizzy. So, let's talk about strategies for slowing down absorption and mitigating that impact.

1. EAT FIBER FIRST.

The best thing for your blood sugar is to start your meal with a serving of fiber. One study found that you can reduce your overall glucose spike by more than 70 percent just by eating fiber first, followed by protein and fat. Starches and sugars should, ideally, come last.[9]

The small intestine is where we absorb all our nutrients, including glucose. **Fiber slows our digestive organs**, preventing our stomach from emptying its contents quickly into the small intestine. Fiber also plays another important role: it forms a literal barrier as it moves through your system, so simple sugars don't get sucked immediately through your intestinal wall into the bloodstream.

You can think of your intestinal wall as a fine-mesh sieve. If you poured a glass of apple juice through it, the liquid would pass easily and leave no residue. But if you were to add some mashed-up apple first? Well, the skins and seeds would clog up the mesh and make any liquid added thereafter take longer to make its way through. The result is a slow drip in the bowl versus an unobstructed stream. If you need a visual learning tool, make the **Raspberry Lime Rickey Curd Tart** (page 111) and see what those raspberries do to your strainer! Fat and protein can have a similar effect on gastric emptying, but they won't form that protective seal (or sludge) around your intestinal barrier.

You'll find plenty of examples of this ethos in ancient culinary traditions. In Japanese culture, for example, it's common to enjoy a bowl of edamame at the beginning of a meal. This means any white rice that follows will be metabolized more slowly.

At home, there are many ways you can tackle fiber first, but one of the easiest is to make a **Simple Starter Salad** (page 81) and enjoy a serving before your main meal. These are some of the only carb-free recipes in the book, and they are intended to fulfill your "fiber first" mantra. Some quicker options that I usually have on hand include a handful of almonds, a few carrot sticks (with hummus, perhaps), or a whole dill pickle.

You can experiment with the order of your food. For example, start your day with 1 cup of white rice for breakfast. The next day, try eating 1 cup of white rice with a whole avocado on top. On Day 3, start your day with a whole avocado, followed by a cup of white rice 15 minutes later. Pay attention to your energy in the hours that follow, and your hunger levels. When I tried this experiment while wearing a CGM, the difference in my blood sugar curves was astonishing. See **DIY Carbivore Blood Sugar Experiments** (page 331) for more ideas.

KEY STRATEGIES TO PUT FIBER FIRST

- Start your meal with a salad or vegetable side.
- If you can't take a few bites of vegetables first, then start with fats and protein before digging into the carbs.
- Avoid the bread basket on an empty stomach.
- Eat sugars (including fruit) last.

2. CHEW YOUR FOOD AND SLOW DOWN.

I know many of us rush through meals, especially at work during the day. But if you're swallowing your food whole, it doesn't matter how many grass-fed meats or plants are on your plate, you're going to have a harder time extracting their nutrients. In particular, our saliva contains enzymes that begin the process of breaking down carbohydrates. The act of chewing also signals to your brain that food is on the way, it's time to get your stomach acid flowing, and to switch into rest-and-digest mode. Even chewing your smoothies and soups helps slow you down and gets your digestive system working properly, though it may sound weird!

Though there's less compelling data on eating speed and blood sugar, common sense dictates that if you put food into your mouth and swallow it more slowly, it will naturally enter your bloodstream at a more moderate clip. Eating slowly also gives your digestive system time to do its job and can have a huge impact on gut health.

KEY STRATEGIES TO EAT MORE MINDFULLY

- Instead of counting bites, try to make sure that whatever is in your mouth becomes mush before swallowing. Don't be afraid to be the last one finished at a meal—make that your GOAL!
- Put down your fork between bites.
- Eat without distractions. No emails. No TV. No books. Just you and your plate and your thoughts. This will also have a wonderful effect on your mental well-being and whole nervous system, even if it's hard to prioritize.
- Say grace! This doesn't have to be religious. Before dinner, my husband and I share three things we're grateful for. It prevents us from diving into a meal mindlessly and, instead, prepares the gut-brain axis for digestion.

3.   ADD A "CARB COMPANION" TO YOUR MEAL.

We've talked about how quickly sugar hits your bloodstream on an empty stomach. But refined starches like pasta, white bread, and rice are not much better in this regard. Without anything else in your system, your body can convert those starches into sugars quickly and easily.

If you abide by tip #1 and eat a salad before your spaghetti, you won't have too much to worry about. But, as a general rule, especially when left to your own devices in the kitchen, it's best to add fat, fiber, and protein—what I call **carb companions**—to your bowl. At restaurants, one of the worst things you can do for your blood sugar is dive right into the bread basket before a meal. But if you must, try to add a classic carb companion: butter, hummus, or another type of dip.

The good news is, carb companions can make your meals even more delicious! Most recipes in this book are designed with built-in carb companions, like the spinach, yogurt, and cheese in **Spanakopita Lasagna** (page 201), bok choy and jammy eggs on top of **Steel Cut Oat Congee** (page 99), or the sausage, shrimp, and Swiss chard in **Quinoa Paella** (page 151). But whenever possible, add more!

One of my favorite tactics is to add a **Nut Crunch or Seed Sprinkle** (page 75) to a carb-y meal. Nuts and seeds are the ultimate carb companions because they are a great source of healthy fat, fiber, AND protein wrapped in one tiny package.

- A fried, jammy, or poached egg
- Canned beans or crunchy chickpeas
- Cheese
- Dollop of yogurt, crème fraîche, sour cream, or whipped cream (or plant-based alternatives)
- Flaked canned fish
- Frozen (thawed) edamame
- Kimchi or sauerkraut
- Nut crunches and seed sprinkles (see page 75)
- Sliced or diced avocado
- Scoop of unsweetened nut butter
- Sliced cooked chicken breast
- Smoked salmon

4. CHOOSE "WHOLE" FOODS OVER PROCESSED FOODS.

An actual whole food is something that hasn't undergone any processing. It's the whole almond, not the almond flour or the almond milk. Choosing to consume foods in this whole, "natural" state will always be better for your blood sugar. Instead of an industrial processor doing all the work, your body will be forced to break down that almond. And this means any carbs will get converted into glucose more slowly.

Even the healthiest smoothie or vegetable soup, if pureed, is not going to give you the full benefit of its fiber-rich ingredients. When we chew our food, we break fiber down into smaller particles. But even if you follow tip #2 to the best of your ability and grind your dinner to mush, you won't be able to do the job of a high-powered blender, which pulverizes the fibers into microscopic bits.

This doesn't mean I don't eat smoothies and pureed soups—I have a few of the latter in this book! But I make sure to eat something more fibrous first (per tip #1) or add some carb companions as a garnish (tip #3).

KEY STRATEGIES TO FORTIFY SOUPS & SMOOTHIES

- **Soups:** Reserve some of the vegetables you're pureeing and add them to the bowl. Garnish with a nut or seed sprinkle (page 42). Drizzle with extra-virgin olive oil and puree with more heart-healthy oil (carb companions).

- **Smoothies:** Add flaxseed meal or almond butter to the base (carb companions). Use less fruit and add some avocado, cauliflower, kale, or zucchini. Garnish with chia seeds and whole fruit (whole foods).
- Remember, fruit purees are not the same as whole fruit. Skip the applesauce, jam, pouches, and pulps. Eat an actual piece of fruit.

5.   EAT MORE, SNACK LESS.

Even when implementing all these best practices, your blood sugar still rises and falls every time you eat—that is the nature of the beast. Each time we consume food, we ask a lot of our metabolism. During the act of digestion, our immune system is put on hold so our hormones can rush into formation and blood can flow to our gut to do all the heavy lifting—sorting, secreting, and absorbing.

The solution isn't to skip meals. Intermittent fasting for too long can put a woman's body into a state of starvation similar to eating too few carbs. Rather, it's to **space out meals—going four to five hours between them without eating** so our organs can catch up.

For our great-grandparents, snacking as a concept did not exist. People ate three meals a day, moved their body plenty in between, and worked up an appetite before dinner. Not only were there no metabolic issues then on the same scale as today, but gut issues were also much rarer.

The **migrating motor complex (MMC)** is our small intestine's street sweeper wave that cleans up after a meal. When it's not working as it should, food remnants and (potentially) unwanted bacteria are left to fester in the long and winding path of our intestinal tract. Our MMC is powered by nerve waves, and they kick in only after **a fasting state of ninety minutes or more**. That means if you're prone to snacking, even if it's a healthy, Carbivore-approved whole food snack like a handful of nuts every hour, your MMC isn't able to clean up fully after your meal. This can contribute to bigger issues, like SIBO, but it can also make your overall digestive system less efficient.

If you're feeding yourself nutritious, well-balanced meals—meaning plates packed with vegetables, healthy fats, whole grains, and protein and free of hidden sugars—on a regular schedule, you shouldn't be facing the types of food cravings that drive snacking. If you find that you become starving two hours after lunch, perhaps you're not having a large or filling enough meal. Or, perhaps, you have bigger fish to fry when it comes to balancing your blood sugar with all the other strategies in this chapter.

Lastly, most packaged snacks are full of added sugar. Often, eating these will make it even less likely that you'll get to the next meal without going back for more snacks. If you have to eat something between meals, choose savory whole foods.

6. DRINK WATER WHEN YOU'RE NOT EATING.

Though water, overall, is the best beverage for your blood sugar, drinking a lot of it during a meal can increase your glucose spikes.[10] Have plenty of water throughout the day, but enjoy it outside of your actual meals. This is also a best practice for your digestive system and ability to stay hydrated. Water dilutes the natural enzymes in your saliva that help break down carbs and has a similar effect when it reaches other digestive organs.

To maximize retention, stop drinking thirty minutes before eating and wait an hour after you're done to drink more. This can be a struggle for some people, especially when you accidentally eat the ghost pepper in your Thai curry. But it's a fairly easy adjustment in the grand scheme of these Carbivore strategies.

7. DON'T HAVE CAFFEINE ON AN EMPTY STOMACH.

You now know to avoid sweeteners in your coffee drinks or matcha lattes, but you may want to also wait until after breakfast to consume your caffeinated beverages to improve your blood sugar response to them.

If you've ever felt a surge of fatigue a few hours after your cup of coffee, it might not be the caffeine wearing off, but your body experiencing a dip in blood sugar. When the rollercoaster comes back down, you might end up more tired than you were when you decided to grab that cup of coffee in the first place.[11] This can be amplified by a bad night's sleep, which makes your morning blood sugar tolerance more volatile (more on this in the next section).

STEP 3: TWEAK YOUR LIFESTYLE TO CREATE BETTER BLOOD SUGAR OUTCOMES

If I've learned anything from my years of health research, it's that your food choices do not happen in a vacuum. So often, they are influenced by what time you went to sleep, how stressful your workday was, or who you're sitting down to eat with. Many habits can help improve blood sugar outcomes (exercising after a meal); others can exacerbate an already unsteady curve (getting a bad night's sleep). If changing *what* or *how* you're eating feels overwhelming, here are some other areas you can focus on.

1. USE YOUR MUSCLES AFTER A MEAL.

Like all heavy-duty machinery, your muscles require a lot of energy. When they kick into gear, any available glucose in your bloodstream gets gobbled up. This is generally why elite athletes can get away with eating more carbs and sugary gels before and during a hard workout: Their muscles are using all that energy quickly.

When I experimented with my continuous glucose monitor, the impact of moving my muscles after a meal was a big "aha" moment. I saw what white rice on an empty stomach did to my blood sugar—sky-high spike. But when I ate the same thing and went for a brisk fifteen-minute walk afterward? Things were steady.

KEY STRATEGIES TO MOVE YOUR BODY MORE

- **Take a lap after lunch:** Move within an hour of eating a carb-heavy meal. It doesn't have to be anything strenuous—a walk around the block, a series of jumping jacks or sun salutations next to your desk, or climbing a few flights of stairs—anything to get moving will do!
- **Add strength training to your regular exercise routine:** Try weight lifting, kettle bells, or any sort of resistance exercise using your body weight, like Pilates. Research in the *International Journal of Cardiology* found that for people with type 2 diabetes, strength training can be even more beneficial than cardio.[12] But it has long-term benefits for all.

---

2. PRIORITIZE SLEEP.

Our bodies experience a cycle of changes every day called a circadian rhythm. Some organs, like your intestines, go dormant overnight. For other organs working the graveyard shift, like your liver, their work is just getting started. **Our blood sugar levels are naturally elevated at night and when we sleep.** This isn't usually problematic, but multiple studies have shown that repeated awakenings during the night, along with insufficient or irregular sleep, can increase glucose intolerance and worsen conditions like diabetes.[13]

Food choices affect sleep quality, and sleep quality can also affect food choices. The day after a poor night's sleep, you will see a halo effect on your blood sugar regulation. A carb-y breakfast that might not ordinarily cause a big blood sugar spike could send you into a tailspin after a night of disrupted sleep. Even though you might be dragging, it becomes even more important to avoid a sugary breakfast or caffeine on an empty stomach.

The impact of diet on sleep is fickle—each individual may have their own Goldilocks issue to sort through. Ultra-low-carb diets can disrupt sleep, leading to a phenomenon called *keto insomnia*. But eating a dinner that causes a big blood sugar surge, especially if there is alcohol involved, will likely also wake you up in the middle of the night when that spike hits.

The sweet spot can be a simple matter of finding the right timing. If low-carb meals disrupt your sleep, try integrating more carbs at dinner time. Don't go to sleep hungry, but also don't eat too close to bedtime, which is not great for your gut and might mean you'll have undigested food hanging out in your intestines overnight. **Eating two to three hours (and not more) before bedtime** seems to be the ideal scenario that works for most people.

KEY STRATEGIES TO GET A BETTER NIGHT'S SLEEP

- **Get sunshine in the morning.** Supplementing with a liquid vitamin D or getting a good dose of natural sunlight in the morning tells our body it's time to start the day. This will also help your sleep hormones (melatonin) kick in by bedtime.
- **Check your phone at the bedroom door, or turn it off.** Try to keep electronic devices out of the bedroom or set them to airplane mode so you're not tempted to mindlessly browse the internet before bed. Using devices can be stimulating for the mind and confuse your circadian rhythm because blue light mimics the sun.
- **Take a hot bath or shower before bed.** A drop in body temperature is a key prelude to sleep. If your internal thermostat is off, one way to hack it is to take a twenty-minute bath or shower. Adding some relaxing lavender bath salts and sipping sleepy tea is a sleep prep triple threat.
- **Have magnesium at night.** In addition to being an essential mineral, magnesium can be helpful as a muscle relaxant and it's been known to promote a better night's sleep as well.

3. ADJUST YOUR DIET ACCORDING TO YOUR MENSTRUAL CYCLE.

Because blood sugar moderation is ruled by the hormone insulin, it can be affected by any other hormonal changes in the body. Unfortunately for women, these changes happen several times a month by the very nature of our design.

A woman's four distinct hormonal phases need to be fed slightly differently to maximize the body's ability to process estrogen, boost progesterone, and make sure you're getting enough of all the other hormones. Alisa Vitti, author of the books *WomanCode* and *In the Flo,* recommends focusing on healthy fats and protein to restore energy during your menstrual period. Even if you've been conditioned to ease any discomfort with a hot water bottle and a box of chocolates, sweets will just add more insult to injury.

During your luteal phase, the lead-up to your period, your blood sugar will naturally be at its highest and most volatile. It's an important time to stick to foods that support the liver—beets, leafy greens, fresh herbs—that can help flush excess hormones more quickly. Any sugar consumed during this time may spike you more than it normally does at other times of the month.

4. DECREASE STRESS.

When experiencing physical or emotional stress, our primary fight-or-flight hormones, cortisol and adrenaline, are released into the bloodstream. The result is higher blood pressure, an increased heart rate, and a rise in blood sugar.

This is a perfectly natural adaptive response. If you're being chased through the jungle by a tiger, you need extra energy to flee. These days, however, we tend to get stuck in a state of stress and agitation, even though there is no immediate threat beyond the passive-aggressive email you just received. Your stress hormones and blood sugar stay surging, and without using your muscles (as you would to flee a big, hungry cat), there's not much else that will bring them down. This is why **having a regular practice to calm the nervous system is so important for overall carb tolerance**.

It's also another big reason that overly restrictive dieting is not the solution. As I always say, **if you're stressing all the time about what you're eating, no amount of kale will make you healthy**. This is especially true when it comes to blood sugar. Use the **Carbivore Symptom & Activity Tracker** (see Resources) to learn how chronic stress may be affecting your reaction to certain foods. If you find that the same meal has very different effects on separate days, your stress levels and sleep (and the negative impact of stress levels on your sleep!) could be the hidden difference.

For some, stress management might be exercising a couple times a week; for others, talk therapy. Self-care can be an Epsom salts bath and a DIY face mask, or a night out with friends and family. Don't underestimate the importance of having stillness in your life and daily rituals to relax the nervous system (like journaling, float tanks, infrared saunas, massages, and other practices that help quiet the mind).

KEY STRATEGIES TO LIMIT EVERYDAY STRESS

- **Try deep belly breathing.** Slowing your breathing can activate the body's parasympathetic nervous system. Breathe in through your nose for four seconds, feeling your belly rise. Hold the breath for four seconds, then exhale through your mouth for six seconds, letting the belly fall.
- **Start a meditation or yoga practice.** Across disciplines, meditation has been studied as a panacea for relieving stress. For IBS sufferers, meditation, yoga, and other relaxation techniques have been shown to be extremely effective for reducing symptoms and alleviating gut anxiety.[14]
- **Create boundaries around your electronic devices.** The constant stimulation from smartphones puts more unconscious stress on your body. Switch your email settings to fetch manually, turn off notifications, stop checking your feeds every five minutes, and designate times for turning off your phone completely.

5. SUPPORT YOUR GUT MICROBIOME.

The trillions of bacteria that comprise our gut microbiome are intimately linked to blood sugar metabolism. For each of us, that mix of critters is more varied and unique than a fingerprint, which means that how we maintain a healthy environment can mean different things. Most people, however, are dealing with a diversity issue thanks to our modern food system. For this reason, it's important not to let blood sugar levels be the sole driver of our health choices. Although a snack of deli meat and cheese might be better for our glucose regulation, eating a whole apple is going to be much less inflammatory for your gut overall.

KEY STRATEGIES TO FEED YOUR GUT CRITTERS

- **Diversify your diet.** Eating many different vegetables and types of fiber on a daily basis is one of the most profound ways to support microbial diversity. Even on a low-FODMAP diet, it's still important to aim for diversity.

- **Use broad-spectrum antibiotics only when absolutely necessary.** Antibiotics can be lifesaving, but they can also be doled out for unnecessary short-term gains. It is also important to buy and consume animal protein that hasn't been raised on antibiotics because eating them affects our guts too.
- **Don't sterilize your life.** Ditch the sanitizing wipes, antimicrobial soaps, harmful household cleaners, and chemical-ridden personal care products for the sake of your long-term gut health and immunity.
- **Filter your water.** Chlorine is a harmful purifier. Like bleach on your floors, these chemicals kill delicate microbes on your skin and in your gut.
- **Buy organic and avoid pesticides.** The pesticides on our crops do something similar once they reach our gut: they kill off microorganisms. Try to buy organic, non-GMO, and pesticide-free produce and grains whenever possible.

6.   MODIFY YOUR ALCOHOL INTAKE.

We talked about sugar. We talked about coffee. But you might be wondering about that other vice: alcohol.

Alcohol, in its most basic form, is not necessarily an enemy to blood sugar. Most distilled liquors—gin, vodka, tequila, whiskey—won't have an effect. It's only when sugary mixers come into play that a cocktail can send your glucose levels sky high. If you're having a sweet drink, it's best to do so on a full stomach with plenty of fiber in your system. Beer is also higher in carbohydrates, so the same rules apply.

Most wines won't impact glucose levels, but beware that some cheaper big-box brands might contain added sugar. You won't see it on the ingredient list, but you may feel it the next day in the form of a massive headache!

Now, all that said, booze can affect blood sugar in more indirect ways, the most significant of which is through sleep. Some people might use alcohol to fall asleep, but since it causes disruptions to your deepest (REM) sleep, people who drink before bed often experience insomnia or wake in the night. This can lead to a vicious cycle where you reach for caffeine first thing on an empty stomach, or a sugary snack to get you through the afternoon.

Then there's simply what alcohol can do to your overall judgment. I know I am less likely to make smart food decisions when I'm under the influence, and if I'm at all hungover, that lack of moderation spills into the next day. It's okay to let off steam and have fun, but as with all of life's pleasures, moderation is key.

7. CELEBRATE SMALL VICTORIES—PERFECTION IS A MYTH!

Anxiety, stress, resentment, fear, obsessiveness, perfectionism, control—these are all things that can torpedo your health journey before it even starts.

You don't need to get a gold star on every single slow carb strategy, or live with your blood sugar in mind 100 percent of the time—80, or even 60, percent is a fantastic improvement and a wonderful place to be. If you're not in control of your circumstances, or need a day to throw caution to the wind, the inevitable blood sugar spikes won't set you back to square one. As I like to say, **tomorrow there will always be more kale**.

THE SWEET SPOT

Every single diet dogma can be abused, misinterpreted, and used for harm instead of good. The same goes for some of the slow carb strategies in this book. If you focus too hard on your blood sugar, you might drift too far away from the foods that support your gut health. On the other side of the coin, if you're someone with IBS and focus too much on foods that don't make you bloated (like white rice), you might be doing damage to your hormones. As with all things, there is a balance to be had.

Although blood sugar is important, it is meaningless if we don't also live an anti-inflammatory lifestyle that takes our gut, individual frailties, and overall hormone health into consideration. Dark rye or pumpernickel bread will cause fewer glucose spikes, but it isn't the best choice for those with celiac disease or someone who might have an inflammatory reaction to gluten. Cheese is a better option than a package of fruit snacks but, potentially, might make someone with lactose intolerance or IBS more miserable. And although bacon, beef, and processed deli meats are likely to keep your glucose levels low, the overwhelming nutritional science says that legumes, whole grains, and plant protein are better for long-term gut and heart health.

If you have diabetes, you'll need to choose a different carb adventure than someone with SIBO. So, **pick and choose which tactics work best for your lifestyle**, and marry them with the amount of carbs that seem to support your body best.

Now that you've learned a few more ways to slow down or offset the carbs on your plate, in the next section we'll focus on the plate itself, including which foods have the best anti-inflammatory impact and how to adapt the recipes in this book for special diets.

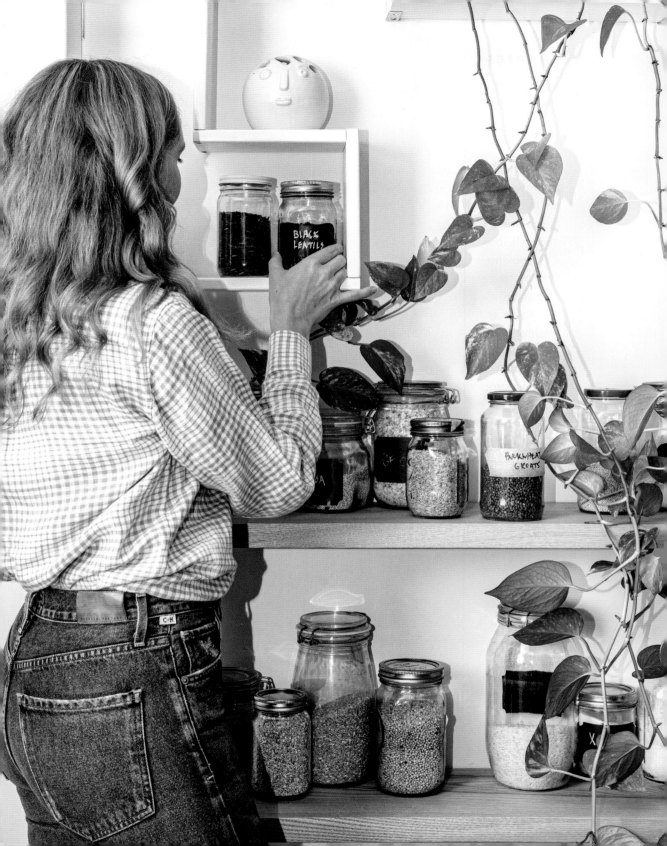

CHAPTER 3

Cooking Like a Carbivore

It's in the kitchen where you will put much of your newfound blood sugar knowledge to work. For many of you, that might require a bit of a learning curve. You may have to rethink your pantry, eschewing certain sugars and flours for new grains like kasha and millet. But the recipes in this book will make this process as fun, painless, and delicious as possible.

Cooking is not an exact science (despite what some chefs may tell you) and the tips in this section provide a great jumping-off point for you to find variety and get to the point where you can "freestyle."

There is no one diet that these recipes follow, but the closest would be the Mediterranean way of eating, which prioritizes anti-inflammatory vegetables, whole grains, legumes, seafood (more so than meat or poultry), fermented dairy, and heart-healthy oils. Populations in this part of the world continue to live longer than others, comprising many of the centenarian areas that make up the "Blue Zones." But there are other global influences with a similar culinary ethos that I've used for inspiration as well.

All recipes are labeled by various dietary restrictions—you'll find the key at the end of this chapter. The book is **completely gluten-free** as this is how I approach my diet. But it is not necessarily a health edict I mean to impose on you. You can find more information on how gluten fits into the carb picture at the end of this chapter, along with recommendations for modifying the recipes if you're a Carbivore who eats wheat.

Because of all the information in Chapters 1 and 2, I haven't included many snacks, sweet breakfasts, or desserts. The sweet recipes in this book are meant to be special-occasion affairs, and even more everyday items like **Violet's Big Blueberry-Oat Muffins** (page 103) should, ideally, not be eaten on an empty stomach. But rest assured that the comfort foods you find here will be less damaging to your blood sugar than most. To get a sense of where a recipe stands on the carb front, I've included a **Carb-O-Meter rating**. You can find an explanation for the levels at the end of this chapter.

Because there are a lot of one-pan or one-pot dinners, I offer suggestions for how to "Make It a Meal" with various sides from the book. That said, with the exception of the main course salads, few dishes won't benefit from adding one of the **Simple Starter Salads** on page 81 to begin. Though most dishes are designed around vegetables, there are also suggestions for how to add "Carb Companions." And because I'm always about making a recipe your own, you'll see some suggestions for other ingredients to use from your pantry in the "Carb Swap" section. Finally, for times of the year when certain produce might not be available, I give substitution suggestions for a "Change of Season" to make these dishes year-round.

Beyond anything, remember that **food is more than just medicine**. Many of you may be facing health challenges that have complicated your relationship with foods you used to love, perhaps through intolerances or ongoing chronic issues. Perhaps mealtime has become a charged affair, and your kitchen a place you resent spending time.

Just remember, cooking can be a source of joy, not stress. Part of healthy living is spending time with friends and family around a table. There is so much more that controls our blood sugar (and general health) than what we eat. **Let the recipes in this book be an opportunity to rediscover food freedom and put that love on the plate for all to share.**

CARBIVORE KITCHEN MANTRAS

Make Vegetables the Star of Your Meal

The ideal Carbivore blue plate special is divided into two sections, with half the real estate dedicated to vegetables, and animal protein and carbs splitting the other half. This doesn't necessarily happen with every meal or recipe, but it's what I strive for to ensure there's maximum nutrient density and fiber to slow your carbs.

Use Meat as a Garnish, Not the Main Event

One of the pitfalls of a low-carb diet is, often, the real estate on your plate that might have been taken up by carbs gets shifted to animal protein. This book focuses on leaner proteins like fish and poultry, and uses little red meat. Try to avoid highly processed deli meats, which have been classified by the World Health Organization as carcinogens.[15] You'll find some bacon and prosciutto here and there (because, hedonism), but buy paleo varieties without added sugar, nitrates, or other additives.

Put Carbs at the Bottom of the Bowl

One way to eat your fat, fiber, and protein first is to make composed bowls and bury the carbs beneath all the other ingredients. It's a more natural way to food sequence and go "slow carb" without driving yourself crazy. If you're making **The Simplest Poke Bowls** (page 123), spread the rice on the bottom of the bowl and pile the cabbage slaw and diced fish on top. You'll be forced to work your way down through the vegetables, fat, and protein to reach the carbs. You can use this method with any type of weeknight carb-based bowl, like **Grilled Skirt Steak & Vermicelli Bowls with Nuoc Cham** (page 198).

Don't Peel Your Veggies

Plants store more fiber in their skin than their fleshy centers. One easy way to up the fiber content of your meals—and save a lot of time in the kitchen!—is to use produce unpeeled. This is the default for all the recipes in this book, especially carrots and potatoes, so leave the skin on unless explicitly told otherwise. This rule can also apply to using a vegetable "nose to tail." Don't toss those broccoli stalks—there's even more delicious fiber in them than the florets!

Develop Resistant Starch

Certain types of starch can actually be beneficial to your blood sugar. In particular, the resistant starch in legumes, potatoes, and unripe bananas cannot be broken down by the digestive system. Instead of being converted into glucose and absorbed into the bloodstream, it passes into the colon, where it feeds your friendly gut bacteria. In many ways, **resistant starch acts in the same way as fiber does in our bodies.** For starchy foods like rice and potatoes, it's possible to develop resistant starch even further by cooking and then cooling these foods to room temperature before eating them. Like sourdough fermentation, this practice falls into the category of **"slow carb"** culinary techniques. When prepared this way, an ingredient that might otherwise cause blood sugar spikes, instead, can improve insulin sensitivity and increase satiety, so you feel less hungry. **Crispy Rice with Spicy Beet Tartare** (page 125), **Crab Cake Twice-Baked Potatoes** (page 223), and **Roasted Sweet Potatoes with Beans & Greens** (page 311) are examples of recipes for which cooking and cooling your carbs to develop resistant starch can be organically part of the dish.

Add Vinegar to Salads & Soups

Vinegar is acetic acid, which has the power to temporarily inactivate the enzyme we need to break down starches into glucose. The acid also activates our muscles to use more glucose. The result of these two phenomena is less glucose in the bloodstream: It enters more slowly and gets used more quickly. This can be a big asset to cooking, as vinegar is a delicious way to add a sour balance to sweet or spicy flavors. But you can also actively consume **1 tablespoon apple cider vinegar diluted in 8 ounces water** before a high-carb meal to improve blood sugar tolerance.

Drinking vinegar before meals isn't a license to have a carb binge every day, but on special occasions, it can allow you to indulge in some birthday cake without suffering the consequences to your sleep, skin, and energy the following day. It also has the added benefit of getting stomach acid flowing, which is important for good digestion (even though you've heard otherwise in many pep-themed ads).

If you're starting a meal with a green salad, using a vinegar-based dressing, like my **Spicy Sesame Dressing** (page 60), **Summer Tomato-Cashew Dressing** (page

59), or **Basic Balsamic Vinaigrette** (page 60), is a great way to do double duty for your blood sugar. I also love using vinegar for finishing soups, like my **Warming Mushroom & Wild Rice Soup** (page 127) or **Greenhouse Gazpacho** (page 256). We can even see this tip at work in the classic carb combination of malt vinegar on fish and chips!

Fresh lemon juice has a similar impact but isn't as effective as vinegar. Still, if you prefer the flavor, it's a wonderful addition to any recipe.

Soak & Sprout Your Grains

Until about a hundred years ago, humans harvested grains and left them in the field until they were ready to process. With this exposure to the weather, at least some of the grains would begin to sprout. Skipping that essential step may be one reason we are unable to digest grains as well as we used to.

The sprouting process increases the bioavailability of some vitamins (including B vitamins, vitamin C, and folate).[16] It also decreases the amount of starch in grains, so they contain fewer carbs and more protein. Though the recipes in this book don't specifically call for sprouted grains, you will gain a leg up by seeking out pre-sprouted store-bought options or by sprouting whole grains yourself before cooking them. The process is simple, but takes a little forethought: Start with a whole grain, like brown rice, with the bran and germ intact, soak it in water overnight, and rinse before using. Although they are not fully sprouted at this stage, these soaked grains often require less liquid to cook and are easier for your body to break down.

Use a Nut Crunch or Seed Sprinkle

The ultimate carb companions, nuts and seeds add healthy fats, fiber, and protein to your plate, along with vitamins and minerals that reduce risk factors for chronic diseases. Health bonus points aside, they are a delicious way to get creative with various spices and low-sugar "candying" techniques, and add a necessary crunch to any dish that needs a little variation in texture (like pureed soups). There are many ancient culinary traditions that use nut and seed sprinkles in carb dishes. For example, dukkah and za'atar in parts of the Middle East, and gomasio in Japan. See page 75 for a range of recipes for these toppings!

Keep Dried Fruit to a Minimum

As you learned in Chapter 1, dried fruit has almost five times the sugar content as the same quantity of fresh fruit because all the water weight has been removed. Although I avoid snacking on dried fruit, there is a place for it in some savory cooking, especially as a way to complement rich stews and smoky spices. When using dried fruit, make sure you have plenty of fiber and protein to offset it. This is common in Middle Eastern cooking, which inspired dishes like my **Spicy Beef Tagine with Apricots & Rosemary** (page 220), **Sweet & Sour Moroccan Chicken-Rice Casserole** (page 119), and **Braised Chickpeas & Broccolini with Golden Raisins** (page 323).

Opt for Berries or Underripe Fruit

Though all whole fruit has the benefit of fiber, some fruits have higher levels of fructose than others. In general, berries tend to be the best option for sugar-to-fiber ratios, followed by cherries, citrus, kiwis, green apples, and underripe bananas. A green mango will have a very different sugar profile than a fully ripe orange-fleshed one. And, in general, the fruits with the highest sugar ratios tend to be pineapple, watermelon, banana, and mango.

Choose Full-Fat Dairy

Though we more commonly think of dairy as a fat or protein, it is also full of carbohydrates, including the sugar lactose! When you remove the fat, the percentage of sugar per ounce increases naturally. This makes skim milk and fat-free yogurt much worse for your blood sugar. Fat also has the upside of decreasing the amount of insulin released after a meal. If you eat dairy, buy whole milk, heavy cream, or full-fat unsweetened Greek yogurt. If you're plant based, choose unsweetened coconut, nut, or seed milk instead of oat milk, which is higher in carbs. Oat milk is great for adding creaminess to dishes with built-in carb companions, but less ideal for adding to coffee or consuming as part of breakfast—avoid it on an empty stomach!

Eat Sourdough Bread

Bread that's made with a true sourdough starter will have fewer carbs and less gluten thanks to the fermentation process. Often, sandwich bread that is called "sourdough" in the supermarket is not true sourdough, so when possible, try to invest in local bakers who use this slow, ancient preparation instead of industrial mixers with half the rise time. If you can find whole wheat, rye, pumpernickel, or seed breads made with sourdough starter, even better. Those who are sensitive to gluten can often tolerate true sourdough, but it is not suitable for those with celiac disease. Luckily, there are plenty of gluten-free sourdough loaves now without wheat flour.

In addition to the health benefits, sourdough has a complex tang and spongy crumb that adds nuance to recipes like **Sheet Pan Chicken BLT Panzanella with Vinegared Tomatoes** (page 243), **Butternut Squash & Leek Stuffing** (page 259), and **Grilled Balsamic Mushroom Melts** (page 253).

Swap Added Sugar for Nature's Candy

Whenever I'm doing a "vice detox" or trying to tamp down my sugar intake, I try to fill my plate with vegetables that are naturally sweet when caramelized, like baked root vegetables, slow-roasted cherry tomatoes, or sautéed sweet corn. Adding cinnamon, clove, and other warming spices can help accentuate those naturally sweet notes. For example, if you want a completely sugar-free option for my **Basic Bitch Kale Salad** (page 85), swap the dried cherries for roasted butternut squash, sweet potato, or beets.

Use 70 Percent or Higher Chocolate

Chocolate with a higher percentage of cacao, anything above 70 percent, is much better for your blood glucose levels because it is lower in sugar. One benefit of making your own candy, like my **PB & J Cups with Crunchy Quinoa** (page 167), is being able to use good quality chocolate.

Halve the Sugar in Baked Goods

If you're going to have dessert, it should be something you'll really enjoy and savor, which is why I'm not a huge fan of "copycat" or "guilt-free" healthy desserts. That said, I find most baking recipes to be overly sweet, especially if you've deprogrammed your tongue from needing a massive amount of sugar. You will find you can reduce the quantity of sugar in most cake, muffin, and quick bread recipes. All the baked goods in this book contain roughly 50 percent less sugar than the average recipe does. You can always add more to taste, but I try to go with the bare minimum to please my palate.

Serve Dessert with a Carb Companion

When balancing blood sugar, I like to focus on what you can add, not just what you need to take away. Keeping that abundance mindset is one way to enjoy healthy hedonism while being mindful of carbs. So, embrace dessert and add a dollop of Greek yogurt, crème fraîche, or whipped cream to your cake. A sprinkle of nuts or seeds works, too. You can also replace some of the regular flour with almond flour since it's higher in fiber and protein and naturally lower in carbs—one of my tricks for **Violet's Big Blueberry-Oat Muffins** (page 103) and **Upside-Down Strawberry-Rhubarb Polenta Cake** (page 293). Both are also even more delicious with a schmear of nut butter or creamy topping.

GETTING TO KNOW YOUR CARB ALL-STARS

Now that you're familiar with some of the Carbivore cooking strategies I use in my recipes, let's talk about the cast of carb characters that are the stars of the show, including their origin stories and health benefits. The recipes in this book are organized by type of carb for those of you who like to menu-plan based on what you have in the pantry, or type of craving. For more on their preparation, see the beginning of each recipe chapter.

Oats

Though we've come to know oats mostly as the base for a quintessential breakfast porridge, they have been used around the world for centuries to create milky drinks, distilled alcoholic beverages, as flour for breads and noodles, and even in bath bombs to soothe rashes and pest bites.

Oats are often referred to as a whole grain, even in more processed forms, because the husk and germ almost always remain intact. Compared to other grains, oats are extremely well balanced: high in protein, lower in carbohydrates, and with healthy amounts of fat and fiber. One cup of oats covers 67 percent of your daily manganese requirement, which helps the body form connective tissue and build sex hormones. And most important for Carbivores, oats play a positive role in your carbohydrate metabolism by slowing gastric emptying and increasing the production of satiety hormones.

You've probably seen some of these claims touted on the back of cereal and granola boxes. But the fiber and protein content of oats improve insulin sensitivity and help lower blood sugar levels only when prepared properly, that is, as part of a balanced meal, like my **Savory Yogurt & Granola Bowls with Avocado & Eggs** (page 94), not in a quick-cooking microwavable packet rife with added sugar. Like other grains, the less processed the oat, the better it will be for your blood sugar. For this reason, steel cut is the best choice.

Though oats are naturally gluten-free, if you're gluten-sensitive or have celiac disease, buy oats that are certified gluten-free, as many producers use the same processing equipment for wheat and other gluten-containing grains.

Rice

The most prolific grain across the world, rice is, perhaps, the carb that's most foundational to global cuisine. **Nearly half of the world's population gets more than half of their daily calories from rice.** There are more than forty thousand different heirloom varieties of rice, grown from the paddies of Thailand and Vietnam to the lowlands of the American South—and each has its own distinctive shape, color, starch content, and flavor.

The main way rice grains are classified is by their length-to-width ratio once cooked. Long-grain rice tends to be drier, fluffier, and more forgiving, which makes it ideal to use in salads and pilafs, where aromatics and spices are added at the beginning of the cooking process. Short- and medium-grain rice, on the other hand, tends to be higher in starch, develops more of a sticky quality, and clumps together when cooked.

The second differentiation is usually color. Other than wild rice (which gets its own explanation), brown rice maintains its color because it's a whole grain, with the fibrous bran, germ, and endosperm intact. Like steel cut oats, any whole-grain rice—which includes black "forbidden" rice from China, purple Thai rice, Himalayan red rice, and many others—has a chewier texture and takes longer to cook. White rice, on the other hand, has had the bran and germ removed, making it quicker cooking and less likely to spoil. Although colorful whole-grain rice has double the nutrient density of white rice, that doesn't mean white rice can't be part of a healthy diet, especially with the right carb companions.

Arguably, the healthiest type of rice is sprouted or germinated brown rice, which is sometimes sold as GABA rice or under its Japanese name, *hatsuga genmai*. The sprouting process makes your grains' nutrients more bioavailable, and with rice, particularly vitamin E, magnesium, B vitamins, potassium, zinc, and the amino acid GABA, a neurotransmitter with calming effects on the brain.

Finally, in a category unto itself, is wild rice. Technically a seed from lake grass, wild rice is indigenous to the American Midwest. High in protein and fiber, with thirty times the amount of antioxidants in white rice, wild rice is the healthiest choice for managing blood sugar. In particular, it is high in manganese and is alkaline-forming, which can help your gut maintain a healthy pH. The high fiber content of wild rice can combat constipation, whereas most white rice tends to be a better choice if you're prone to diarrhea or struggle with gut issues and need something that's easier to process.

Millet

Though it is common in many parts of the world, millet is most prevalent in West African cuisine, where each different variety has its own preparation. Teff, the slightest of millet seeds, is often ground into flour and used in flatbreads, such as the Ethiopian staple injera. Fonio, which is now making its presence better known on American supermarket shelves, is perfect for a quick-cooking pilaf. Like many ancient grains, millet is low on the glycemic index and high in iron, zinc, and antioxidants. It separates itself from the rest of the field with certain amino acids that are not found in other grains.

Quinoa

Quinoa is an Andean plant originally grown by the Inca in parts of Peru, Chile, and Bolivia, who called it the mother of all grains. In the last two decades, quinoa has become a staple "superfood" of American wellness culture, largely due to its reputation as a complete protein, meaning it contains all the amino acids necessary to build tissue and transport nutrients to our cells that our bodies don't produce on their own.

Buckwheat

Earthy, moody buckwheat is central to many cultures across the globe, from the craggy Northern European coast of Brittany and its savory, square *galette bretonne*

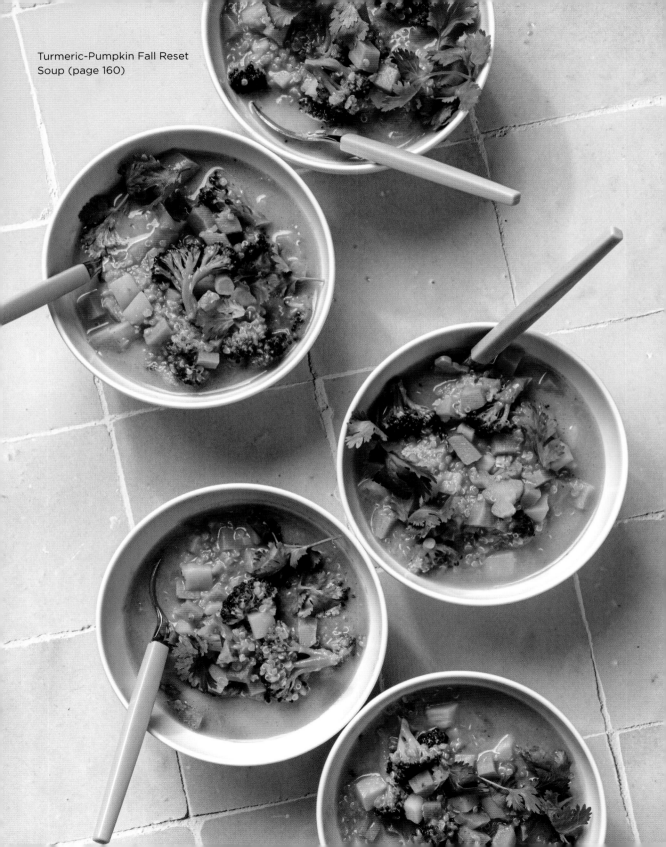

Turmeric-Pumpkin Fall Reset
Soup (page 160)

to the shorelines of Japan, where buckwheat flour has been pulled into soba noodles since the Middle Ages. But buckwheat is, perhaps, the most integral to the cuisines and economies of Eastern Europe and Russia. There, buckwheat groats are eaten whole in breakfast porridge and pilafs, like my **Kasha Pilaf with Mushrooms, Bacon & Greens** (page 162), and baked into sweet and savory loaves, like in my **Black Sesame–Buckwheat Banana Bread** (page 164).

Buckwheat's rich color reflects the bevy of important nutrients it contains: zinc, potassium, manganese, and B vitamins. It has significantly more protein and fiber than many of the healthiest grains (looking at you, oats) and is naturally gluten-free. It is a perfect example of a complex carbohydrate that slows digestion and helps keep blood sugar levels stable longer. From a sustainability standpoint, buckwheat is just as nutritious for the soil as it is for the humans and livestock that consume it.

Pasta

Noodles span continents, come shaped like bow ties, ears, or sheets, and can be made from wheat, mung beans, sweet potato, rice, corn, buckwheat, quinoa, legumes—really any carb in this book! As author Jen Lin-Liu discovered while researching *On the Noodle Road: From Beijing to Rome, with Love and Pasta,* the earliest Chinese noodles were actually formed from bread dough and thrown into a wok full of boiling water to cook.

From a health standpoint, pasta, by definition, is a processed food and so will carry the nutritional merits only of whatever flour it was created from. Red lentil or buckwheat noodles will have more protein, antioxidants, and fiber than a regular wheat or white rice noodle. But in terms of your blood sugar, the carb impact is negligible, because no matter what, your body will break down the flours quickly—that is, unless there is something else in the mix to slow it down.

The healthiest way to enjoy noodles is tossed with plenty of carb companions. Whether it's green vegetables as in **Green Curry Ramen with Eggplant & Green Beans** (page 181) or **Spanakopita Lasagna** (page 201), lean protein, like the hunks of fish in **Cod & Orzo Arrabbiata** (page 178) or **Salmon & Broccoli Noodle Casserole** (page 188), fat-rich nut or seed butters in **Creamy Sesame Noodle Salad with Smashed Cucumbers** (page 183), or even a modest helping of gooey melted cheese in a more indulgent **Spinach-Artichoke Dip Mac & Cheese** (page 173).

At the end of the day, noodles are comfort food. So start with a green salad, embrace a little hedonism along with your veggies, and make them count.

Potatoes

One reason the humble potato has been so prized for centuries is its unmatched nutritional yield per acre. Potatoes contain nearly every important vitamin, but the majority of their nutritional value is in the skin, so it's important to leave it on!

The flesh has another important health feature, though: resistant starch. This starch is not fully absorbed by your body and becomes fast food for beneficial butyrate-producing bacteria in your gut once it reaches the large intestine. Studies have shown that butyrate can reduce inflammation in the colon and lower cancer risk. This type of bacteria is also essential for maintaining a healthy digestive system and avoiding acute issues like IBS or SIBO.

Potato starch has been shown to reduce insulin resistance and improve blood sugar control. Though potato starch can be bought as a powdered by-product and whisked into beverages, soups, and baked goods, you can increase the amount of naturally occurring resistant starch in potatoes by boiling them and then cooling them in the fridge for an hour or overnight before eating or using them in a recipe.

Although all potatoes have fiber, protein, and antioxidants, certain varieties make a stronger showing in certain categories. Russets are the highest in protein. Red potatoes are the most nutrient dense and possess high levels of quercetin, a flavonoid with anticancer and anti-inflammatory properties, and choline, an essential nutrient for women in their childbearing years. Colorful options, like blue and sweet potatoes, have the best mineral profile, including most of your daily values of copper, magnesium, manganese, phosphorus, and potassium.

Bread

Since wheat was domesticated in ancient times, bread dough was the glue that held whole societies together. It has been used nub to crumb for centuries as a culinary jack-of-all-trades, thickening and binding, adding texture or creaminess, stretching a meal of fresh produce from one mouth to four, or hiding in the background of a dip, if only to make more of it for your crust to plunge into. And yet today, we scoop out our bagels and make flatbread out of cauliflower. I can picture the ancient Egyptians rolling in their sarcophagi!

Bread can be part of a healthy diet if not eaten on an empty stomach straight from the basket before a meal. In fact, so many of our iconic bread pairings include built-in carb companions: pita and hummus, melted cheese in a grilled sandwich, bagels with lox and a schmear.

In terms of what your bread is made from, there is not a huge difference between white and wheat bread when it comes to blood sugar, though anything with whole seeds inside or on top (like in multi-grain bread) helps. Rather, the healthiest varieties are some of the oldest: fermented from a sourdough starter or using whole grains like rye berries instead of refined, milled flour—the darker, the better. Sprouted-grain breads contain even less starch and more bioavailable minerals. Sourdough bread is similarly a better choice for your blood sugar as the fermentation process involves bacteria eating away at the carb count and gluten.

Non-celiac gluten sensitivity has risen to epic proportions in the last decade, spurring numerous theories as to why people are reacting to a protein in wheat that has been our culinary lifeline for centuries. One potential reason is this: Over the years, wheat has been hybridized to withstand increased levels of pesticides, most notably glyphosate, the main ingredient in Roundup. This chemical is as disruptive to beneficial flora in our gut as it is to pests in nature.

The gluten protein itself has posed a risk in the autoimmune era because of molecular mimicry, a phenomenon that occurs when a foreign player is so structurally similar to your body's own tissues that when your immune system creates antibodies to attack the invader, it mistakenly attacks your body in the process. Gluten is structurally similar to a number of your body's tissues, particularly the thyroid gland, making it both a contributing factor for autoimmune thyroid diseases and an ingredient that fans the flames of those already struggling with high thyroid antibody counts. Because I fall under this category, all recipes in this book were tested using gluten-free bread. That said, many commercial gluten-free options are made with refined flours, gums, and stabilizers and, often, have added sugar in them. So, if you tolerate wheat and can buy freshly baked sourdough from a specialized baker, that is usually a healthier option than a highly processed gluten-free loaf with ten-plus items on the ingredient list.

Corn

The two varieties of corn that we've come to know in our kitchen are sweet corn, the whole cobs (that have the juice!), and field corn, which is ground into starch, flour, meal, and grits, or used whole for popcorn. Sweet corn is typically thought of as a vegetable and used as such, grilled or steamed whole and slathered with butter, or sautéed with other summer vegetables in a succotash (see **Summer Squash Succotash Enchiladas,** page 285). Field corn by-products are pantry items that we more typically think of as part of the grain family—a traditional carb, if you will.

Though the way it's been bred over time has upped the sugar content, sweet corn still has a healthy amount of dietary fiber to offset it, along with high levels of vitamin A and antioxidants. That means more food for the good gut bacteria in your large intestine. In fact, because it's not uncommon to find whole corn kernels in your stool, it's also a great transit test to see how well your gut motility is working. Ideally, you'd want to see those kernels hit the toilet between twenty-four and thirty-six hours after eating them if your bowels are moving well.

When used as a grain, corn undergoes various types of processing. One of the most ancient techniques is nixtamalization, which is a method of soaking maize in an alkaline solution—usually limewater—that was used by Indigenous Peoples of Mesoamerica, like the Mayans. And like many centuries-old "slow carb" practices, it not only makes the corn easier to work with, but also more nutritious. The soaking process increases the bioavailability of nutrients like calcium and niacin, and the alkaline solution ensures that no mold or mycotoxins can develop. Today, the process is still commonly used on hominy, which is then ground into masa for corn tortillas, arepas, and tamales.

Unfortunately, about 90 percent of American-grown field corn is genetically engineered (GMO). There are many people who argue that these modifications pose no issue for the human body. But many GMO crops were designed to produce their own insecticide, called Bt toxin, which kills insects by destroying the lining of their digestive tracts. Studies have shown that this action is also effective on human cells, damaging the intestines and causing leaky gut. For this reason, I recommend investing in high quality cornmeal, masa, and polenta from smaller producers who grow non-GMO heirloom varietals, especially blue-, red-, or pink-hued. See the Resources section for some of my favorites.

Legumes

Legumes, also known as pulses, are one of the world's oldest superfoods and were the strongest constant in the diet of every centenarian population studied in Dan Buettner's *The Blue Zones Solution: Eating and Living Like the World's Healthiest People.* They are also in a carb category unto themselves.

Beans, peas, and lentils—among the many other varieties—are high in starch, but also have two to three times more protein than wheat and rice. What sets legumes apart, though, is that so much of their starch content is "resistant starch," which acts similarly to dietary fiber in the body (and legumes have a lot of that, too).

Of course, one person's pleasure is another person's pain. Having written recipes for the IBS and SIBO community, I know legumes can be a big pitfall that leads to unwanted bloating and discomfort for some. Usually, this is a sign of a larger imbalance. If you've lost all your butyrate-producing bacteria (due to overuse of antibiotics or an unhealthy diet), you can eat all the beans in the world and they're just going to make you miserable.

This isn't a lifelong sentence, however. Gas is a natural by-product of all that good fermentation that's happening in your gut when you eat legumes. The key is to ramp up your intake carefully so the bloating doesn't get uncomfortable. After a period of gut healing and gradual integration, eventually, a big bowl of chili or **Lazy-Day Dal** (page 309) won't affect you the way it used to.

There are hundreds of varieties of pulses grown around the globe, and due to their nutrient density and affordability, they are often mixed with other starches as built-in carb companions: rice and beans in Central America; mujaddara, a rice and lentil pilaf from the Middle East; and, of course, the most humble and delicious of Anglo lunches, beans on toast.

NAVIGATING CARB CONSUMPTION FOR YOUR DIETARY RESTRICTIONS

As I mentioned at the end of Chapter 2, it's important to consider your individual body and digestive system when tackling the recipes in this book. We all have different tolerances and restrictions. Here are a few examples of how the recipes can be interpreted for different diets.

Adapting Recipes If You Eat Wheat

Although for many people eating gluten-free is a better choice, there are also plenty of ways to be unhealthy on a gluten-free diet. If you tolerate wheat, feel free to use any bread or pasta you like in these recipes. Regular soy sauce can be substituted for gluten-free tamari. And gluten-containing whole grains, like farro, barley, or bulgur wheat, can be substituted in many of the recipes calling for quinoa, millet, or kasha. The one place where substitutions won't work perfectly is in baked goods. Gluten-free flours often have different densities than wheat flour, so a one-to-one swap will work only if the ingredient called for is an all-purpose gluten-free baking flour. All other flours should be used as specified.

Adapting Recipes for a Paleo Diet

The majority of the Spuds chapter is paleo and, in many other cases, you can remove the grains and still enjoy a recipe. For pasta dishes, substitute zucchini noodles, cassava flour pasta, or kelp noodles for gluten-free pasta. Shirataki noodles can also work in place of rice noodles or ramen.

For rice recipes, cauliflower rice will work in most quick cooking stir-fries or pilafs but is less ideal for a casserole or risotto. In the Corn chapter, Siete brand almond flour or cassava tortillas can replace corn tortillas. In all cases, plant-based cheese, milk, yogurt, and butter can be substituted for regular dairy.

Adapting Recipes for IBS, SIBO, or a Low-FODMAP Diet

For those with certain types of gut issues, like SIBO and IBS, tons of fiber is just going to make you miserable. For many, the solution is a low-carb approach to eating, like the low-FODMAP diet, which includes many starchy ingredients we embrace in this book, but limits certain carbohydrates in vegetables and fruits. A short-term (eight weeks maximum) stint on this diet can reduce gut inflammation and allow the tight junctions in our intestinal lining to repair. And this, eventually, has a positive halo effect on our large intestine's microbiome—and our blood sugar.

You'll find recipes that can be adapted for the low-FODMAP diet noted on the dietary restriction key. Since gluten-free grains like quinoa, millet, rice, and oats, along with potatoes and flint corn, are all naturally low in FODMAPs, there are many recipes you can use as a guide and swap out high-FODMAP veggies for a different carb companion.

If you fall into this camp, be mindful that certain strategies in Chapter 2 might not be the best fit for you. For example, starter salads could prove too much for your digestive system, and so you might be better off incorporating vegetables in their pureed form, even if it isn't as beneficial for your blood sugar. Some of the lifestyle tips, like walking after a meal or drinking vinegar in water before eating, are better options in those cases.

CARB-O-METER RATINGS

No one likes to be bogged down counting macros, so I've created a simple cheat sheet to help you determine whether a recipe can be enjoyed with abandon or requires some of the carb-mitigating tactics laid out in Chapter 2 to prevent a blood sugar spike.

CARB LEVEL 1

These recipes are predominantly made up of fat, fiber-rich plants, and protein. They may contain some carbs as an accent, but are balanced enough that you can enjoy a serving or two without having to worry about the impact on your blood sugar.

CARB LEVEL 2

Moderate-carb recipes, like those in Level 2, are starch heavy, but predominantly savory. They may already include carb companions, yet would still benefit from a few of the strategies for carb mitigation, like beginning your meal with a green salad or moving for ten minutes after eating.

CARB LEVEL 3

The recipes in this tier are more special-occasion (and often sweet) dishes that warrant being mindful of your portions. Avoid eating on an empty stomach.

RECIPE DIETARY RESTRICTION KEY			
GF	Gluten Free	Vgt	Vegetarian / Plant-Based
LF	Low-FODMAP	V	Vegan
DF	Dairy-Free	SF	No Added Sugar
P	Paleo		

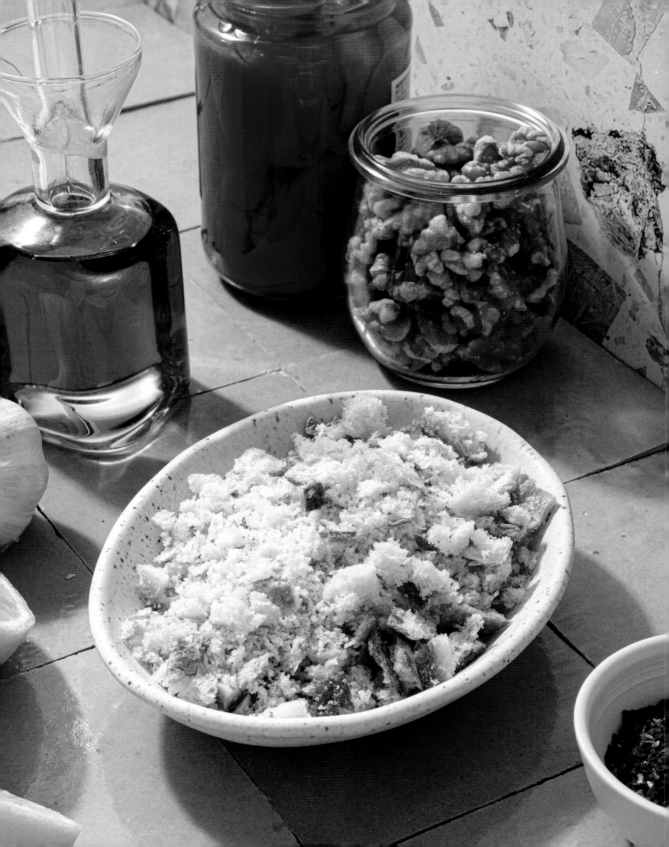

PART TWO

THE RECIPES

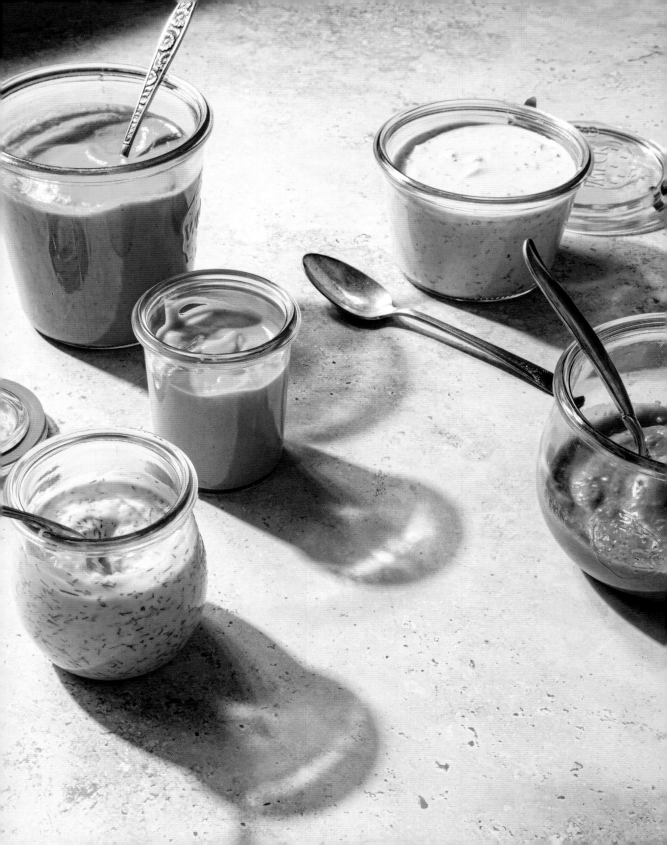

CARB COMPANIONS

Sauces, Condiments, Toppings & Starters

• • •

Summer Tomato-Cashew Dressing

Basic Balsamic Vinaigrette

Spicy Sesame Dressing

Creamy Caper Dressing

Liquid Gold Turmeric-Tahini Dressing

Caesar-ish Dressing

Lemon Poppy Vinaigrette

Kefir Green Goddess Dressing

Ginger-Walnut Sauce

Low-Fructose BBQ Sauce

Harissa Yogurt

Chipotle-Tahini Sauce

Tarragon-Chive Tartar Sauce

Dill Aioli

Arugula-Almond Pesto

Cilantro-Sriracha Mayo

Charlie's Magic Grill Marinade

Sugar-Free Ginger Applesauce

Raspberry-Chia Jam

Nut Crunches & Seed Sprinkles, 5 Ways

Simple Starter Salads, 4 Ways

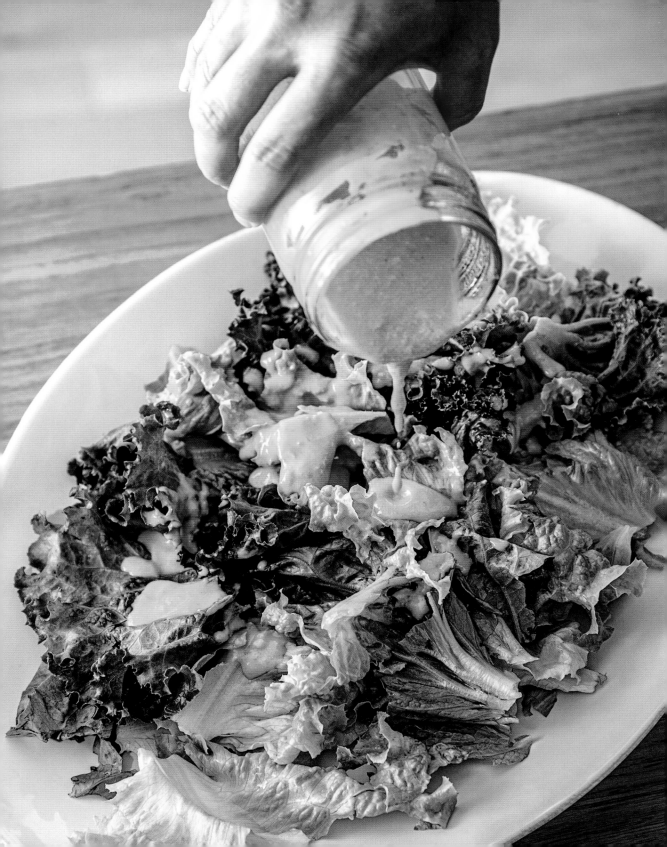

Summer Tomato-Cashew Dressing

I have a bit of an over-buying problem when it comes to tomatoes, so they often find their way not only into my salads, but also the dressings. This bright stunner of a sauce evolved from a vegan tomato soup I make that uses cashews as the thickener. Tomatoes carry their own lovely acidity, but are punched up here by cider vinegar. If you don't have a high-speed blender, soak the cashews in boiling water for ten minutes before using. The dressing tastes wonderful warm or at room temperature and can double as a sauce for anything that comes off the grill. You can also use it as a substitute for the dressing in my **Roasted Cauliflower Salad with Quinoa, Arugula & Creamy Romesco Dressing** (page 146).

MAKES 1 CUP

- 1 medium heirloom tomato (8 ounces), cut into wedges
- 1 small shallot, thinly sliced
- 2 tablespoons raw cashews
- ¼ cup extra-virgin olive oil
- ½ teaspoon sea salt
- ¼ teaspoon red pepper flakes (optional)
- 1 tablespoon apple cider vinegar

1 In a small saucepan over medium heat, combine the tomato, shallot, cashews, oil, salt, and red pepper flakes (if using). Cook, stirring occasionally, until the tomato softens and the shallot is translucent, about 4 minutes.

2 Off the heat, stir in the vinegar, scraping up any browned bits from the bottom. Transfer the contents of the pan to a high-speed blender and puree until smooth. Taste for seasoning, and add more salt, as needed. If the dressing is too thick, add a little water, 1 tablespoon at a time, to thin it to your desired consistency. Refrigerate in an airtight container for up to 1 week.

GF DF P Vgt V SF

Basic Balsamic Vinaigrette

This back-pocket dressing uses the proper technique for emulsifying vinegar into oil. Consider it a step up from your usual mason jar shake, with double the creaminess for half the bicep effort. True balsamic vinegar doesn't have any added sugar, but is naturally sweet thanks to the grapes it was fermented from. Many commercial balsamic vinegars, however, are made quickly in a lab with flavor additives, including grape concentrate. If you use balsamic often, it's worth investing in an authentic Italian-made product.

MAKES ¾ CUP

¼   cup balsamic vinegar

2   tablespoons Dijon mustard

½   teaspoon sea salt

½   cup extra-virgin olive oil

In a small bowl or liquid measuring cup, whisk together the vinegar, mustard, and salt until smooth. Add **1 teaspoon oil** and whisk vigorously until combined. Repeat twice more with another teaspoon of oil. Once the oil is assimilating easily, slowly drizzle in the remaining oil, whisking throughout. Taste for seasoning, and add more salt or oil, as needed. Refrigerate in an airtight container for up to 1 month.

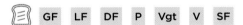

GF   LF   DF   P   Vgt   V   SF

Spicy Sesame Dressing

I often use this dressing on pasta as a nut-free alternative to peanut noodles (see **Creamy Sesame Noodle Salad with Smashed Cucumbers**, page 183) or as a side salad topper. Gochugaru is a mild Korean chili flake often used in kimchi. If you're replacing it, use 2 teaspoons sriracha or sambal olek, or ¼ to ½ teaspoon red pepper flakes.

MAKES ½ CUP

¼   cup tahini

2   tablespoons rice vinegar

2   tablespoons gluten-free tamari or soy sauce

1   tablespoon toasted sesame oil

1   tablespoon sesame seeds

1   teaspoon gochugaru (see headnote)

¼   teaspoon sea salt

In a small bowl or liquid measuring cup, whisk together the tahini, vinegar, tamari, sesame oil, sesame seeds, gochugaru, and salt. Add **2 tablespoons water** and whisk until smooth and the consistency of ranch dressing. Taste for seasoning, and add more salt or spice, as needed. Refrigerate in an airtight container for up to 1 month.

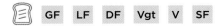

GF   LF   DF   Vgt   V   SF

Creamy Caper Dressing

Capers and seafood are a match made in heaven, so I often use this dressing as an adjunct to salads with shrimp or fish, like the **Seared Tuna Niçoise-ish Salad** (page 215). Because it's mayo based (but not overly weighed down by it), this dressing is also a healthier option to drizzle on a wedge salad (no offense to ranch or blue cheese). It also happens to be one of my favorites for dipping **Stuffed Artichokes with Italian Stallion Breadcrumbs** (page 261).

MAKES 1 CUP

2	tablespoons Dijon mustard
2	tablespoons mayonnaise
6	tablespoons capers (from one 3-ounce jar)
¼	cup tightly packed fresh parsley leaves
¼	cup fresh lemon juice (from 2 lemons)
¼	teaspoon sea salt
½	cup extra-virgin olive oil

In a small food processor or blender, pulse the mustard, mayonnaise, capers, parsley, lemon juice, and salt until finely chopped. With the machine running, slowly stream in the oil and puree until smooth. Taste for seasoning, and add more salt, as needed. Refrigerate in an airtight container for up to 1 week.

GF LF DF P Vgt SF   V use plant-based mayo

Liquid Gold Turmeric-Tahini Dressing

When you mix together lemon and tahini, you'll find my favorite example of culinary magic (what some people might call "science"). The mixture immediately seizes up into a paste, but when you add water, the tahini becomes pale, opaque, and creamy. If you add less water, you get the easiest five-ingredient dip for crudités (lazy cook's hummus!). But this iteration is thinned into a sauce, with anti-inflammatory turmeric to give it even more of a golden sheen. I like using it on **Basic Bitch Kale Salad** (page 85), but any salad greens will work.

MAKES ½ CUP

- ¼ cup tahini
- ¼ cup fresh lemon juice (from 2 lemons)
- 1 teaspoon honey or maple syrup
- ½ teaspoon sea salt
- ¾ teaspoon ground turmeric

In a medium bowl, whisk together the tahini, lemon juice, honey, salt, and turmeric. The mixture will seize up—don't worry! Add **2 tablespoons water** to the sauce and continue whisking until it resembles the consistency of ranch dressing. Add more water, as needed, to thin the sauce. Taste for seasoning, and add more salt, as needed. Refrigerate in an airtight container for up to 2 weeks.

  GF **DF** **P** **Vgt**  **LF** **V** use maple syrup **SF** omit sweetener

Caesar-ish Dressing

If raw egg yolk freaks you out, you can cheat by making a classic Caesar dressing with mayonnaise. It is, essentially, the same base ingredients, just preserved differently. My version is dairy-free but still packed with the requisite anchovies, since they are high in selenium and omega-3 fatty acids, but low in mercury. A dream carb companion.

MAKES ½ CUP

4   oil-packed
      anchovy fillets, or
      1 tablespoon anchovy
      paste

1   garlic clove

¼   cup fresh lemon juice
      (from 2 lemons)

2   tablespoons
      mayonnaise

1   tablespoon Dijon
      mustard

¼   teaspoon sea salt

¼   cup extra-virgin
      olive oil

In a small food processor, combine the anchovies, garlic, lemon juice, mayonnaise, mustard, and salt. Pulse until smooth. Stream in the oil slowly, pulsing to combine. If you don't have a food processor, mince the anchovies and garlic by hand and whisk into the remaining ingredients. Taste for seasoning, and add more salt or lemon juice, as needed. Refrigerate in an airtight container for up to 1 week.

GF   DF   P   SF   LF   omit garlic   **Vgt**   omit anchovies

Lemon Poppy Vinaigrette

One of my favorite trashy salads—the kind with dressing that makes the lettuce taste like candy—is from a place called Cowgirl in Manhattan. The lemon poppy seed dressing is addictively delicious. And now that I'm a Carbivore, I know that statement is not hyperbole thanks to all the sugar in it! My version uses a little maple syrup, but the sugar is offset by equal parts poppy seeds for fiber. I like this vinaigrette best on bitter or peppery lettuces like the arugula and radicchio found in my **Back-Pocket Tricolore Salad** (page 82).

MAKES ⅔ CUP

- ¼ cup fresh lemon juice (from 2 lemons)
- 2 tablespoons Dijon mustard
- 2 teaspoons maple syrup
- 2 teaspoons poppy seeds
- ½ teaspoon sea salt
- ¼ cup extra-virgin olive oil

In a small bowl, whisk together the lemon juice, mustard, maple syrup, poppy seeds, and salt until smooth. While whisking, slowly stream in the oil until it incorporates easily. Taste for seasoning, and add more salt, as needed. Refrigerate in an airtight container for up to 2 weeks.

GF   LF   DF   P   Vgt   V   SF   omit sweetener

Kefir Green Goddess Dressing

I adapted this gut-friendly dressing from my book *The Wellness Project*, where I discovered that the probiotic-rich drinkable yogurt, kefir, is the perfect texture for a creamy sauce that mimics ranch dressing. I try to buy the lactose-free variety of kefir, but if you can't find it at all, use ⅓ cup full-fat plain yogurt and ⅓ cup water. Any combinations of soft green herbs will work in this dressing, and miraculously, the yogurt is an excellent preservative, so the vibrant green color will keep.

MAKES 1 ½ CUPS

⅔	cup packed mixed fresh herbs (dill, basil, mint, parsley, chives)
½	avocado
1	garlic clove
2	tablespoons fresh lemon juice (from 1 lemon)
⅔	cup plain unsweetened kefir or plant-based alternative (see headnote)
¾	teaspoon sea salt

In a small food processor or blender, puree the herbs, avocado, garlic, lemon juice, kefir, salt, and **¼ cup water** until smooth. Add more water, 1 tablespoon at a time, until the dressing consistency resembles ranch. Taste for seasoning, and add more salt, as needed. Refrigerate in an airtight container for up to 1 week.

 GF **Vgt** **SF** **DF** **P** **V** use plant-based kefir or yogurt

Ginger-Walnut Sauce

Walnuts act as a thickener in this sauce (much like a nut butter) and also lend a subtle buttery flavor that pairs nicely with the spicy ginger and salty miso paste. Other than as a dipping sauce for the **Prelude-to-Summer Rolls** (page 131), you can use it as a salad dressing or topper for rice noodles.

MAKES ¾ CUP

⅓ cup raw walnuts

One 3-inch piece fresh ginger, peeled and roughly chopped

1 garlic clove

2 tablespoons fresh lime juice (from 1 or 2 limes)

2 tablespoons rice vinegar

2 tablespoons gluten-free tamari, soy sauce, or coconut aminos

2 tablespoons white miso paste

2 teaspoons maple syrup

½ teaspoon sea salt

⅓ cup extra-virgin olive oil

In a small food processor, pulse the walnuts, ginger, and garlic until finely chopped. Add the lime juice, vinegar, tamari, miso, maple syrup, and salt. Puree until smooth. Pulsing continuously, drizzle in the oil until the dressing consistency is between a vinaigrette and a pesto—you don't want the sauce too thin. Refrigerate in an airtight container for up to 2 weeks.

GF   DF   Vgt   V

LF   omit garlic   SF   omit maple syrup

Low-Fructose BBQ Sauce

Barbecue sauce (and ketchup, which often provides the base) is one of the most sugar-laden condiments on the shelf. But you need *some* sweetness to create that harmony of smoky spices, punchy vinegar, rich tomato, and heat. So, although I didn't eliminate the sugar entirely from this homemade version, it's definitely downgraded to more of a background vocal than the lead melody. We keep this sauce on hand for grilled salmon, steak, or chicken wings. And it works well in the **BBQ Chicken Thighs with Black-Eyed Peas & Collards** (page 303).

MAKES 2 CUPS

1   teaspoon extra-virgin olive oil

One 6-ounce can tomato paste

1   tablespoon onion powder

1   tablespoon garlic powder

1   tablespoon smoked paprika

2   teaspoons ground cumin

1   teaspoon sea salt

¼   teaspoon cayenne pepper (optional)

One 14-ounce can tomato sauce

2   tablespoons apple cider vinegar

2   tablespoons maple syrup

1   tablespoon gluten-free tamari, soy sauce, or coconut aminos

1   teaspoon Dijon mustard

❶ In a saucepan over medium-low heat, combine the oil, tomato paste, onion powder, garlic powder, smoked paprika, cumin, salt, and cayenne (if using). Stir to combine fully and cook until the tomato paste has darkened and caramelized, 2 to 3 minutes. If the tomato paste is sticking to the bottom of the pan, stir in **1 to 2 tablespoons water**, scraping up any browned bits from the bottom.

❷ Whisk in the tomato sauce, vinegar, maple syrup, tamari, and mustard. Bring to a gentle simmer and cook over medium heat until the tomato sauce has lost its acidity and the flavors become complex, about 10 minutes.

❸ Transfer the BBQ sauce to an airtight container and refrigerate for up to 1 month.

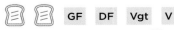

GF DF Vgt V

LF omit garlic and onion powder   **P** use coconut aminos

Harissa Yogurt

This sauce, which combines a spicy North African red pepper paste with full-fat plain yogurt, is so easy it feels like cheating. It's a terrific last-minute dip to serve with crackers and carrots, or as a sauce for more elaborate homemade treats like **Millet & Zucchini Cakes** (page 145) or **Parsnip-Potato Latkes** (page 225). The spicy yogurt can also serve as a schmear at the bottom of your breakfast bowl (see page 94).

MAKES 1 CUP

1   cup full-fat plain Greek or regular yogurt

¼   cup chopped fresh mint

2   tablespoons harissa paste

¼   teaspoon sea salt

In a medium bowl, stir together the yogurt, mint, harissa, and salt until combined. Taste for seasoning, and add more salt or harissa, as needed. Refrigerate in an airtight container for up to 2 weeks.

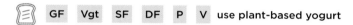 GF Vgt SF DF P V use plant-based yogurt

Chipotle-Tahini Sauce

Though tahini is most popular in Middle Eastern cooking, I've found it to be a perfect creamy base for sauces influenced by other cuisines, like this spicy, lime-y Southwestern number. If you're sensitive to heat, start with one or two chipotles before adding more. I use this sauce on my **Roasted Sweet Potatoes with Beans & Greens** (page 311), but it also tastes fantastic on any kind of taco or as a salad dressing with romaine lettuce.

MAKES 1 CUP

½   cup tahini

½   cup fresh lime juice (from 6 to 8 limes)

1   large garlic clove

2 or 3 chipotle chiles (from a can of chipotles in adobo sauce)

1 ½   teaspoons sea salt

In a small food processor or blender, combine the tahini, lime juice, garlic, chipotles (see headnote), salt, and **1 cup water**. Puree until smooth. Taste for seasoning, and add more salt, as needed. Refrigerate in an airtight container for up to 1 week.

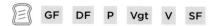 GF DF P Vgt V SF

Tarragon-Chive Tartar Sauce

This is a French-y take on tartar sauce using anise-forward tarragon and cornichons instead of relish. In addition to **Mom's Millet Flour Fish Fry** (page 159), you can serve this sauce with poached shrimp (mayo dippers are always better than sugary cocktail sauce), crab cakes, and all manner of crispy potatoes.

MAKES 1 ½ CUPS

1   cup mayonnaise

2   tablespoons roughly chopped capers

2   tablespoons finely chopped cornichons

2   tablespoons finely chopped fresh chives

2   tablespoons finely chopped fresh tarragon

2   tablespoons Dijon mustard

Grated zest of 1 lemon

1   tablespoon fresh lemon juice

In a small bowl, stir together the mayonnaise, capers, cornichons, chives, tarragon, mustard, lemon zest, and lemon juice. Refrigerate in an airtight container for up to 1 week.

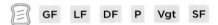 GF   LF   DF   P   Vgt   SF

Dill Aioli

It feels a little too fashionable in the culinary world to be a "dill girl" these days, but I will pile on anyway, since it is one of my beloved stand-alone herbs to flavor a creamy dipping sauce. This aioli works well as a slightly less time-consuming alternative to tartar sauce with crispy fish dishes like **Mom's Millet Flour Fish Fry** (page 159), but it is also my go-to dipper for **Hemp-Crusted Chicken Tenders** (page 136).

MAKES ½ CUP

½   cup mayonnaise

¼   cup finely chopped fresh dill

1   tablespoon Dijon mustard

1   tablespoon fresh lemon juice

1   small garlic clove, minced or pushed through a press

Sea salt

In a medium bowl, whisk together the mayonnaise, dill, mustard, lemon juice, and garlic until smooth. Taste for seasoning, and add salt, as needed. Refrigerate in an airtight container for up to 1 week.

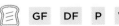 GF   DF   P   Vgt   SF   V   use plant-based mayo

Arugula-Almond Pesto

When pine nuts started to get absurdly expensive a decade or so ago, I began substituting whole almonds in my pesto. And when supermarkets started replacing big bunches of herbs with teeny tiny little plastic clamshells, well, I started using arugula as my green of choice! This pesto is peppery, garlicky, and bright. You can add parmesan for more nuttiness, but I think it tastes fresher without the cheese. I like using this pesto to liven up a veggie sandwich (see **Grilled Balsamic Mushroom Melts**, page 253), as a pizza topper, or as a mix-in, in the case of **Pesto Socca with Antipasti Salad** (page 318), as a simple pasta sauce, and as a condiment for fish or chicken.

MAKES 1 SCANT CUP

- 4 cups packed arugula
- 1 large garlic clove
- ¼ cup almonds
- 1 tablespoon fresh lemon juice
- ½ cup extra-virgin olive oil
- ½ teaspoon sea salt

In a food processor or blender, combine the arugula, garlic, almonds, lemon juice, oil, and salt and puree until smooth. Add more oil, as needed, to create a creamy texture. Refrigerate in an airtight container for up to 1 week.

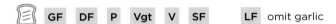

GF   DF   P   Vgt   V   SF   LF omit garlic

Cilantro-Sriracha Mayo

This easy semi-homemade condiment will give your fries and burgers a kick in the pants. It is the perfect complement to **Ginger-Salmon Burgers** (page 249), an alternative sauce option for **Sweet Potato & Cabbage Rosti with Kimchi Aioli** (page 231), and definitely a dipper for **Hemp-Crusted Chicken Tenders** (page 136). You can even mix it with canned fish for a twist on tuna salad.

MAKES ½ CUP

- ½ cup mayonnaise
- ¼ cup finely chopped fresh cilantro
- 1 tablespoon fresh lime juice
- 1 tablespoon sriracha or hot sauce

In a small bowl, stir together the mayonnaise, cilantro, lime juice, and sriracha. Taste for seasoning, and add more sriracha, as needed. Refrigerate in an airtight container for up to 1 week.

 GF   DF   P   Vgt   SF   LF use LF hot sauce

Charlie's Magic Grill Marinade

My husband is the grill guy. If that sounds like a gender cliché, I will follow it by saying he went pescatarian a few years ago (like my dad) and grills meat only on my behalf. A few times a month, he'll take it upon himself to make me a steak, marinated in some combination of vinegar, tamari, natural sweetener, and Dijon. The marinade is rather magical because it also lends an umami depth to vegetables, especially mushrooms, which is what he'll prepare for himself, either on the grill or tossed on a sheet pan and roasted in the oven. His original version uses more honey than this recipe, so feel free to up it if you want the acid offset further with sweetness. For obvious Carbivore reasons, I've kept it minimal!

MAKES ½ CUP

- 2 tablespoons balsamic or red wine vinegar
- 2 tablespoons Dijon mustard
- 2 tablespoons gluten-free tamari, soy sauce, or coconut aminos
- 2 tablespoons extra-virgin olive oil
- 1 teaspoon honey or maple syrup
- 1 teaspoon sea salt

In a mason jar or liquid measuring cup, whisk together the vinegar, mustard, tamari, oil, honey, and salt until well blended. Refrigerate in an airtight container for up to 1 month.

GF   DF   Vgt

P use coconut aminos   LF   **V** use maple syrup

Sugar-Free Ginger Applesauce

This applesauce uses the power of natural sugars and zippy fresh ginger to add a hint of spice. It's on the chunky side, since we know that whole foods are better for your blood sugar than pulverized ones. But if you like a smoother consistency, use an immersion or standard blender to achieve your desired texture. This applesauce can be used in baking, much like store-bought options, or as a semisweet condiment for **Parsnip-Potato Latkes** (page 225). If you don't mind an even coarser texture, leave the skins on the apples!

MAKES 4 CUPS

4   large Honeycrisp or Pink Lady apples (about 2 pounds), peeled, cored, and cut into 1- to 2-inch chunks

1   tablespoon grated fresh ginger

Pinch sea salt

❶ In a large lidded heavy-bottomed pot over medium-high heat, combine the apples and ½ cup water. Bring to a boil, then reduce the heat to medium-low to maintain a simmer. Cover the pot and cook until the apples are tender, about 15 minutes. Use the back of a wooden spoon or a potato masher to begin breaking up the apples.

❷ Continue to cook for 40 minutes more until the apples are very soft, using your wooden spoon or potato masher to mash the apples further every 10 minutes or so. Stir in the ginger and salt.

❸ Let cool, then transfer to a resealable mason jar. The applesauce will keep for up to 2 weeks in the refrigerator.

GF   DF   P   Vgt   V   SF

Raspberry-Chia Jam

Like my **Sugar-Free Ginger Applesauce** (page 72), this jam uses no added sweetener (unless you want it to!) and relies on the gelatinous texture of chia seeds to thicken the fruit compote into a syrupy consistency. You can substitute any berry in this recipe, but note that frozen options lend the jam more depth of color. Enjoy it on buttered toast and as a topping for steel cut oatmeal, or in my **PB & J Cups with Crunchy Quinoa** (page 167).

MAKES ½ CUP

- 12 ounces fresh or frozen raspberries (about 3 cups)
- 2 tablespoons chia seeds
- 1 tablespoon fresh lemon juice
- 1 to 3 teaspoons honey or maple syrup (optional)

❶ In a small saucepan over medium heat, cook the raspberries, stirring occasionally, until the berries begin to release their juices and bubble, about 5 minutes. Use a spoon to break apart the raspberries as they cook until you get a coarse puree.

❷ Off the heat, stir in the chia seeds and lemon juice until well mixed. Taste the jam for sweetness—I like this jam tart. Stir in the honey (if using), to taste. Set aside to cool—the seeds will plump and thicken the jam as it sits.

❸ Stir a few more times to redistribute the seeds, then transfer the jam to an airtight container and refrigerate for up to 2 weeks, or freeze for later. Thaw overnight in the refrigerator before using.

GF DF P Vgt

LF V use maple syrup   SF omit sweetener

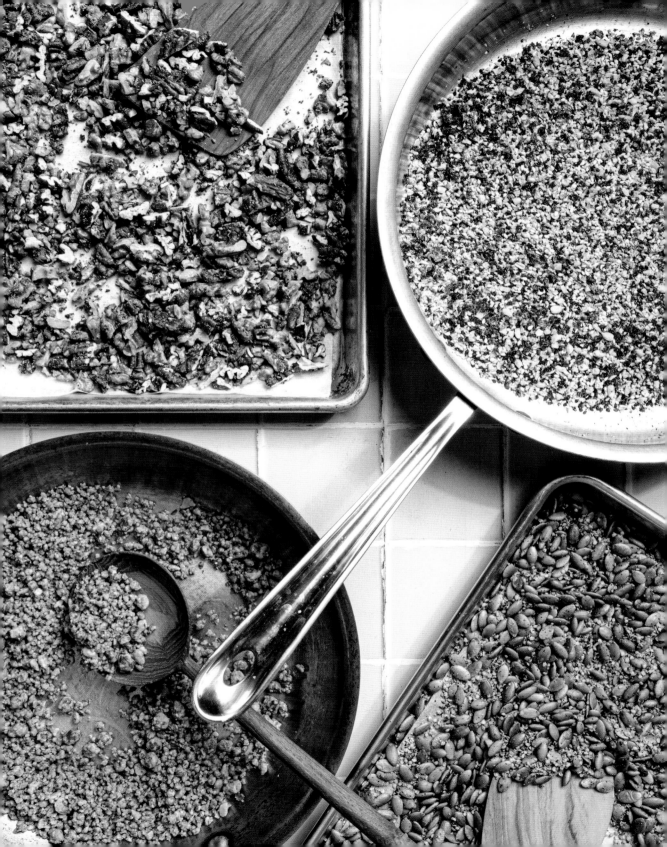

Nut Crunches & Seed Sprinkles, 5 Ways

These mixes add gourmet flair to even the simplest salad or weeknight supper. Make a batch of each and store them in airtight jars on the counter for up to a month, or up to 6 months in the fridge, so you always have them handy. The ultimate carb companions, each of these crunches and sprinkles is included in several recipes in the book so you won't be at a loss for how to use them. Of course, making them from scratch will add time to your prep process, so again, it's a better strategy to have them around to offset any carb-o-loading at a moment's notice.

Salty Sesame-Sunflower Gomasio

Gomasio is a Japanese condiment of toasted sesame seeds and salt that's often sprinkled over white rice. You can find it in the spice or Asian foods section of many grocery stores, but I like making my own so I can add other nutritious ingredients, like sunflower seeds and dried sushi nori. The latter gives the seed sprinkle a subtle umami quality and infusion of iodine, which is essential for good thyroid health. You can leave the seaweed out for seed purists. I love sprinkling this gomasio on **The Simplest Poke Bowls** (page 123), **Ginger-Scallion Chicken Soba Noodle Soup** (page 196), and **Crispy Rice with Spicy Beet Tartare** (page 125).

MAKES ¾ CUP

- ¼ cup raw black sesame seeds
- ¼ cup raw white sesame seeds
- ¼ cup raw sunflower seeds
- 1 sheet sushi nori, or 1 tablespoon dulse flakes (optional)
- ½ teaspoon sea salt

❶ In a small skillet over low heat, toast the black and white sesame seeds and sunflower seeds until fragrant, about 2 minutes. Set aside.

❷ Make sure the nori (if using) is completely dry, then tear it roughly into pieces. Transfer the nori to a small food processor and pulse a few times until the seaweed becomes fine crumbs. Add the sesame-sunflower seed mixture (still warm, preferably) and the salt. Pulse one or two times until everything is combined—you want to see all the seeds and don't want them overly broken down. Taste for seasoning and add more salt, as needed.

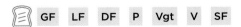 GF LF DF P Vgt V SF

Tangy Peanut-Cashew Crunch

In addition to tasting delicious on many dishes, this is my favorite crunch to have around as an elevated bar snack. The lime juice, cayenne, and shredded coconut give the peanuts a Thai flair. Crumble it over my **Minty Green Rice Pilaf with Chiles & Peanuts** (page 134), **Braised Coconut-Lime Sweet Potatoes & Bok Choy** (page 226), or **Peanut & Lime Slaw** (page 83). Feel free to use all peanuts or all cashews if you have only one type of nut on hand. You can omit the scant amount of sugar, but it helps the coconut adhere to the nuts.

MAKES 2 CUPS

3 tablespoons fresh lime juice (from 2 or 3 limes)

Grated zest of 2 limes

2 teaspoons honey or maple syrup

1 teaspoon sea salt

½ teaspoon cayenne pepper

2 cups raw unsalted peanuts, roughly chopped

1 cup raw unsalted cashews, roughly chopped

⅓ cup unsweetened shredded coconut

❶ Preheat the oven to 250°F. Line a rimmed sheet pan with parchment paper.

❷ In a medium bowl, whisk together the lime juice, lime zest, honey, salt, and cayenne until combined. Add the peanuts, cashews, and coconut. Stir until the nuts are evenly coated. Transfer the nuts to the prepared sheet pan and arrange in an even layer. Bake until the nuts are fragrant, dry, and beginning to darken, about 20 minutes.

❸ Toss the nuts to redistribute and let cool completely on the pan.

GF   DF   P   Vgt

LF   use maple syrup; sub peanuts for cashews   V   use maple syrup

Anise-y Pine Nut–Almond Crunch

I consider this nutty crunch an Italian interpretation of dukkah, using fennel seeds, dried herbs, and red pepper flakes. And it makes me feel better when I use it on my Carbivore lazy dinner of choice: spaghetti and tomato sauce (with a starter salad, duh). It pairs well with other ingredients that have a hint of anise, like the fennel in **Spring Potato-Leek Soup with Asparagus** (page 209) and **Seared Scallops with White Beans, Watercress & Kefir Green Goddess Dressing** (page 321), or the basil in **Crispy Polenta Cakes with Eggplant–Cherry Tomato Caponata** (page 272).

MAKES 1 CUP

- ½   cup unsalted almonds
- ½   cup pine nuts
- 1   teaspoon fennel seeds
- 1   teaspoon fresh oregano, rosemary, or thyme leaves, or ¼ teaspoon dried
- ½   teaspoon sea salt
- ¼   teaspoon red pepper flakes

❶ In a small food processor, pulse the almonds, pine nuts, fennel seeds, oregano, salt, and red pepper flakes until the nuts are coarsely chopped. Alternatively, chop everything by hand.

❷ Transfer the nut mixture to a small dry skillet and place it over medium-low heat. Toast the nut mixture, stirring occasionally, until very lightly browned and fragrant, about 2 minutes.

❸ Let the nuts cool completely before storing.

GF   LF   DF   P   Vgt   V   SF

Maple Walnut–Pecan Spice Brittle

Though this "brittle" doesn't use much sugar (just a teaspoon of maple syrup), it's amplified by warming cinnamon and ground ginger. It's my go-to nut crunch for the holiday season, adding texture to fall salads like my **Brussels Sprouts & Wild Rice Salad** (page 139) or even **Basic Bitch Kale Salad** (page 85). It would also be a wonderful adjunct to anything with similar spices, like **Carrot Cake Baked Steel Cut Oats** (page 96) or **Year-Round Fruit & Almond Crisp** (page 106), especially if made with apples or pears.

MAKES 2 CUPS

1   cup raw walnuts, roughly chopped

1   cup raw pecans, roughly chopped

1   tablespoon poppy seeds

1   teaspoon maple syrup

½   teaspoon sea salt

½   teaspoon ground cinnamon

½   teaspoon ground ginger

❶ Preheat the oven to 300°F. Line a rimmed sheet pan with parchment paper.

❷ In a medium bowl, stir together the walnuts, pecans, poppy seeds, maple syrup, salt, cinnamon, and ginger until evenly coated. Transfer the nuts to the prepared sheet pan and arrange in an even layer. Bake until the nuts are fragrant, dry, and beginning to darken, about 20 minutes.

❸ Let cool completely on the pan.

GF   LF   DF   P   Vgt   V

Smoky Pumpkin-Hemp Sprinkles

Pumpkin seeds are high in magnesium, selenium, and zinc—all important nutrients for thyroid hormone production. Flavored with chili powder, cumin, and coriander, this seed mixture is great as a topper for a variety of cuisines: Moroccan, Middle Eastern, Mexican, even Indian. Here are some of my favorite dishes to use it in: **Smashed Chickpea Shakshuka with Summer Tomatoes** (page 306), **Seedy "Avocado Toast" Arepas** (page 282), **Greenhouse Gazpacho** (page 256), and **Big Leaf Lettuces with Summer Tomato-Cashew Dressing** (page 81). If you don't feel like turning on the oven, toast the seeds in a dry pan over medium-low heat until golden brown, about 5 minutes.

MAKES 1 ½ CUPS

1	cup raw pumpkin seeds
½	cup hemp seeds
1	teaspoon chili powder
1	teaspoon ground cumin (whole seeds work too)
½	teaspoon ground coriander
¼	teaspoon sea salt
1	tablespoon extra-virgin olive or avocado oil

❶ Preheat the oven to 350°F. Line a rimmed sheet pan with parchment paper.

❷ In a medium bowl, toss together the pumpkin seeds, hemp seeds, chili powder, cumin, coriander, salt, and oil until evenly coated. Transfer the seeds to the prepared sheet pan and arrange in an even layer. Bake until the seeds are fragrant and golden, about 10 minutes—you don't want them to get any darker!

GF   LF   DF   P   Vgt   V   SF

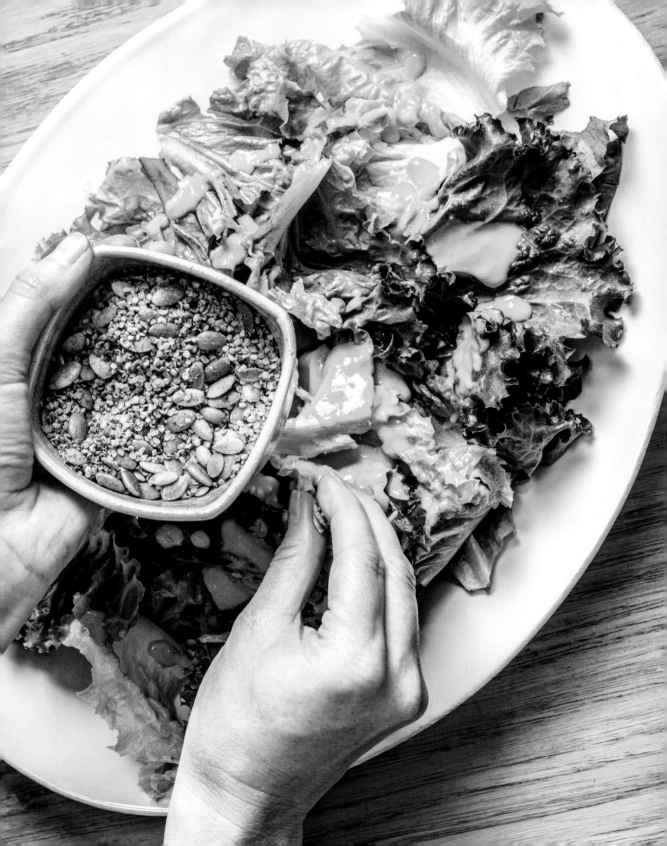

Simple Starter Salads, 4 Ways

Throwing together a green salad to munch on before your carb-centric meal doesn't have to be a complicated affair—just use your favorite greens and one of the dressings from earlier in this chapter. That said, I've decided to give you a few simple recipes to get a little more creative or make a larger portion for company.

Big Leaf Lettuces with Summer Tomato-Cashew Dressing

In my household, we try to reduce waste by buying whole heads of lettuce instead of mixes that come in a plastic clamshell. But for pure quality reasons, these big leaf lettuces tend to last longer, stay crisper, and look much more gorgeous on a platter or plate. I love letting the lettuce shine by using a thicker dressing drizzled on top, and finishing the plate with one of my seed sprinkles. If the Southwestern combo doesn't do it for you, try the following: **Spicy Sesame Dressing** (page 60) + **Salty Sesame–Sunflower Gomasio** (page 75); **Basic Balsamic Vinaigrette** (page 60) or **Kefir Green Goddess Dressing** (page 65) + **Anise-y Pine Nut–Almond Crunch** (page 77); **Lemon Poppy Vinaigrette** (page 64) + **Maple Walnut–Pecan Spice Brittle** (page 78).

MAKES 4 SERVINGS

1   head Little Gem, Boston, or Bibb lettuce

1   head red leaf lettuce

⅓   cup **Summer Tomato-Cashew Dressing** (page 59)

⅓   cup **Smoky Pumpkin-Hemp Sprinkles** (page 79)

2   tablespoons chopped fresh chives (optional)

Separate the lettuce leaves from the stalk. Rinse thoroughly and dry in a salad spinner. Using clean hands, tear the lettuces roughly. Feel free to leave the small inner leaves intact. Arrange the leaves on a large platter and drizzle with the dressing. Garnish with the pumpkin-hemp sprinkles and the chives (if using). Serve immediately.

GF DF P Vgt V SF

Back-Pocket Tricolore Salad with Lemon Poppy Vinaigrette

This green salad is like a good pair of blue jeans. It can flatter pretty much any culinary outfit. The trio of bitter radicchio, peppery arugula, and crunchy romaine lettuce is an easy mix to throw together at the beginning of the week. You can always substitute endive for a more traditional tricolore combo, and add ½ cup thinly sliced veggies, depending on the season: roasted beets (fall), Brussels sprouts (winter), sugar snap peas (spring), avocado or tomato (summer).

MAKES 8 SIDE SERVINGS

5   ounces baby arugula (about 4 cups, packed)

½   medium head radicchio (8 ounces), thinly sliced (about 2 cups)

1   heart of romaine lettuce, thinly sliced (about 3 cups)

⅔   cup **Lemon Poppy Vinaigrette** (page 64)

2   tablespoons toasted sunflower seeds, chopped almonds, or walnuts (optional)

In a large bowl, toss together the arugula, radicchio, romaine, and ⅓ **cup vinaigrette** to combine. Taste for seasoning and add more dressing, as needed. Garnish with sunflower seeds (if using) to serve.

GF   LF   DF   P   Vgt   V

Peanut & Lime Slaw

Though the base is just cabbage, carrots, and scallions, you can add any of your favorite crunchy vegetables—like radishes, cucumbers, sugar snap peas, or bell peppers—to this make-ahead slaw. Fish sauce gives the mayo-free dressing a Southeast Asian funk that pairs well with the fresh mint and chopped peanuts. If you have time to make the **Tangy Peanut-Cashew Crunch** (page 76), it adds even more bold flavor to this simple side.

MAKES 4 SERVINGS

1	small head napa cabbage (1 pound), thinly sliced
2	medium carrots, shredded (about 2 cups)
1	bunch scallions, thinly sliced
¼	cup chopped fresh mint leaves
2	tablespoons fish sauce
2	tablespoons rice vinegar
2	tablespoons fresh lime juice (from 1 or 2 limes)
2	tablespoons avocado oil
½	teaspoon sea salt
½	cup salted peanuts, chopped, or **Tangy Peanut-Cashew Crunch** (page 76)

In a large bowl, combine the cabbage, carrots, scallions, mint, fish sauce, vinegar, lime juice, oil, and salt. Toss until well combined. Taste for seasoning and adjust the salt, as needed. Garnish with the peanuts before serving.

  GF DF P SF

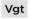

LF green scallions only   Vgt V sub tamari for fish sauce

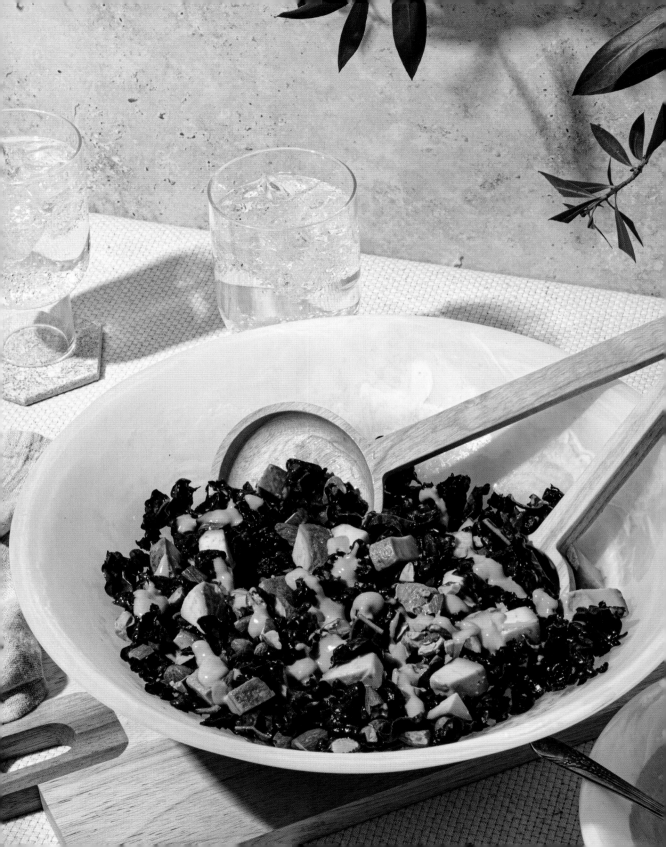

Basic Bitch Kale Salad with Liquid Gold Turmeric-Tahini Dressing

Massaged kale salad had a big moment in the late aughts, and has since become a little overdone on restaurant menus. But like most basic things, it's ubiquitous because it's delicious. The simplest version of this salad would just include the greens, lemon, olive oil, salt, and garlic. It's a dressing in and of itself; however, the addition of creamy tahini takes it up a notch, as do add-ins like avocado and chopped nuts. If you can find tamari almonds, they add even more umami to the salad. But any nut will work, as will many of the crunches or sprinkles in the previous section. Other possible additions include diced roasted beets or roasted sweet potato if you want to substitute the dried fruit for another type of nature's candy.

MAKES 4 SERVINGS

- 1 bunch Lacinato kale
- 1 garlic clove
  Fine sea salt
- 1 tablespoon fresh lemon juice
- 1 tablespoon extra-virgin olive oil
- 1 avocado, cubed
- ¼ cup almonds, roughly chopped
- 2 tablespoons dried cherries or dried cranberries (optional)
- ½ cup **Liquid Gold Turmeric-Tahini Dressing** (page 62)

❶ **Prepare the kale:** Remove the thick stem from the center of the kale leaves by carefully tearing away the bottom part of the leaf and then grabbing hold of the stem. Pull up along the stem. The leaf should come away intact, aside from the center vein where the stem once was. Stack the kale leaves, with the largest at the bottom and smallest at the top. Roll the leaves widthwise into a cigar shape and thinly slice them—the result will be beautiful ribbons of kale. Transfer to a large bowl.

❷ **Make the garlic paste:** Mince the garlic on a work surface, gather it into a pile, and sprinkle with salt. Keep mincing, rendering the garlic even finer, then begin scraping the garlic with your knife. The knife should be flush with the work surface. Put pressure on the blade as you draw it over the surface of the garlic, forming a paste—10 or so strokes should do it. Transfer the garlic to the bowl with the kale.

❸ **Marinate the kale:** To the bowl, add the lemon juice, oil, and ¼ teaspoon salt. Using clean hands, toss the kale until it's coated well in the lemon-oil mixture—don't be afraid to give it a deep tissue massage!

❹ **Assemble the salad:** Transfer the kale to a serving dish. Top with the avocado, almonds, and dried cherries (if using). Drizzle with the tahini dressing to serve.

 GF DF P Vgt V SF omit dried fruit

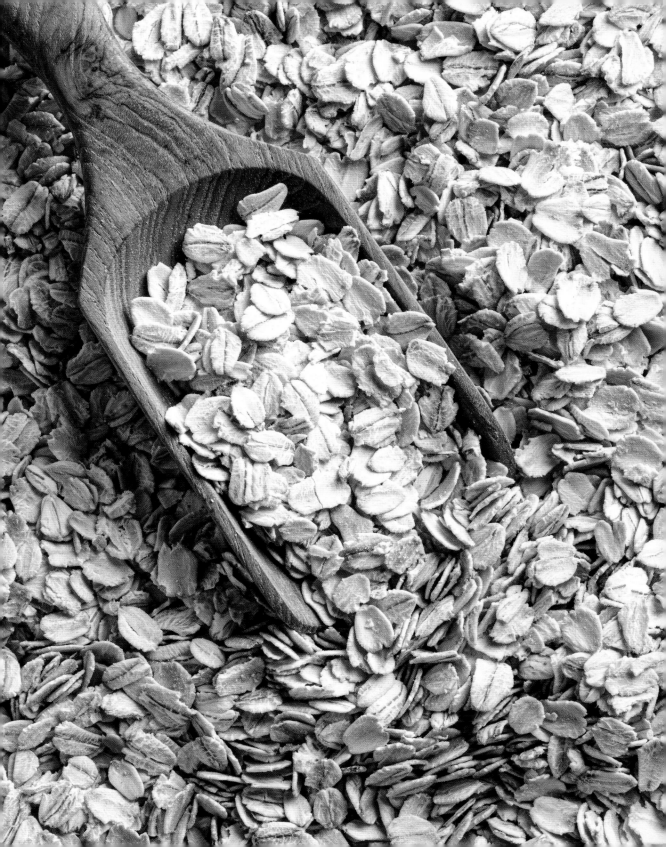

OATS

• • •

Sweet & Savory Granola, 3 Ways

Savory Yogurt & Granola Bowls with Avocado & Eggs

Lemon Poppy Overnight Oats

Carrot Cake Baked Steel Cut Oats

Steel Cut Oat Congee with Bok Choy

Dijon Turkey Meat Loaf with Spinach

Ham & Cheese Dutch Baby with Peas

Violet's Big Blueberry-Oat Muffins

Year-Round Fruit & Almond Crisp

Ginger-Pear Cake with Oat Crumble

Raspberry Lime Rickey Curd Tart

TYPES & PREPARATION TIPS

If you are gluten intolerant or have celiac disease, buy certified gluten-free oats. Though oats are naturally gluten-free, they are often prepared in a facility with wheat-based products.

Steel Cut Oats

Popular preparation methods: absorption

Ratio: 1 cup steel cut oats to 3 cups liquid

Cook time: 25 to 40 minutes

The less processed the oat, the better it is for your blood sugar. Though you can buy whole groats (the entire kernel), the more common variety is steel cut, which is exactly what it sounds like: pieces of the whole groats cut into smaller, more manageable sizes. Even when simmered for a long period, as in my **Steel Cut Oat Congee with Bok Choy** (page 99), steel cut oats maintain their shape and bite. This might be an acquired texture, but certainly a refreshing one if you've never been a fan of Dickensian, overly mushy gruel—in which case, turn immediately to page 96 and make my **Carrot Cake Baked Steel Cut Oats**.

Rolled Oats

Popular preparation method: absorption

Ratio: 1 cup whole rolled oats to 2 cups liquid

Cook time: 5 to 10 minutes

Unlike steel cut oats, rolled oats are pre-steamed, softening the groats enough to be flattened between steel rollers. These tiny oat pancakes (like oat tostones!) are what most people picture when they think of oats. There are several varieties at the grocery store: "whole rolled" and "old-fashioned" oats are interchangeable terms. Both are on the thicker side and maintain some of their original chew, whereas "quick cooking" or "instant" oats are pressed even thinner to reduce cooking time. As with all grains (and plants, in general), the trade-off for more processing and convenience is your body doesn't have to work as hard to break down food into usable energy (which can lead to blood sugar spikes). For this reason, I use only steel cut or whole rolled oats and try to add seeds, nuts, and whole fruit or vegetables to each recipe. Rolled oats are also my favorite whole-grain swap for breadcrumbs as a binder.

Oat Flour

Light, airy, and subtly sweet, oat flour is one of my favorite alternatives for gluten-free baking. You can make your own by pulsing rolled oats in a food processor, but you'll find that the industrially made options have a much fluffier texture. Its flavor is incredibly versatile for both sweet (**Violet's Big Blueberry-Oat Muffins**, page 103) and savory (**Ham & Cheese Dutch Baby with Peas**, page 102) recipes. Especially when combined with vanilla and maple syrup to bring out its buttery crumb, like in my **Raspberry Lime Rickey Curd Tart** crust (page 111), oat flour melts in your mouth like a shortbread cookie.

Oat Milk

Though higher in readily accessible sugars than nut milks, oat milk has risen to the top of the nondairy beverage category because of its creamy texture. Although I try to opt for one of the lower-carb nut milks when making smoothies or adding a splash to my morning tea, oat milk is wonderful for baking or enjoying alongside other ingredients with more built-in fiber and fat, like in the batter of my **Ginger-Pear Cake with Oat Crumble** (page 109).

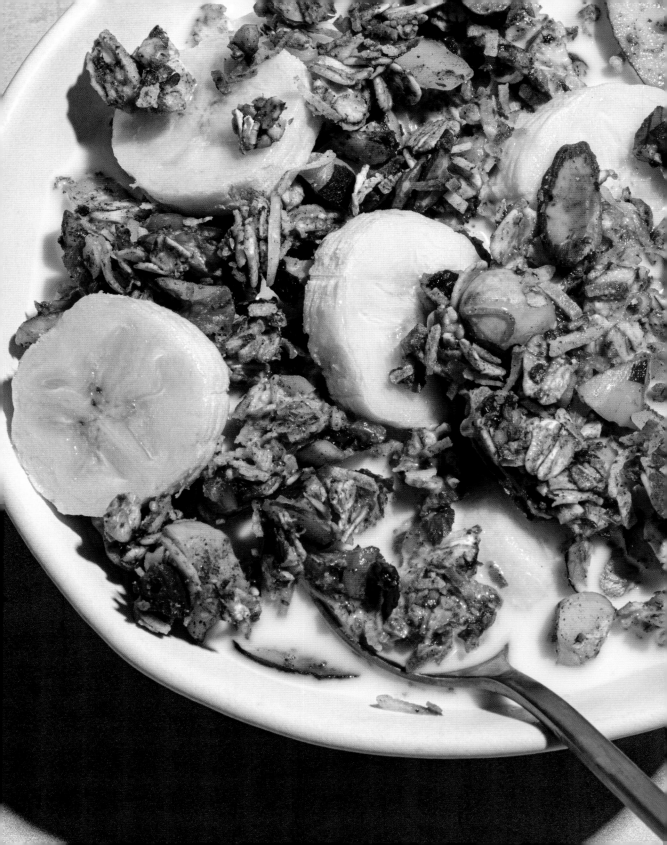

Sweet & Savory Granola, 3 Ways

Most packaged granolas have as many grams of sugar per serving as a cookie, which is not ideal for getting off to the right start in the morning. If you're a die-hard granola-with-milk eater, making your own granola lets you dial down the sweetener and up the fiber. But better yet, opt for one of my two savory options, which can be munched on by the handful as a snack, sprinkled over salads, or eaten with yogurt (see page 94) for breakfast.

Banana–Nut Crunch Granola

One of my readers (hi, Tara!) sent me her recipe for a granola that doesn't use any added sugar at all, just a mashed (very ripe) banana. The flavor—somewhere between a banana chip and a granola—brought me right back to the Nut & Honey Crunch cereal I ate as a kid. The banana gives the oats a slight chew, so the granola is a great candidate to eat with some nut milk and fresh berries. Often-overlooked, the Brazil nuts in this breakfast are an excellent source of selenium, which is an important ingredient for thyroid health.

MAKES 2 ½ CUPS

- 1   tablespoon flaxseed meal
- 1   medium (very ripe) banana
- 1   tablespoon maple syrup (optional)
- 1   tablespoon vanilla extract
- 2   teaspoons ground cinnamon
- ½   teaspoon sea salt
- 1   cup whole rolled oats
- ½   cup finely chopped raw walnuts or pecans (or a mix)
- ½   cup finely chopped raw almonds
- ½   cup finely chopped Brazil nuts
- ½   cup unsweetened finely shredded coconut

1. Preheat the oven to 325°F. Line a rimmed sheet pan with parchment paper.

2. In a medium bowl, whisk together the flaxseed meal with **2 tablespoons water**. Let sit for 5 minutes.

3. Add the banana and mash it thoroughly with a fork until there are no large clumps. Stir in the maple syrup (if using), vanilla, cinnamon, and salt until smooth. Fold in the oats, walnuts, almonds, Brazil nuts, and coconut. Transfer the granola to the prepared sheet pan and spread it into an even layer.

4. Bake for 40 minutes, stirring once halfway through, or until the banana bits are fully dry and the oats are lightly browned. Let the granola cool completely on the pan, then break it apart into large clumps. Store in an airtight container at room temperature for up to 2 weeks.

GF   DF   Vgt   V   LF   safe serving: ¾ cup   SF   omit sweetener

Seed Cracker Granola

At times, I've worried that savory granola might be the culinary equivalent of trying to "make fetch happen," but every person who's tried this seed cracker version falls in love immediately. The combination of caraway and cumin seeds adds a fabulous Middle Eastern flavor, and the quinoa, sunflower seeds, and chia seeds give it an addictive crunch.

MAKES 3 CUPS

- 1 cup whole rolled oats
- ½ cup uncooked quinoa or millet
- ½ cup raw sunflower or pumpkin seeds (or a mix)
- 2 tablespoons hemp seeds
- 2 tablespoons chia seeds
- 2 teaspoons caraway seeds
- 1 teaspoon cumin seeds
- 1 teaspoon paprika
- ½ teaspoon sea salt
- 1 large egg white
- 1 tablespoon extra-virgin olive oil
- 1 tablespoon maple syrup or honey

❶ Preheat the oven to 325°F. Line a rimmed sheet pan with parchment paper.

❷ In a medium bowl, stir together the oats, quinoa, sunflower seeds, hemp seeds, chia seeds, caraway seeds, cumin seeds, paprika, and salt until well mixed. Add the egg white, oil, and maple syrup and stir until the oats and seeds are coated well.

❸ Arrange the granola on the prepared sheet pan in an even, compact layer, packing down the granola with the back of a spoon so it almost looks like a big cracker.

❹ Bake for 20 to 30 minutes until the oat mixture is lightly browned and hardened. If you smell burning at any point, immediately remove the pan from the oven and turn down the heat. Let the granola cool completely on the pan, then break it apart into large clumps.

❺ Store in an airtight container for up to a month on the counter, or for many months refrigerated.

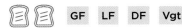 **GF LF DF Vgt**   **V** use flax egg (see page 91, step 2)

Everything Bagel Granola

Variation: *Sub **poppy seeds** for chia seeds, and **sesame seeds** for hemp seeds; use **½ teaspoon onion powder** and **½ teaspoon garlic powder** instead of cumin and caraway seeds.*

GF DF Vgt   **V** use flax egg (see page 91, step 2)

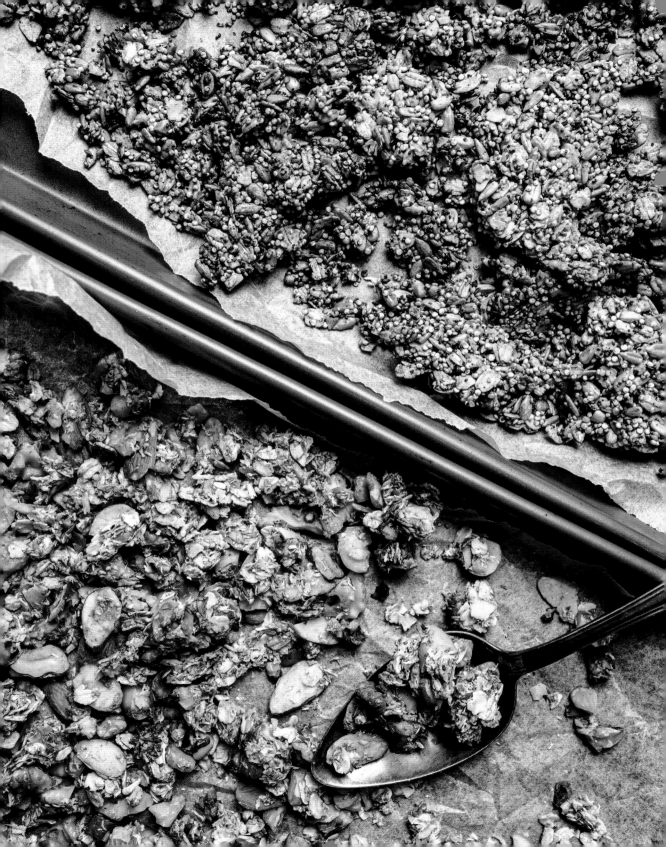

Savory Yogurt & Granola Bowls with Avocado & Eggs

This quick-fix breakfast is a sugar-free alternative to the usual yogurt, fruit, and granola bowl. All you need are two make-ahead elements—spicy **Harissa Yogurt** (page 68) and **Seed Cracker Granola** (page 92)—and the rest comes together in minutes. Slather yogurt at the bottom of your bowl, then top with a sliced avocado, a fried (or poached) egg, and a handful of granola. It's a rich, spicy, satisfying start to the day that's full of protein and healthy fat to keep your blood sugar steady and skip the mid-morning scaries.

MAKES 2 SERVINGS

½ cup **Harissa Yogurt** (page 68)

1 avocado, thinly sliced

Extra-virgin olive oil

2 large eggs

Sea salt and Aleppo pepper

½ cup **Seed Cracker Granola** (page 92) or **Everything Bagel Granola** (page 92)

Fresh cilantro or mint leaves (optional)

❶ Divide the **harissa yogurt** between two bowls, using the back of a spoon to create a tasteful schmear.

❷ Arrange half an avocado in each bowl, fanning out the slices.

❸ Right before you're ready to eat, prepare the eggs: In a large (12-inch or bigger) cast-iron skillet, heat a generous layer (about ¼ inch) of oil over medium-high heat. Crack each egg into the skillet, keeping them on separate sides as much as possible. Cook until the bottoms are set and beginning to crisp slightly, about 2 minutes, then turn off the heat. Tilt the pan toward you and, using a spoon, baste the tops of the egg whites with the hot oil. Do this a few times over each egg until all the whites are cooked through. Using a spatula, transfer the eggs to each bowl.

❹ Sprinkle the eggs and avocado with a little salt and pepper.

❺ Crumble the granola over the top and garnish with cilantro (if using). Serve immediately.

  GF **Vgt**  **DF** use plant-based yogurt

Lemon Poppy Overnight Oats

Having breakfast in the fridge, already made, doubles my chances of actually eating something in the morning. Overnight oats are such a great strategy in this regard. As they sit, the grains rehydrate into something not quite as fluffy as regular stovetop oatmeal, but not a far cry from it either. Raw oats contain high levels of resistant starch that you lose in the cooking process, so even though we are using rolled oats for this instead of steel cut, we get that added blood sugar protection. The poppy seeds add crunch and the chia seeds plump to give the oats more body—and both add fiber and fat. Zesty lemon pairs beautifully with the acidity of the yogurt—another companion to slow our carbs' roll! If you want more, top the oats with fresh berries, shredded coconut, or toasted walnuts.

CARB SWAP: To make this with steel cut oats, double the milk and bring to a boil with the oats. Cook for 1 minute, then remove from the heat and add the remaining ingredients.

MAKES 4 SERVINGS

1 cup whole rolled oats

¼ cup chia seeds

2 tablespoons poppy seeds

Pinch sea salt

1 cup unsweetened almond milk

½ cup unsweetened coconut yogurt or full-fat plain Greek yogurt (4 ounces)

Grated zest of 1 lemon

¼ cup lemon juice (from 1 or 2 lemons)

2 tablespoons maple syrup or raw honey

2 tablespoons cashew or almond butter

½ teaspoon vanilla extract

❶ In a medium bowl, stir together the oats, chia seeds, poppy seeds, and salt until well combined. Add the almond milk, yogurt, lemon zest, lemon juice, maple syrup, nut butter, and vanilla and whisk until smooth.

❷ Transfer the oat mixture to a mason jar or resealable container and refrigerate overnight, or for at least 8 hours. You can also divide the mixture into individual portions to make it easier to grab and go.

❸ Keep refrigerated until ready to eat, up to 1 week. For warm oatmeal, pop the bowl in the microwave for 30 seconds.

GF **Vgt** **LF** use coconut yogurt, almond butter, maple syrup

DF **V** use coconut yogurt **SF** omit sweetener

Carrot Cake Baked Steel Cut Oats

The one downside to steel cut oats is that they take longer to cook. I'd argue that the pro column far outweighs this one gripe, especially when there are hands-off ways to prepare them like, say, in the oven. This oatmeal is a fantastic dump-and-stir recipe inspired by a beloved cake. Even though it is a sweet breakfast, you get the added blood sugar benefit of vegetables in your bowl, in addition to walnuts and cinnamon. It's perfect to make for the week ahead or as part of a brunch spread. Refrigerate any leftover portions and reheat with a splash of plant-based milk. This recipe is purposefully not too sweet, especially if you skip the raisins. You can always add a drizzle of maple syrup—just try to add another carb companion to steady your glucose curve, like almond butter, fresh berries, or plain yogurt.

MAKES 6 TO 8 SERVINGS

2 large carrots, unpeeled, coarsely grated (about 1 cup)

2 ½ cups unsweetened almond milk

3 tablespoons maple syrup

1 large egg

3 tablespoons melted coconut oil

2 teaspoons vanilla extract

1 cup steel cut oats

½ cup flaxseed meal (optional)

2 teaspoons ground cinnamon

1 teaspoon baking powder

¼ teaspoon fine sea salt

½ cup raw walnuts, finely chopped

2 tablespoons raisins (optional)

❶ Preheat the oven to 350°F. Line a 9 × 13-inch baking dish with parchment paper.

❷ In a large bowl, whisk together the carrots, almond milk, maple syrup, egg, melted coconut oil, and vanilla to blend. If your milk is cold, the coconut oil might seize up—do your best to whisk out any large lumps, but don't stress about it! It will melt in the oven.

❸ Stir in the oats, flaxseed meal (if using), cinnamon, baking powder, and salt. Fold in the walnuts and raisins (if using). Transfer to the prepared baking dish and spread evenly.

❹ Bake the oatmeal for 50 minutes, or until the top is set and turning golden brown around the edges. Let cool for a few minutes before serving, or store covered in the refrigerator for up to a week.

GF   LF   DF   Vgt

V omit egg   SF omit maple syrup and raisins

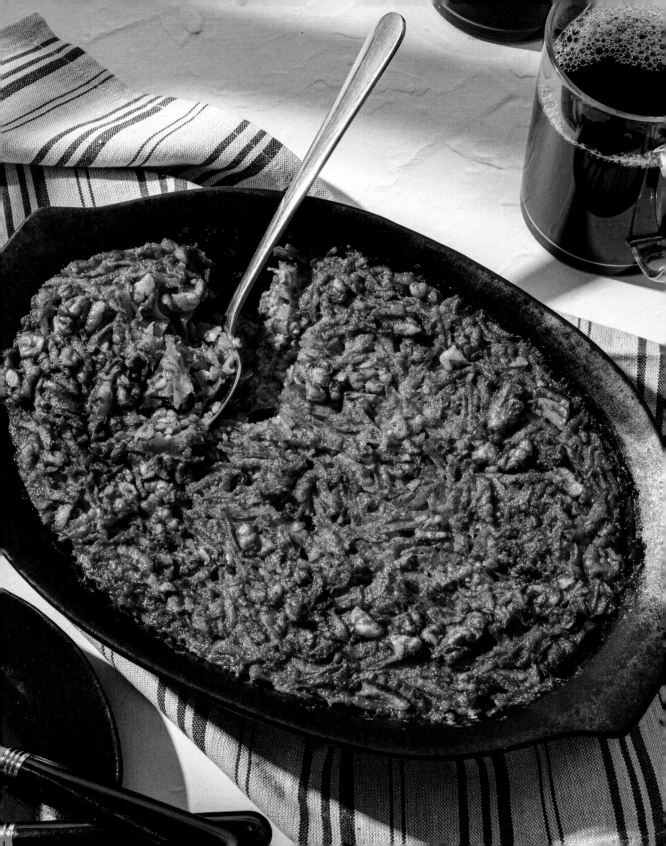

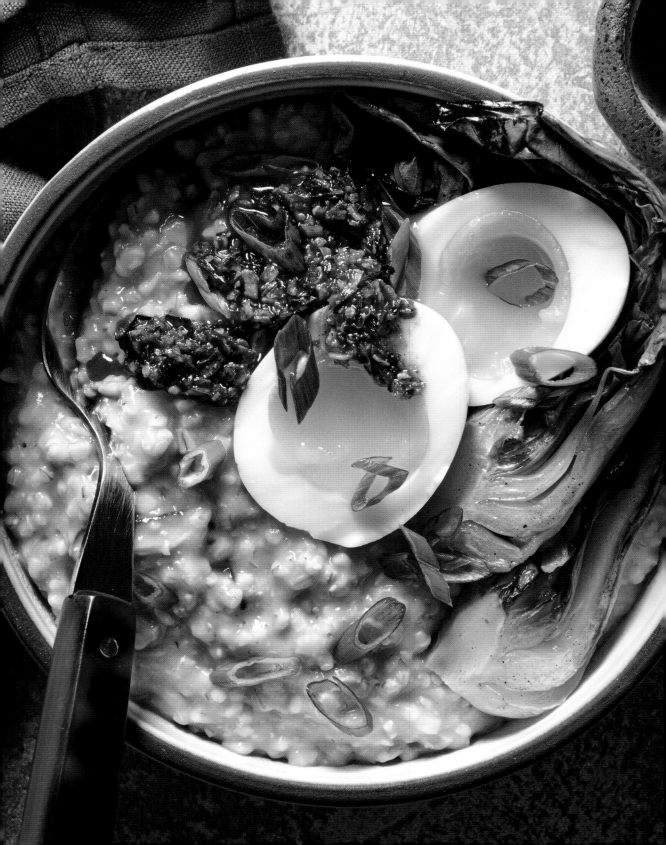

Steel Cut Oat Congee with Bok Choy

Congee is often used in Chinese medicine as a way to give the digestive system a day off. Usually made with rice and a high ratio of water to grain, the thick porridge is easy for your gut to assimilate and helps you stay hydrated when nothing else is staying down. Because I'm already a huge fan of congee as a savory breakfast, I subbed in steel cut oats, which are higher in fiber than white rice and will keep you fuller longer. If you're not plant based, feel free to add a few chicken thighs instead of (or in addition to) the mushrooms. They'll be fork-tender by the time the oats are and can be shredded and added back to the pot.

MAKES 4 SERVINGS

6	cups chicken or vegetable broth, preferably homemade
1	cup steel cut oats
4	shiitake mushrooms, thinly sliced
1	tablespoon minced fresh ginger
4	scallions, thinly sliced, white and green parts separated
	Sea salt
4	large eggs
1	tablespoon avocado oil
2	baby bok choy, thinly sliced
	Gluten-free tamari or soy sauce
	Chili crisp (optional)

❶ In a large stockpot or Dutch oven over high heat, combine the broth, oats, mushrooms, ginger, white scallions, and **1 teaspoon salt** and bring to a boil. Adjust the heat to medium-low and cook, uncovered, stirring occasionally, until the oats are soft and the broth is thick and starchy, 40 to 50 minutes. Remove from the heat.

❷ Meanwhile, make the eggs: Prepare a large bowl of ice water and set aside. Bring a large saucepan full of water to a boil over medium-high heat. Using a slotted spoon, one at a time, carefully lower the eggs into the water. Cook for 6 ½ minutes, adjusting the heat to maintain a gentle boil. Transfer the eggs to the ice water and chill until just slightly warm, about 2 minutes. Peel and set aside.

❸ Make the bok choy: In a small skillet, heat the oil over medium-high heat. Add the bok choy and stir-fry until wilted but still crunchy, about 3 minutes. Season lightly with salt.

❹ Ladle the congee into bowls and top with the green scallions, halved jammy eggs, and bok choy. Or, store each element separately in airtight containers for later. They'll keep for up to a week.

❺ To serve, garnish with a drizzle of tamari and some chili crisp (if using).

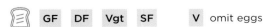 **GF** **DF** **Vgt** **SF**   **V** omit eggs

LF sub 1 carrot, diced, for mushrooms; use LF stock; green scallions only

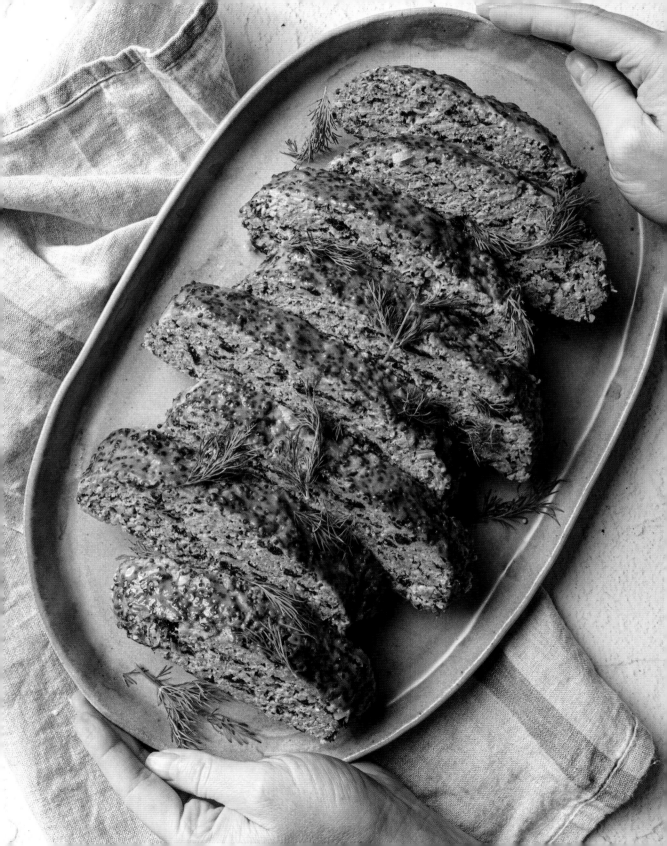

Dijon Turkey Meat Loaf with Spinach

I was raised to have reverence for the blue plate special—that perfect trinity of protein, veg, and carbs. It was how my mother approached every homemade meal, and now I know she was ahead of her time from a nutrition (not just a comfort) standpoint. Unfortunately, I am usually too harried by 6 p.m. to make three separate dishes for dinner—which is where recipes like this meat loaf come in. Packed with spinach and whole oats, it is, essentially, a blue plate special in one bite. The oats completely melt away in this dish, but keep the meat mixture light and tender. Instead of a sugary ketchup-y coating, I opt for a homemade honey mustard-esque condiment with just a hint of sweetness.

MAKES 6 SERVINGS

Glaze

¼ cup Dijon mustard

2 tablespoons whole-grain mustard

1 tablespoon honey or maple syrup

Loaf

½ cup whole rolled oats

2 large eggs

1 large shallot, minced

2 garlic cloves, minced

1 tablespoon Dijon mustard

1 tablespoon whole-grain mustard

1 tablespoon gluten-free tamari

1 teaspoon smoked paprika

1 teaspoon sea salt

One 10-ounce package frozen chopped spinach, thawed

2 pounds ground dark meat turkey

❶ Preheat the oven to 350°F. Line a baking sheet with parchment paper.

❷ **Make the glaze:** In a medium bowl, whisk together the Dijon and whole-grain mustards and honey. Set aside.

❸ **Make the loaf:** In a large bowl, mix the oats, eggs, shallot, garlic, Dijon and whole-grain mustards, tamari, smoked paprika, and salt.

❹ Working over the sink, gather the thawed spinach in a clean kitchen towel and squeeze until all the water is removed. You should have a baseball-size wad of spinach as a result. Add the spinach to the oat mixture.

❺ With clean hands, fold in the ground turkey until the oat-spinach mixture is evenly distributed. Form the meat into an oval loaf (roughly 10 inches long × 6 inches wide × 1 ½ inches high) on the prepared baking sheet. Slather the top and sides evenly with the glaze.

❻ Bake for 50 minutes to 1 hour until the top has caramelized and the bottom has formed a crust, or until internal temperature reaches 160°F. Let the meat loaf stand at room temperature for 10 minutes before slicing.

 GF **DF** **LF** omit shallot and garlic; use maple syrup **SF** omit sweetener

Ham & Cheese Dutch Baby with Peas

What's referred to as a "Dutch baby" in the United States is quite different from the pancakes *(pannenkoeken)* you'll find in the Netherlands, where my husband and I spent six weeks during the nascence of this book. When we first tried the country's signature breakfast, instead of the puffed skillet creations I was used to, we got thin crepe-like pancakes that were wider in diameter than most dinner plates with the toppings baked in. I fell in love with the spongy texture immediately and the potential for delicious savory add-ins. This version with thick-cut deli ham, nutty Gouda, and peas is one of my favorites.

MAKES 2 TO 4 SERVINGS

4 large eggs

⅔ cup unsweetened oat or almond milk

½ cup oat flour

¼ cup brown or white rice flour

Sea salt

2 tablespoons extra-virgin olive or avocado oil

4 ounces ham (from about 4 thicker-cut deli slices), thinly sliced, divided

⅓ cup grated Gouda or Gruyère cheese

⅓ cup fresh or frozen sweet peas

¼ cup chopped fresh chives or basil

2 tablespoons unsalted butter or grass-fed ghee

2 cups baby arugula

2 teaspoons fresh lemon juice

① Preheat the oven to 450°F. Place a large (12- to 15-inch) oven-safe cast-iron skillet in the oven while you prepare the batter.

② In a blender, combine the eggs, milk, oat flour, rice flour, **½ teaspoon salt**, and the oil. Blend until the batter is smooth and frothy.

③ In a medium bowl, combine half of the ham, the cheese, peas, and half the herbs.

④ Remove the hot skillet from the oven and add the butter, swirling it around until the skillet is nicely coated. Pour the batter into the skillet. Quickly sprinkle the ham mixture over the top of the pancake, covering the outside edges as well. Reserve the bowl.

⑤ Bake the pancake for 15 to 20 minutes, or until fully golden brown on top and slightly puffed, like a frittata (don't worry if it's not soufflé-like). You want to avoid opening the door while baking. Wait until the 15-minute mark to check. Remove the Dutch baby from the oven.

⑥ In the reserved bowl, toss together the arugula, remaining ham, remaining herbs, and lemon juice. Season lightly with salt. To serve, cut the Dutch baby into slices and divide among plates, then top with a handful of the arugula salad.

GF   SF   LF omit peas   DF omit cheese   Vgt omit ham

Violet's Big Blueberry-Oat Muffins

These muffins, which are inspired by my favorite fictional human fruit, Violet Beauregarde, may not be big in stature, but they are big on blueberry—which is the only size that matters, in my opinion. Whole blueberries are pureed into the batter and plopped throughout the muffins, allowing you to pack way more antioxidants into the mix without ending up with an overly wet, weighed-down muffin. You can use fresh fruit, but frozen blueberries, for whatever reason, hold their color better in the batter, which turns a lovely (dare I say . . .) violet hue. Noted earlier, muffins are, essentially, cupcakes with better branding. Even though these have less sugar and more fiber than most, they should be considered a treat.

MAKES 12 MUFFINS

2 cups (10 ounces) frozen blueberries, thawed

1 ¾ cups oat flour

¾ cup almond flour

2 teaspoons baking powder

½ teaspoon ground cinnamon

¼ teaspoon sea salt

½ cup unsweetened oat or almond milk

½ cup melted coconut oil or avocado oil

3 large eggs, at room temperature

¼ cup maple syrup

2 teaspoons vanilla extract

1 ½ cups whole rolled oats

Streusel

½ cup whole rolled oats

¼ cup almond flour

2 tablespoons coconut sugar or maple syrup

2 tablespoons unrefined coconut oil or unsalted butter, chilled (you want it solid)

Pinch sea salt

❶ Preheat the oven to 375°F. Line a standard muffin tin with paper liners.

❷ **Make the muffins:** Place the thawed blueberries in a fine-mesh strainer and drain thoroughly. Set aside.

❸ In a blender, combine the oat flour, almond flour, baking powder, cinnamon, and salt. Pulse once or twice to mix the dry ingredients. Add the milk, melted coconut oil, eggs, maple syrup, and vanilla. Puree on medium speed until a batter forms, scraping down the sides with a spatula, if needed.

❹ Add half of the thawed blueberries and blend until the mixture turns purple. Remove the blender bowl from the base and add the remaining blueberries along with the rolled oats. Using a spoon, stir to combine.

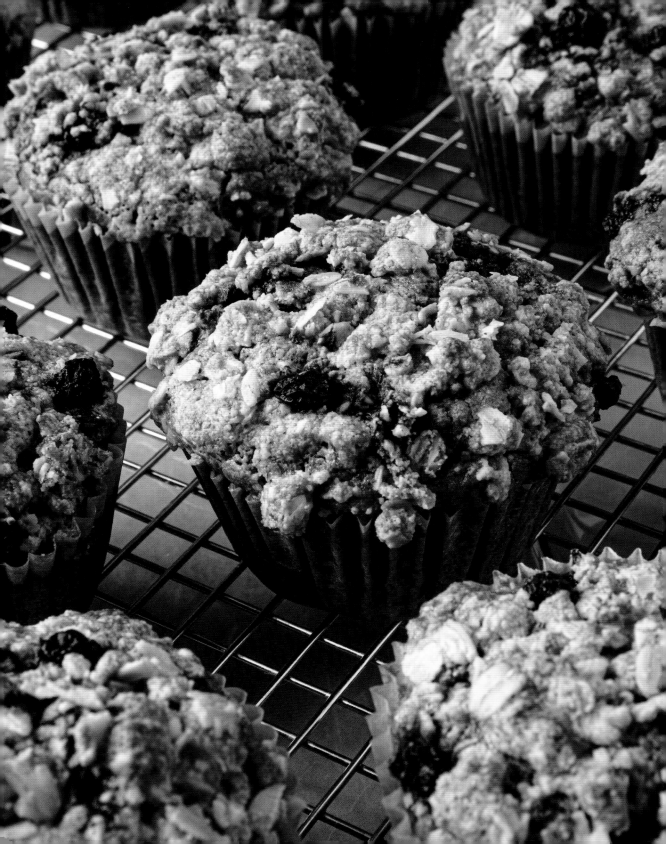

⑤ Make the streusel: In a medium bowl, combine the oats, almond flour, coconut sugar, coconut oil, and salt. Using a fork, mash the streusel together until coarse crumbs form. If it feels too sticky, pop the streusel in the fridge or freezer for a few minutes to firm up.

⑥ Divide the blueberry batter evenly among the muffin liners, filling them nearly to the top. Top each with a dollop of streusel, doing your best to have it not be one clump.

⑦ Bake the muffins for about 20 minutes, or until golden brown and a toothpick inserted into the center comes out clean. Remove from oven, and let cool completely in the tin.

GF **LF** **DF** **Vgt**   **V** use flax eggs (see page 91, step 2)

Year-Round Fruit & Almond Crisp

My last-minute dinner party dessert of choice is always a fruit crisp or crumble. The latter part of the formula is really all you need to master, and then the fruit can vary depending on the season. That said, I've designed this recipe to work with frozen fruit that defies the seasons! My preferred combination is a mix of berries because they're the friendliest fruit for your blood sugar. Other than blueberries, raspberries, and strawberries, you can also use frozen cherries or peaches. Fresh fruit, of course, works as well, especially green apples and pears.

MAKES 6 SERVINGS

Fruit

2	pounds frozen fruit (see headnote)
2	tablespoons arrowroot or corn starch
2	teaspoons fresh lemon juice
2	teaspoons maple syrup

Crisp

½	cup whole rolled oats
⅓	cup raw almonds, roughly chopped
¼	cup coconut sugar or maple syrup
¼	cup flaxseed meal
¼	cup finely shredded unsweetened coconut
½	teaspoon ground cinnamon
½	teaspoon sea salt
¼	cup unrefined coconut oil, chilled
¼	cup almond butter
	Vanilla ice cream or coconut yogurt (optional)

❶ Preheat the oven to 375°F.

❷ **Make the fruit:** In a 9 × 13-inch casserole dish or equivalent, toss together the fruit, arrowroot starch, lemon juice, and maple syrup until well combined. Arrange in an even layer.

❸ **Make the crisp:** In a large bowl, stir together the oats, almonds, coconut sugar, flaxseed meal, coconut, cinnamon, and salt until combined. Add the (solid) coconut oil and almond butter. Using a fork, mash the crumble together until you get pea-size clumps. If the coconut oil is melting, pop the bowl into the fridge for 10 minutes until everything clumps together. Spoon the topping over the fruit—feel free to create quite a pile in the center, as some of it will sink.

❹ Bake until the topping is golden brown and the fruit is bubbling, 30 to 40 minutes. Serve warm with vanilla ice cream or coconut yogurt, if desired.

GF   DF   Vgt

LF use blueberries, strawberries, or raspberries   **V** serve with coconut yogurt

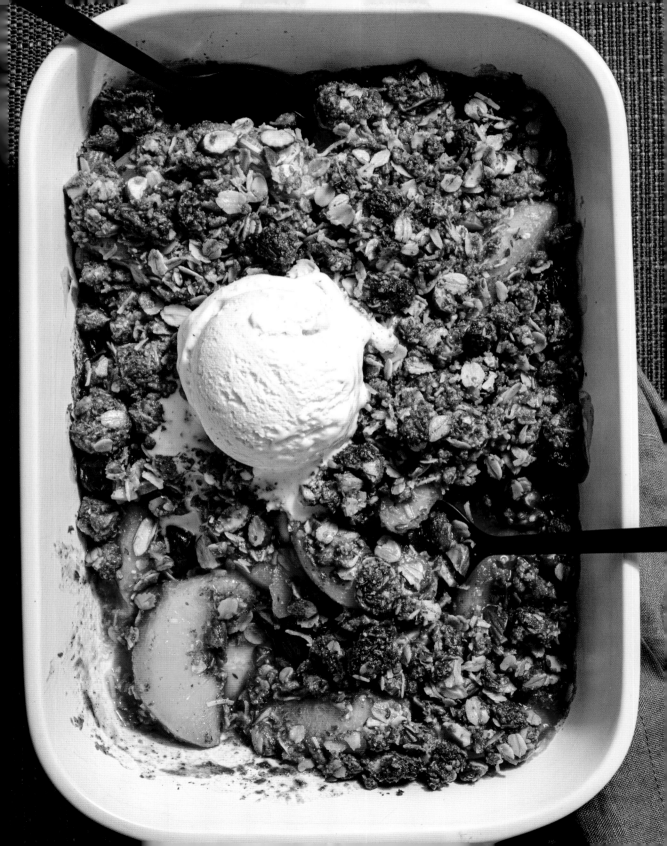

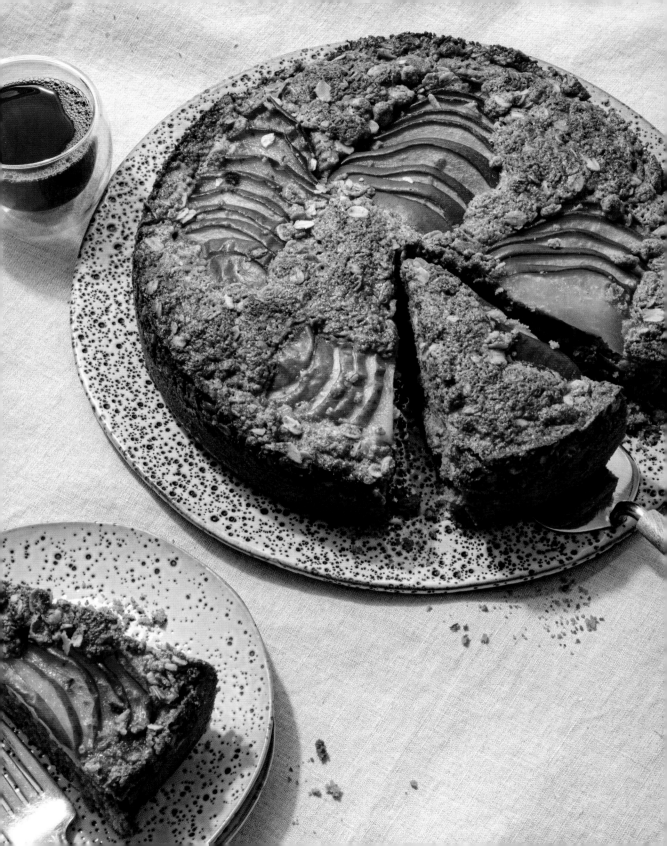

Ginger-Pear Cake with Oat Crumble

The Lapine family Thanksgiving is a large potluck affair, with most people contributing one dish every year. When my husband entered the mix, thus began the ever-important search for his signature item. After a few tries, he made Pamela Salzman's apple crumb cake, and it was the winner. This incredible fall cake is inspired by Charlie's borrowed recipe, using pears as the fruit topper and lots of fresh ginger. It's a moist, stick-to-the-roof-of-your-mouth kind of cake (and, yes, gluten-free!). Oat flour is one of my favorites for baking because it has a subtle sweetness that complements the vanilla and maple syrup. But I also use whole oats here to retain more fiber in the crumble. If you're throwing caution to the wind on the sugar front, candied ginger is a fun addition to the oat topping. You can offset the carbs by serving sour cream, crème fraîche, or unsweetened yogurt on top.

CHANGE OF SEASON: Omit the cinnamon and use fresh sliced peaches instead of pears. Apples also work in fall months.

MAKES ONE 9-INCH CAKE

Crumble

¼ cup coconut sugar

½ cup oat flour

½ cup whole rolled oats

1 teaspoon baking powder

¼ teaspoon sea salt

¼ cup almond butter

¼ cup coconut oil, chilled

Cake

½ cup extra-virgin olive oil or melted coconut oil

½ cup coconut sugar or maple syrup

2 large eggs, at room temperature

1 tablespoon grated fresh ginger

1 tablespoon fresh lemon juice or apple cider vinegar

¾ cup unsweetened oat or almond milk

1 teaspoon vanilla extract

2 ½ cups oat flour

1 teaspoon baking powder

1 teaspoon ground cinnamon

1 teaspoon ground ginger

½ teaspoon baking soda

½ teaspoon sea salt

2 small Bosc pears (or similar)

❶ Adjust an oven rack to the center position and preheat the oven to 375°F. Grease a 9-inch round springform pan with oil and line the bottom with parchment paper.

❷ **Make the crumble:** In a medium bowl, stir together the coconut sugar, oat flour, rolled oats, baking powder, and salt until combined. Add the almond butter and coconut oil. Using a fork or clean hands, mash the oil and nut butter into the dry ingredients until fine clumps form. Refrigerate the crumble in the bowl to keep cool.

3 **Make the cake:** In a large bowl, whisk together the oil, coconut sugar, eggs, fresh ginger, lemon juice, milk, and vanilla until smooth. Stir in the oat flour, baking powder, cinnamon, ground ginger, baking soda, and salt until just combined. Pour the batter into the prepared pan and spread it evenly.

4 Halve the pears lengthwise and remove the core and stems. Thinly slice each half (keeping them together like an accordion). Fan the slices of the pear halves onto the cake—you want this to look tidy, but don't worry, the crumble will cover any messiness.

5 Sprinkle the crumble over the pears, leaving a few of the fanned pieces exposed.

6 Bake on the center rack until a toothpick inserted into the center comes out clean, 45 to 50 minutes. Let the cake cool in the pan for 10 minutes. Run a knife around the edges to loosen the cake and remove the outer ring. Cool completely before serving.

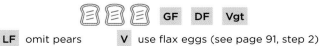

GF   **DF**   **Vgt**

LF omit pears   **V** use flax eggs (see page 91, step 2)

Raspberry Lime Rickey Curd Tart

Although I don't have dessert that often at home, when I am in Paris, I have a gluten-free tart or macaron after every meal. You'd think my energy levels would reflect this rollercoaster of sugar, but my biggest learning is always how good I feel and how little weight I put on. French pastry, though rich and decadent, is so much less sweet than what you'll find in the cookie aisle in the United States. More important, my favorite *tart au citron* uses butter, eggs, and whipped cream to its advantage as carb companions.

This version is similarly full of healthy fat, but can be made completely dairy-free. The curd is a nod to key lime pie, but also laced with raspberries. The oat flour–based shortbread crust is much more user friendly than pie dough: You simply press it into the pan like play dough. The tart keeps well in the fridge for a few days, so it's a good option for making ahead for a spring holiday. Adorn it as simply or elaborately as you like with whipped cream piped on the sides, lime slivers, and, certainly, lots of whole raspberries for fiber (and to hide any imperfections).

CHANGE OF SEASON: Grapefruit, blood orange, or Meyer lemon can be substituted for the lime. Strawberries or blueberries can be swapped for raspberries.

MAKES ONE 8-INCH TART

Crust

1	cup oat flour
½	cup white rice flour or all-purpose gluten-free flour
2	tablespoons tapioca flour or starch
¼	teaspoon fine sea salt
2	tablespoons maple syrup or honey
1	teaspoon vanilla extract
6	tablespoons unsalted butter, chilled, diced

Curd

3	large eggs
¼	cup maple syrup or honey
¼	cup unrefined coconut oil (solid at room temperature)
8	ounces fresh or frozen raspberries, completely thawed
	Grated zest of 4 limes
½	cup fresh lime juice (from 6 to 8 limes)

To serve (optional)

Fresh raspberries

Thinly sliced lime wedges or grated lime zest

Whipped cream, crème fraîche, or plant-based alternative

① Preheat the oven to 350°F. Line the (removable) bottom of an 8-inch tart pan with parchment paper. Grease the sides with **oil or butter**. Set a fine-mesh strainer over a heatproof bowl or 4-cup measuring cup.

② **Make the crust:** In a food processor, pulse the oat flour, rice flour, tapioca flour, and salt until combined. Drizzle in the maple syrup and vanilla, and scatter the butter pieces on top. Pulse until the butter is incorporated and a sticky dough forms. If the dough is still crumbly or not forming, add **1 tablespoon cold water** and continue to pulse.

③ Transfer the dough to the center of the prepared tart pan. Using greased palms, press the dough into an even crust. It's easier to focus on the sides first, then finish the middle, and even out everything. A cup measure is helpful for pressing the crust flat and ensuring an even wall along the sides.

④ Place the tart pan on a rimmed sheet pan and bake for about 20 minutes until firm and golden brown. Press the bottom of the crust gently with the back of a spoon or measuring cup to compact it. Set aside to cool in the pan.

⑤ **Make the curd:** While the crust bakes, in a medium saucepan, whisk the eggs and maple syrup until smooth. Place the pan over medium-low heat. Add the coconut oil and raspberries. Cook, whisking occasionally and breaking apart the raspberries, until the oil melts and the raspberries are falling apart, about 3 minutes. Add the lime zest and lime juice and continue cooking, whisking gently, until the mixture begins to thicken enough to coat the back of a spoon, about 5 minutes. It may feel like nothing is happening, but as soon as gentle bubbles form, the curd will thicken quickly. Remove from the heat immediately and continue whisking to avoid any clumps.

⑥ Carefully strain the curd through the prepared sieve into the bowl. It helps to whisk the solids in the sieve to usher out all the curd. Discard the solids. Transfer the strained curd to the cooked crust and smooth into an even layer with a spatula. Let cool at room temperature, or in the refrigerator, until the filling sets. This can be done a few days in advance.

⑦ If desired, decorate the tart with raspberries, thinly sliced lime wedges, and piped whipped cream. Cut into slices and serve.

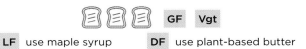

GF **Vgt**

LF use maple syrup   **DF** use plant-based butter

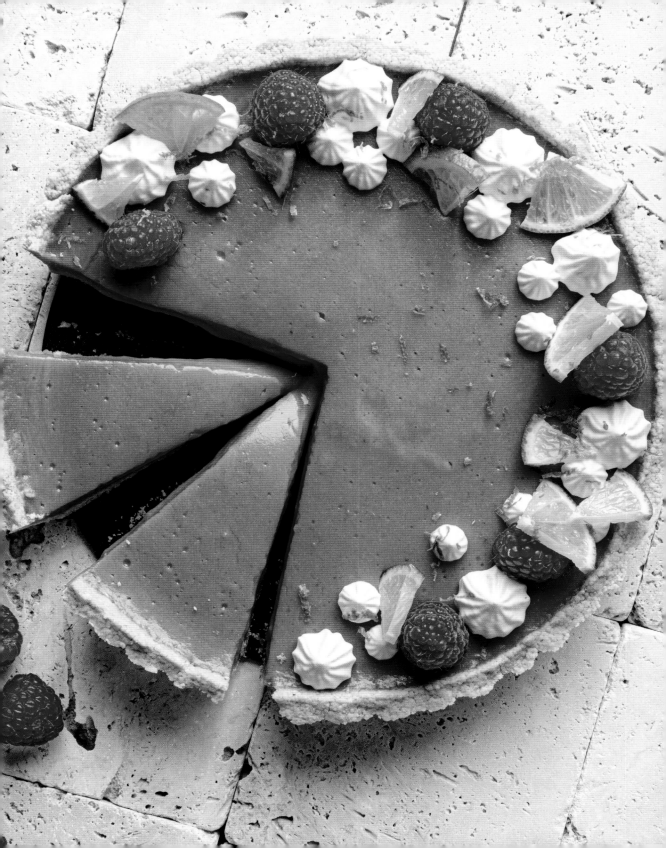

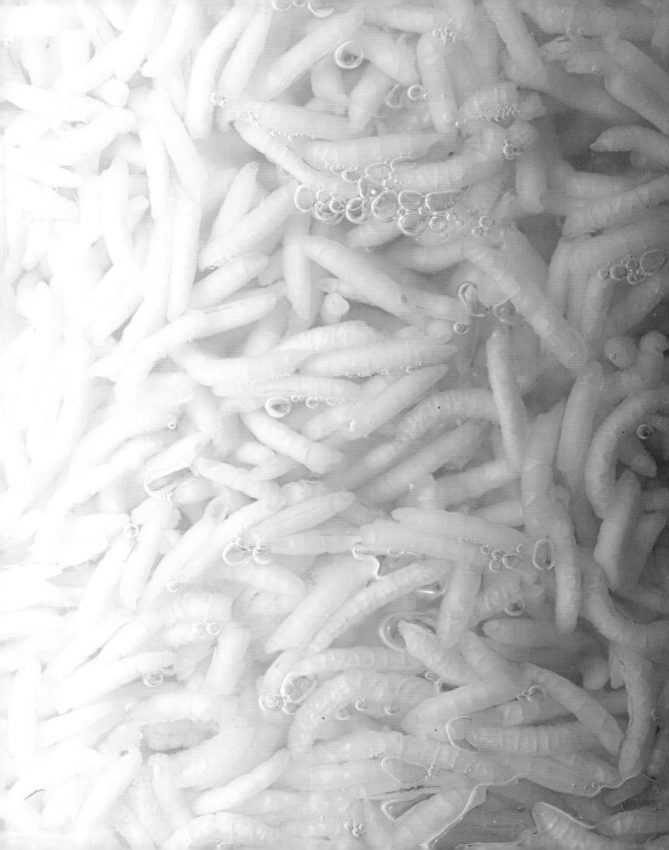

RICE

. . .

Sweet & Sour Moroccan Chicken-Rice Casserole

Miso–Red Curry Black Rice with Kale & Delicata Squash

Low-Sugar Sushi Rice

The Simplest Poke Bowls

Crispy Rice with Spicy Beet Tartare

Warming Mushroom & Wild Rice Soup

Oven Risotto with Shrimp, Asparagus & Peas

Prelude-to-Summer Rolls with Ginger-Walnut Sauce

Kimchi & Cashew Fried Brown Rice

Minty Green Rice Pilaf with Chiles & Peanuts

Hemp-Crusted Chicken Tenders with Dill Aioli

Brussels Sprouts & Wild Rice Salad with
Maple Walnut–Pecan Spice Brittle

TYPES & PREPARATION TIPS

I've given typical cooking times, but because every rice variety is slightly different, it's best to defer to the package directions when using the absorption method.

Wild Rice

Popular preparation method: boiled in a large pot of salted water (like pasta)

Cook time: 45 minutes to 1 hour

Wild rice takes a long time to cook and requires more water than brown rice, so it's best boiled in a large pot like you cook pasta, or added to soups with lots of liquid, like my **Warming Mushroom & Wild Rice Soup** (page 127). You'll know the rice is done when the outer bran splits and the tender, fluffy grain within is exposed. Wild rice is lovely in hearty fall salads, like **Brussels Sprouts & Wild Rice Salad with Maple Walnut–Pecan Spice Brittle** (page 139) as part of a holiday spread.

Brown Rice

Popular preparation method: absorption

Ratio: 1 cup brown rice to 2 cups liquid

Cook time: 40 to 45 minutes

Chewier, more dense, and less fluffy than white rice, brown rice is available in all lengths and many varietals. Because cooking it can add prep time to a weeknight meal, I prefer to make a big batch of brown rice in advance and use it in meals for the week ahead. For this reason, I particularly love using short-grain brown rice in stir-fries like **Kimchi & Cashew Fried Brown Rice** (page 133), since slightly dried-out grains work best. Premade brown rice would also be a perfect carb swap in the **Roasted Cauliflower Salad with Quinoa, Arugula & Creamy Romesco Dressing** (page 146).

Black or Forbidden Rice

Popular preparation method: absorption

Ratio: 1 cup black rice to 2 cups liquid

Cook time: 30 to 35 minutes

With even more powerful antioxidant effects than blueberries, black rice is a wonderful option when you want to stick with a whole grain but switch up the texture and flavor (and save 10 minutes of cook time while you're at it). The "forbidden" name stems from its nutritional value in traditional Chinese medicine as it was once reserved only for the elite, allowing them to prosper, whereas the hoi polloi were prohibited from eating it. When black rice cooks, it blossoms into a deep purple color that looks stunning in salads like my **Miso-Red Curry Black Rice with Kale & Delicata Squash** (page 120). It also makes for a moody rice pudding or porridge.

Arborio Rice

Popular preparation method: risotto

Cook time: 35 minutes to 1 hour

Short-grained and high in starch, Arborio rice is perfect for adding creaminess and bulk to dishes without using dairy. Though it can be used in Spanish paella in a pinch (instead of Bomba rice), it's most commonly known for making Italian risotto, where the grains are slowly coaxed into releasing their starch (see **Oven Risotto with Shrimp, Asparagus & Peas**, page 128). It is also my preferred rice for casseroles because the starch allows you to skip that obligatory cream-of-whatever soup. You can see what I mean in the **Sweet & Sour Moroccan Chicken-Rice Casserole** (page 119).

Sushi Rice

Popular preparation method: absorption

Ratio: 1 cup sushi rice to 1 $\frac{1}{2}$ cups liquid

Cook time: 20 to 25 minutes

Sushi chefs dedicate years of training to the simple art of making sushi rice, one of the trickier varieties to cook. Best results are typically achieved after rinsing the rice thoroughly to get rid of excess starch, then soaking it for 10 minutes in its cooking water. Though the starch adds some of that sticky quality, most prepared sushi rice is seasoned with sugar and vinegar to encourage it to cling together further. I tried to get a similar texture without all the added sweetener in my **Low-Sugar Sushi Rice** (page 121), which forms the basis for **The Simplest Poke Bowls** (page 123) and **Crispy Rice with Spicy Beet Tartare** (page 125).

Long-Grain White Rice (Jasmine & Basmati)

Popular preparation methods: absorption or pilaf

Ratio: 1 cup white rice to 1 $\frac{1}{2}$ cups liquid

Cook time: 15 minutes

Even though it lacks the fiber content of unrefined rice, white rice is still the most consumed variety across the world and the ultimate culinary chameleon. I prefer to buy varieties that have personality and fragrance. Jasmine rice, produced most commonly in Thailand, is floral, soft, and a bit more moist than basmati rice, which has a firmer, drier texture and nuttier scent. I prefer jasmine rice for my **Minty Green Rice Pilaf with Chiles & Peanuts** (page 134) and basmati or Carolina rice for my **Gazpacho Rice & Bean Pilaf** (page 317).

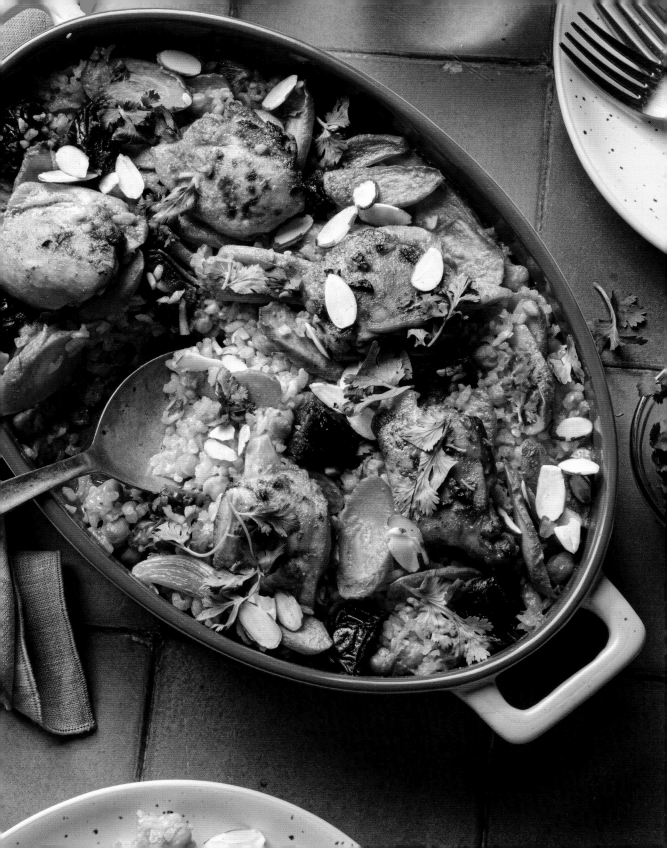

Sweet & Sour Moroccan Chicken-Rice Casserole

If there's one dish I have become known for, it would be the chicken and rice casserole (CRC). And this Moroccan-inspired CRC might be the best one yet. The Arborio rice plumps perfectly in the same amount of time it takes for chicken thighs to become juicy and tender in a marinade of turmeric, cumin, and ground ginger. Moroccan tagines usually include a dried fruit—in this case, I use dates—and coupled with the hit of acid from fresh lemon juice, the sweet and sour base is reminiscent of a chicken Marbella casserole. Though this recipe has some added sugar, it's balanced by fiber-rich chickpeas, carrots, and almonds.

MAKES 4 SERVINGS

¼ cup fresh lemon juice

¼ cup extra-virgin olive oil

2 garlic cloves, minced

2 teaspoons honey

1½ teaspoons ground turmeric

1 teaspoon ground cumin

1 teaspoon ground ginger

Sea salt

1 pound boneless, skinless chicken thighs, cut into 2 pieces

1 cup Arborio rice

One 15-ounce can chickpeas, rinsed and drained, or 2 cups cooked

4 medium carrots (about ¾ pound), sliced on a diagonal

2 medium shallots, quartered

3 ounces pitted dates (about 6), halved widthwise

2 cups chicken stock

2 tablespoons sliced or slivered almonds

2 tablespoons chopped fresh cilantro or mint leaves

❶ In a large bowl, whisk together the lemon juice, oil, garlic, honey, turmeric, cumin, ginger, and **1 teaspoon salt**. Add the chicken and toss until fully coated in the marinade. Refrigerate to marinate for at least 30 minutes while you prep the other ingredients, or cover and chill overnight.

❷ Preheat the oven to 400°F.

❸ Remove the chicken from the marinade, shaking off the excess, and transfer to a plate. To the marinade, add the rice, chickpeas, carrots, shallots, dates, and **½ teaspoon salt** and stir until well distributed. Pour in the stock and stir to combine. Transfer the rice mixture to a 15-inch ovenproof skillet or a 9 × 13-inch casserole dish and arrange in an even layer. Nestle the chicken thighs in the rice mixture.

❹ Bake for 45 minutes, or until the rice is tender and most of the liquid is absorbed. Garnish with the almonds and cilantro and serve straight from the pan.

GF **DF** **SF** omit honey and dates

Miso–Red Curry Black Rice with Kale & Delicata Squash

Though I usually have both miso paste and red curry in my fridge at all times, I would have never thought to combine them until Heidi Swanson's wonderful cookbook *Super Natural Every Day* came into my life. I use this sauce all the time now on roasted potatoes and winter squash, and even baked fish or chicken. Combined with the earthy black rice and bright massaged kale, you'll get the most flavorful grain salad with minimal effort. The sweet delicata is an apt pairing for the salty, spicy paste, and it's one of the lower-maintenance winter squash options because you don't have to remove the skin. Even though the kale is dressed ahead, this dish can sit in the fridge for a few days if you want to make it in advance as a vegetarian lunch or side dish.

MAKES 4 SERVINGS

¼   cup white miso paste

¼   cup extra-virgin olive oil, divided

2   tablespoons Thai red curry paste

2   medium delicata squash, seeded and thinly sliced

1   cup black or forbidden rice

     Sea salt

1   bunch kale, tough stems removed, thinly sliced

2   tablespoons fresh lemon juice (from 1 lemon)

¼   cup toasted pepitas or pumpkin seeds

¼   cup chopped fresh cilantro

❶ Preheat the oven to 425°F. Line a baking sheet with parchment paper.

❷ In a medium bowl, whisk together the miso, **3 tablespoons oil**, and curry paste until smooth. On the prepared baking sheet, toss the delicata with ¼ cup of the miso–red curry paste, then arrange in an even layer. Bake for about 25 minutes, or until the squash is caramelized and soft.

❸ In the meantime, in a lidded saucepan, combine the rice with **1 ¾ cups water** and **½ teaspoon salt**. Bring to a boil over high heat, cover the pan, reduce the heat to low, and cook until the liquid is absorbed, about 30 minutes, or according to the package directions. Set aside, covered.

❹ While the rice cooks, in a large bowl, toss together the kale, lemon juice, remaining **1 tablespoon oil**, and **½ teaspoon salt** and massage until wilted.

❺ Add the cooked squash, rice, and remaining miso–red curry paste to the bowl with the kale and toss until well combined. Garnish with the pepitas and cilantro, and serve warm or at room temperature.

  GF   DF   Vgt   V   SF   LF   omit red curry

Low-Sugar Sushi Rice

The sushi rice at most restaurants in the United States has a lot of added sugar, which, when combined with those simple carbs, doesn't do your blood glucose levels any favors. Still, that slight bit of sweetness complements the vinegar in seasoned sushi rice. This recipe strikes a happy medium. You can use table sugar, but I like using maple syrup or honey because those sweeteners are naturally sticky, which helps when you're trying to mold your rice into handrolls or sushi. I used to eat plain sushi rice as my sick-day comfort food, but now that I know better, I try to offset it with lots of vegetables and protein, like in **The Simplest Poke Bowls** (page 123) or **Crispy Rice with Spicy Beet Tartare** (page 125). If you do serve the rice on its own, add a sliced avocado and a nice dusting of **Salty Sesame–Sunflower Gomasio** (page 75) or sesame seeds.

MAKES 4 CUPS

1 cup sushi rice

1 tablespoon rice vinegar

1 teaspoon gluten-free tamari or soy sauce

1 teaspoon maple syrup or honey

½ teaspoon sea salt

Salty Sesame-Sunflower Gomasio (page 75) or sesame seeds (optional)

❶ Place the rice in a fine-mesh sieve and rinse it under cold water until the water runs clear. Tap the sieve a few times to get out as much water as possible. Place the clean rice into a medium lidded saucepan and pour in **1 ½ cups water**. Let sit for 10 minutes, then bring to a boil over high heat, cover the pan, and reduce the heat to low. Simmer, covered, for 20 minutes, or until all the liquid is absorbed. Remove from the heat and let stand for 10 minutes.

❷ Meanwhile, in a small bowl, whisk together the vinegar, tamari, maple syrup, and salt until the sweetener is fully incorporated. Pour the seasoning over the rice and fluff with a fork to mix well. Taste and add more salt, as needed, especially if the rice tastes too acidic.

❸ Garnish with the gomasio (if using) to serve.

 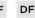 **GF** **DF** **Vgt** **V**   **LF** use maple syrup   **SF** omit sweetener

Rice

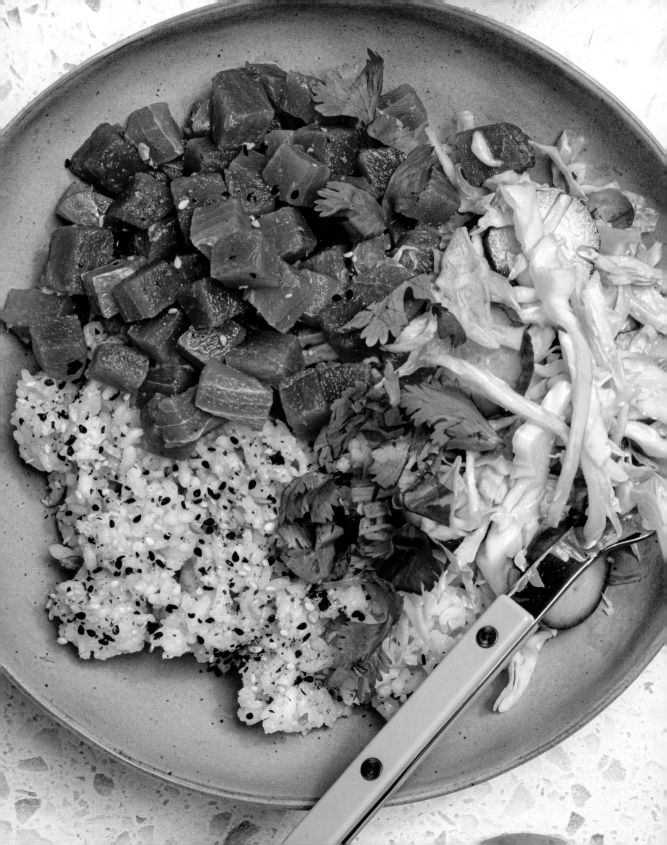

The Simplest Poke Bowls

When the weather gets unbearably hot, poke bowls are the go-to in our house. The sushi rice is the only element that needs any form of heat, and since I crave this carb year-round, it is a sacrifice I am more than willing to make. Poke is a main fixture of Native Hawaiian cuisine and includes some variety of raw diced fish (often marinated), white rice, and various garnishes. This version is about as user friendly as it gets. As with all Carbivore recipes, the rice is intentionally proportioned to take up less real estate than the vegetables and fresh fish. Along with cabbage, cilantro is one of nature's best chelating agents, helping your liver usher out heavy metals from high-mercury fish. To make this vegan, simply swap the **Spicy Beet Tartare** (page 125) made with a plant-based mayo for the fish.

MAKES 4 SERVINGS

Poke bowls

1 ¼ pounds sushi-grade tuna steaks or salmon fillets, skin removed, finely diced

1 small head cabbage, finely shredded (8 cups)

4 small Kirby or Persian cucumbers (about ¾ pound), sliced

3 tablespoons rice vinegar

2 tablespoons gluten-free tamari or soy sauce

1 tablespoon toasted sesame oil

1 teaspoon sea salt

4 cups **Low-Sugar Sushi Rice** (page 121)

1 avocado, diced (optional)

⅓ cup roughly chopped fresh cilantro

¼ cup **Salty Sesame-Sunflower Gomasio** (page 75), or 4 teaspoons sesame seeds

Ponzu sauce

¼ cup gluten-free tamari or soy sauce

¼ cup fresh lemon juice

1 teaspoon sriracha (optional)

Sea salt

❶ In a large bowl, combine the cabbage, cucumbers, vinegar, tamari, sesame oil, and salt. Mix until well combined. Set aside while you prepare the remaining ingredients, tossing occasionally to recoat the vegetables.

❷ **Make the ponzu:** In a small bowl, whisk together the tamari, lemon juice, and sriracha (if using). Taste for seasoning, and add salt, as needed.

❸ To serve, divide the rice among four bowls. Spoon the cabbage-cucumber mixture into one quadrant, the diced fish into another, and the avocado (if using) into a third. Garnish with the cilantro, gomasio, and a spoonful of ponzu. Serve the remaining sauce on the side.

 GF **DF**

LF omit avocado and sriracha   **SF** sub diced jalapeño for sriracha

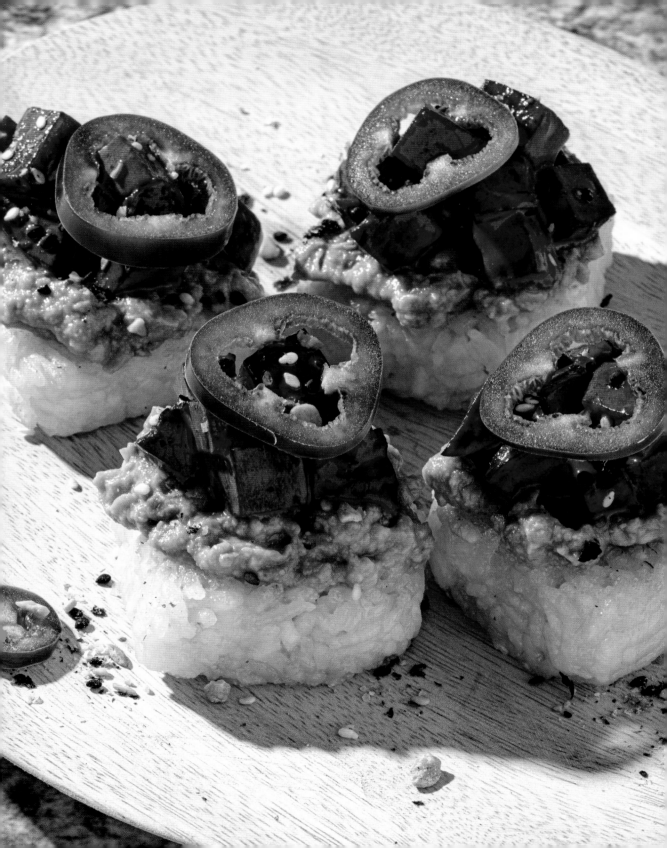

Crispy Rice with Spicy Beet Tartare

I thought there was nothing more delicious than a spicy tuna roll until the day I tasted that delicious filling perched atop a piece of crispy rice. Usually, I try to keep things simple, but this is one of those moments that is worth the extra effort—and it's nothing to be intimidated by. As a twist on the traditional tuna, I use roasted beets (which also taste great as a topping for **The Simplest Poke Bowls**, page 123). You can, of course, substitute 8 ounces fresh tuna or salmon in the spicy mayo mixture. To cut prep time, roast the beets in advance. It's a fun special-occasion meal for the family served alongside a green salad with **Spicy Sesame Dressing** (page 60).

MAKES 12 BITES

12 ounces red beets (about 4 medium)

Sea salt

4 cups **Low-Sugar Sushi Rice** (page 121)

2 tablespoons Japanese Kewpie mayonnaise, or regular mayonnaise mixed with 1 teaspoon rice vinegar

2 teaspoons sriracha

2 teaspoons gluten-free tamari

1 teaspoon toasted sesame oil

Avocado oil

White rice flour or all-purpose gluten-free flour

1 avocado, mashed

2 tablespoons **Salty Sesame-Sunflower Gomasio** (page 75) or sesame seeds

1 jalapeño, seeded and thinly sliced

① Preheat the oven to 375°F. Line an 8-inch square pan with parchment paper.

② Arrange two aluminum foil squares on a work surface and divide the beets between them. Season the beets generously with salt, then wrap them tightly in the foil. Transfer the packets to a sheet pan and roast until the beets are tender and their skin has become opaque and scaly, about 1 hour. Open the foil and let the beets cool until safe to handle. Using your fingers, remove and discard the beets' outer skins. Finely dice the beets (the smaller, the better) and set aside.

③ Place the sushi rice in the prepared pan and spread it into an even layer. Top the rice with a second piece of parchment. Using clean hands, press the rice down with full force to compact it into a firm sheet. You can use a measuring cup to tamp it down and even the edges. Refrigerate the rice in the pan for at least 1 hour, or overnight. Everything up to this point can be done several days ahead, covered, and refrigerated.

④ To make the beet tartare, in a medium bowl, whisk together the mayonnaise, sriracha, tamari, and sesame oil. Stir in the diced beets. Taste for seasoning, and add more heat or salt, as needed.

Rice

⑤ Lightly grease a knife with avocado oil and use it to cut the rice into 12 even rectangles—or whatever shape speaks to you!

⑥ Sprinkle a thin layer of flour onto a plate. Dredge each piece of rice lightly in the flour on both sides. Use your fingers to pack in any loose grains around the edges so it's a tight package.

⑦ Place a large nonstick skillet over medium-high heat. When the pan is hot, add a thin layer (about ⅛ inch) of avocado oil. Working in batches, add the rice cakes to the skillet and pan-fry for 2 minutes per side, or until golden brown. Transfer to paper towels.

⑧ To serve, top each crispy rice bite with a spoonful of mashed avocado, followed by the beet tartare. Sprinkle with gomasio and garnish each with a slice of jalapeño.

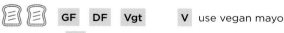

GF **DF** **Vgt**   **V** use vegan mayo

SF sub hot sauce for sriracha

Warming Mushroom & Wild Rice Soup

Growing up, mushroom barley soup was a staple fall comfort, so after giving up gluten, I started making versions with wild rice. Instead of whisking in a béchamel, I simply puree half the soup and add it back to the pot (I use the same trick in my **Creamless Corn & Shrimp Chowder** (page 277). If you're intimidated by the amount of chopping, take a shortcut by pulsing the onion, carrots, and celery in a food processor. Cabbage is a stealth carb companion in this recipe. Not only is it full of fiber, but it's also one of nature's best sources of L-glutamine, a key amino acid for healing leaky gut.

CARB COMPANIONS: Add a dollop of full-fat plain yogurt, crème fraîche, or sour cream.

MAKES 4 SERVINGS

2	tablespoons extra-virgin olive oil
1	small sweet onion, diced
2	medium carrots (4 ounces), diced
2	medium celery stalks, diced
2	cups shredded green cabbage
1	pound cremini mushrooms, stemmed, chopped
2	garlic cloves, minced
2	teaspoons paprika
1/4	teaspoon red pepper flakes
1/2	cup wild rice, rinsed
1/2	cup dry white wine
1	tablespoon gluten-free tamari
1	teaspoon sea salt
6	cups vegetable stock
2	teaspoons apple cider vinegar
2	tablespoons chopped fresh chives

❶ In a large lidded stockpot or Dutch oven, heat the oil over a medium flame. Add the onion, carrots, celery, and cabbage and sauté, about 7 minutes.

❷ Add the mushrooms, garlic, paprika, and red pepper flakes and cook, stirring occasionally, until the mushrooms have softened, about 5 minutes. Stir in the wild rice, wine, tamari, and salt. Cook for about 3 minutes until the wine has all but cooked off. Pour in the stock and bring to a boil. Turn the heat to medium-low, cover the pot, and simmer for 45 minutes, or until the rice is tender.

❸ Off the heat, using an immersion blender, puree half the soup in the pot, or transfer 4 cups of soup to a standard blender to puree, then reincorporate into the pot. You want the broth to be cloudy and creamy looking but still have plenty of whole vegetables and rice. Stir in the vinegar and taste for seasoning, adding more salt, as needed. Ladle the soup into bowls and garnish with a sprinkle of chives and any of the suggested carb companions.

GF DF Vgt V SF

Oven Risotto with Shrimp, Asparagus & Peas

I used to think risotto was the perfect dish to impress a love interest. You can hang out in the kitchen and drink wine while the rice slowly plumps, and then he/she/they slowly falls in love with you because of your ability to stir a starch. Now that I'm in my late thirties, I truly have no one left in my life who I need to impress with my "skills," which is why I often now take the path of least resistance. In this case, oven risotto. Instead of ladling liquid and stirring every five minutes, the rice bakes undisturbed in the oven. The shrimp and asparagus get stirred in toward the end, which allows them to maintain maximum bite and vibrancy. Despite the shortcuts, the resulting bowl is so delicious your friends and family will shower you with praise anyway.

---

*MAKE IT A MEAL: Serve with **Smoky Cauliflower Wedges** (page 250) or **Grilled Romaine with Parmesan Pangritata & Caesar-ish Dressing** (page 255).*

MAKES 4 SERVINGS

3 ½ cups chicken or fish stock, divided

1 cup Arborio rice

1 medium leek, halved, rinsed, and thinly sliced

Sea salt

2 tablespoons extra-virgin olive oil

½ cup dry white wine

1 pound peeled, deveined shrimp

1 bunch asparagus, trimmed, cut into ½-inch pieces (about 2 cups)

1 cup frozen sweet peas

Grated zest of 1 lemon

2 tablespoons fresh lemon juice

¼ cup finely chopped fresh chives

❶ Preheat the oven to 350°F.

❷ In a medium Dutch oven or lidded ovenproof heavy-bottomed pot, bring **3 cups stock** to just shy of simmering over high heat. Stir the rice and leek into the steaming-hot stock, along with **½ teaspoon salt** and the oil. Cover the pot and transfer to the oven. Bake for 20 to 30 minutes until most of the liquid is absorbed and the rice is al dente.

❸ Add the wine, the remaining **½ cup stock, ½ teaspoon salt**, the shrimp, and asparagus to the rice. Stir for a minute or two to warm the raw ingredients until the shrimp begin turning pink. Bake, uncovered, for 5 to 7 minutes until the shrimp are curled and the asparagus is tender.

❹ Add the peas, lemon zest and juice, and half the chives, stirring until the peas are thawed, 30 seconds to 1 minute. Taste for seasoning, and add more salt, as needed.

❺ Serve immediately, garnished with the remaining chives.

GF DF SF   Vgt V omit shrimp; use vegetable stock

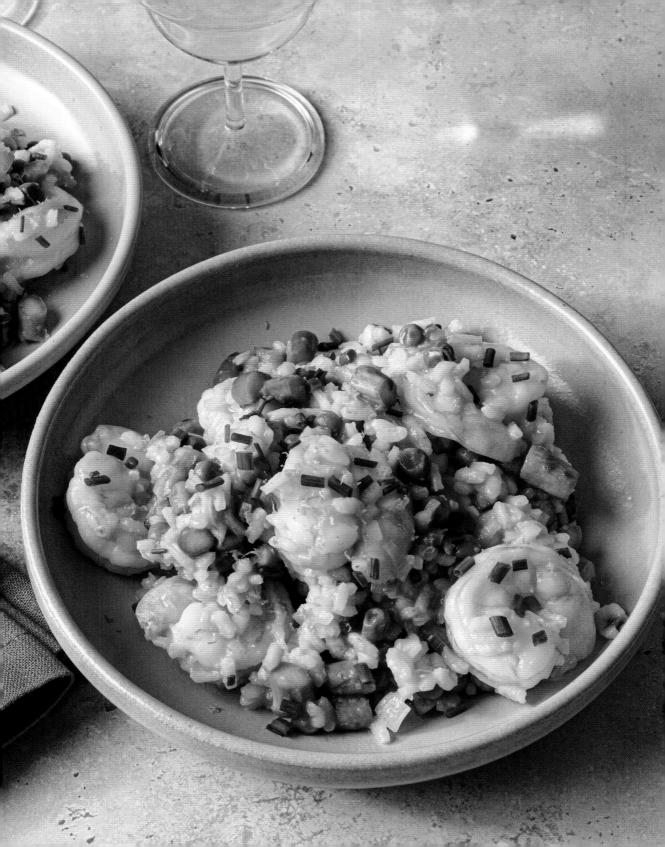

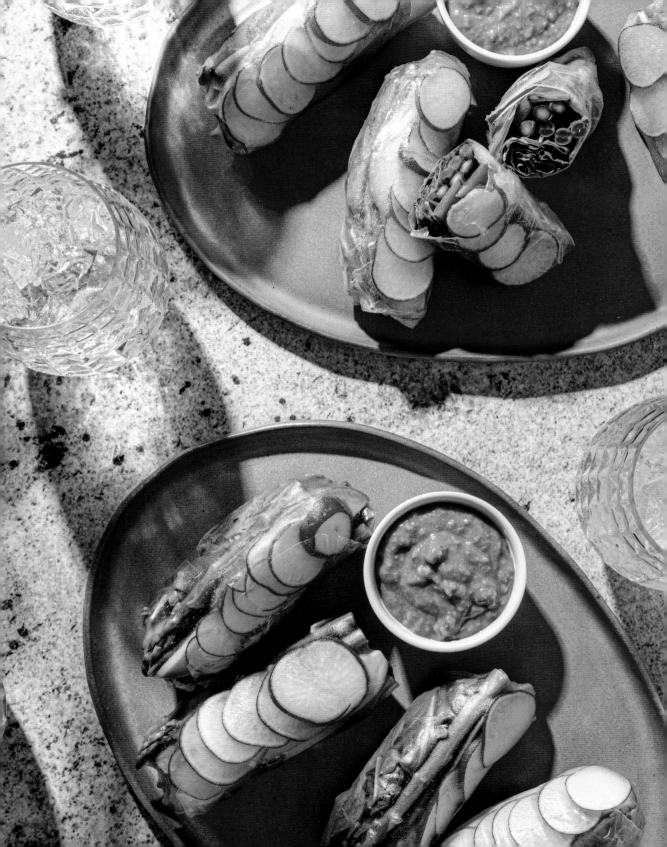

Prelude-to-Summer Rolls with Ginger-Walnut Sauce

Along with salads, summer rolls are one of my preferred ways to eat raw vegetables. I omit the usual vermicelli here and, instead, pack in a slew of spring vegetables, which makes the rice paper–to-fiber ratio a huge Carbivore win. If you can't find green beans, asparagus, or snap peas, try julienned cucumber or red bell pepper. Any big leaf lettuce or baby spinach would also work well in place of the arugula, but I love the peppery bite when paired with the ginger-walnut dipping sauce. Other nontraditional dipping options from this book include **Chipotle-Tahini Sauce** (page 68) and **Spicy Sesame Dressing** (page 60). If you want more protein, poached shrimp (halved lengthwise) can be added to the rolls. Lastly, the rolling gets easier with practice—don't be discouraged if the first one is a bit oddly shaped or messy. If you're making these ahead, wrap them in a wet paper towel to keep them moist and store in an airtight container.

CARB SWAP: Roughly chop all the vegetables and toss them together with 8 ounces cooked rice noodles and the sauce for a cold noodle salad!

MAKES 12 ROLLS

6   red radishes, thinly sliced

2   avocados, sliced

1   bunch asparagus, trimmed

4   ounces green beans, trimmed

4   ounces sugar snap peas, trimmed

1   cup fresh mint or basil leaves (or a mix)

5   ounces baby arugula (about 4 cups, packed)

Twelve 8-inch rice paper spring roll wrappers

Ginger-Walnut Sauce (page 66)

❶ Arrange the radishes, avocados, asparagus, green beans, snap peas, mint, and arugula in neat piles on a plate.

❷ Meanwhile, heat **4 cups water** in a kettle until just shy of boiling. Pour a shallow layer of water into a baking dish and keep the remaining kettle water handy, in case the water in the dish begins to cool.

❸ When the water is safe to touch, dip one spring roll wrapper in the hot water to coat on both sides, shaking off any excess. Immediately place it on a clean work surface. Wait about 15 seconds for the wrapper to soften. In the center, place a few radish slices in a line parallel to your work surface, followed by 2 avocado slices, 2 asparagus spears,

2 green beans, 2 snap peas, and a few mint leaves, arranging all the veggies parallel to the edge of your work surface. If the veggies are too long, snap them in half with your fingers. You want at least 1 inch on either side of the wrapper, widthwise, to play with. Finally, add a small handful of arugula.

④ Fold in the short sides of the wrapper. Fold over the long flap closest to you and pull it tight around the vegetable pile so it seals with the paper on the other side. Then, roll up the whole thing like a neat burrito. It's easiest to do this in one motion, holding in the veggies with your fingers as you roll so you have a tight package. Repeat with the remaining wrappers and fillings. If your roll tears, have no fear. You can double wrap. Simply repeat with a second skin.

⑤ Halve each roll and serve with the **Ginger-Walnut Sauce**.

GF   DF   Vgt   V   SF

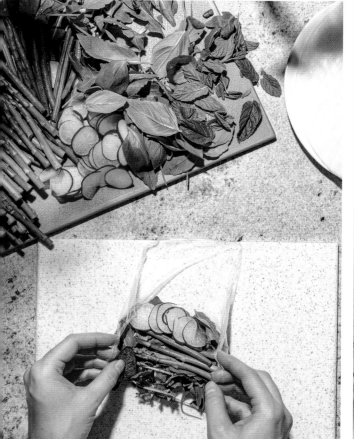
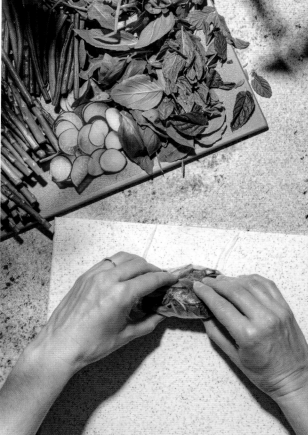

Kimchi & Cashew Fried Brown Rice

The trick to any type of fried rice is beginning with days-old leftover grains. When the rice is dry, it simultaneously soaks up all the flavors of whatever aromatics you add, while remaining nicely toasted. This recipe relies on "pantry vegetables"—the ones that keep forever in your crisper drawer—and the slightly spicy Korean fermented cabbage, kimchi. I save a portion of the raw kimchi to serve as a condiment to maintain the probiotic benefits, while the rest gets caramelized with the other vegetables and provides acid and heat to the fried rice base.

MAKES 4 SERVINGS

3 tablespoons avocado oil or coconut oil, divided

½ cup roughly chopped raw cashews

1 large shallot, sliced

2 medium carrots, thinly sliced

2 cups shredded napa, savoy, or green cabbage

4 scallions, thinly sliced, white and green parts separated

1 ½ cups roughly chopped kimchi (no need to drain), divided

Sea salt

3 cups cooked short-grain brown rice (from 1 cup dried)

4 large eggs, beaten

2 tablespoons gluten-free tamari or soy sauce

2 teaspoons toasted sesame oil

1 tablespoon sesame seeds

1 In a nonstick wok or large skillet, heat **1 tablespoon avocado oil** over medium-high heat. Add the cashews and cook until golden brown and fragrant, 3 minutes. Transfer the nuts to a bowl.

2 Increase the heat to high and add the remaining **2 tablespoons avocado oil**, along with the shallot, carrots, cabbage, and white scallions. Stir-fry until the vegetables soften and are beginning to caramelize, about 7 minutes. Add **1 cup kimchi** and continue to stir-fry until the liquid evaporates, 2 minutes. Season the vegetables lightly with salt.

3 Add the rice and continue to stir-fry for 2 to 3 minutes. Push the fried rice to the side of the pan to create a well in the center. Pour the eggs into the well and cook, undisturbed, for 1 to 2 minutes, until an omelet forms on the bottom. Stir, keeping the eggs in the center of the skillet, to redistribute any uncooked egg, until you have a thick scramble. Toss the fried rice with the egg.

4 Off the heat, stir in the tamari, sesame oil, sesame seeds, half the green scallions, and half the cashews. Transfer the fried rice to bowls and garnish each serving with **2 tablespoons kimchi**, a sprinkle of green scallions, and crispy cashews.

GF   DF   Vgt   SF   V   omit eggs

Minty Green Rice Pilaf with Chiles & Peanuts

Arroz verde, which is a staple of Mexican cuisine, is an iconic pilaf. The base includes cilantro, parsley, green chiles, onions, and garlic. Since the flavors are similar in Southeast Asian cooking, I've given my version a Thai influence with fresh mint, ginger, lime juice, and crunchy peanuts. The beauty of pilafs is that you can add lots of additional fiber to offset the grains, so in addition to the herb slurry, this rice is also packed with green beans and peppers. If you don't have time to make the peanut-cashew crunch, plain nuts are fine, but it certainly adds some major pilaf pizzazz!

---

*MAKE IT A MEAL: Serve as a side for **Chicken Satay Meatballs** (page 155), or as a vegetarian main alongside **Peanut & Lime Slaw** (page 83).*

MAKES 4 SERVINGS

- 1 cup roughly chopped fresh cilantro
- 1 cup loosely packed fresh mint leaves
- 1 ¾ cups chicken or vegetable stock
- 1 small jalapeño or Thai chile, seeded if sensitive to heat
- One 2-inch piece fresh ginger, peeled
- 1 teaspoon sea salt
- 1 tablespoon avocado or coconut oil
- 1 green bell pepper, thinly sliced
- 1 shallot, sliced
- 1 garlic clove, minced
- 1 cup jasmine white rice
- 8 ounces green beans, cut into 1-inch pieces
- 2 tablespoons fresh lime juice
- ⅓ cup chopped salted peanuts, cashews, or **Tangy Peanut-Cashew Crunch** (page 76)

❶ Reserve 1 tablespoon each of cilantro and mint and place the remaining herbs in a blender. Pour in the stock and add the chile, ginger, and salt. Puree until smooth.

❷ In a medium Dutch oven or lidded saucepan, heat the oil over a medium flame. Add the bell pepper, shallot, and garlic and sauté until soft and beginning to caramelize, about 5 minutes. Stir in the rice and toast, stirring occasionally, for about 2 minutes.

❸ Stir in the green beans and herb broth from the blender to combine. Bring to a boil, then reduce the heat to low, cover the pot, and cook for 15 minutes, or until the liquid is absorbed and the rice is tender.

❹ Turn off the heat and let the rice stand, covered, for 10 minutes. Remove the lid, add the lime juice, and fluff with a fork. Garnish with the nuts and the reserved herbs.

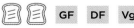 **GF** **DF** **Vgt** **V** **SF** **LF** omit garlic and shallot

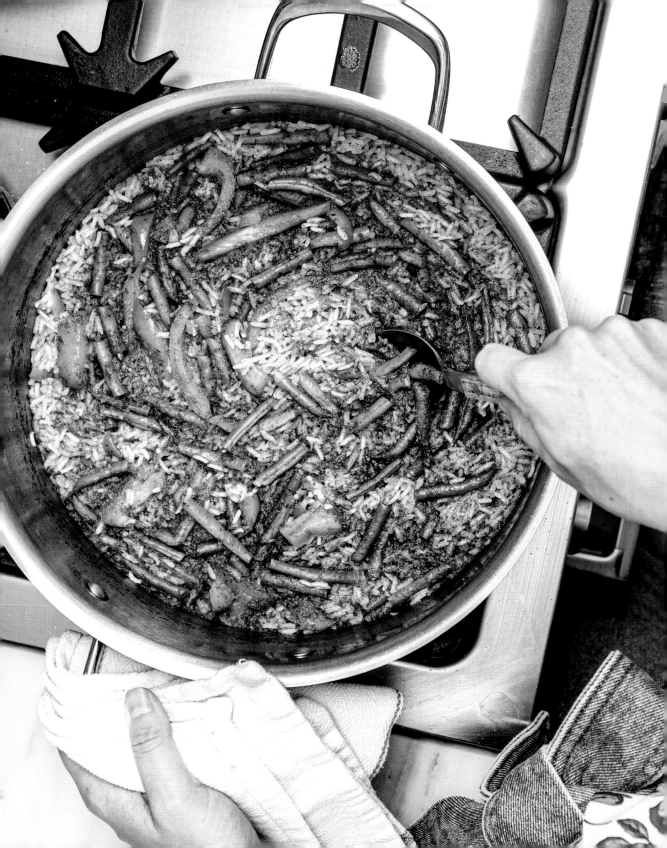

Hemp-Crusted Chicken Tenders with Dill Aioli

I haven't eaten cereal for breakfast since I was a teenager, but I often buy it as a cheater's gluten-free breading for crispy chicken or fish. Since brown rice crisps (what they call off-brand Rice Krispies) have built-in crunch, it doesn't require you to do any double dredging. To make the crust more Carbivore friendly, I cut the rice cereal with hemp seeds, which are high in fiber, have a complete plant-based protein, and have an ideal ratio of omega-6 to omega-3 fatty acids. In terms of dipping, I chose aioli as my carb companion, adding healthy fat and protein instead of the simple sugars in ketchup or honey mustard.

MAKES 4 SERVINGS

Extra-virgin olive oil

2 cups brown rice crisps cereal

1 cup hemp seeds

1 teaspoon paprika

Sea salt

¼ cup Dijon mustard

¼ cup mayonnaise or full-fat plain Greek yogurt

2 pounds chicken breasts

1 cup **Dill Aioli** (page 69)

❶ Preheat the oven to 425°F. Line 2 baking sheets with parchment paper and brush them with oil.

❷ In a small food processor, pulse the cereal, hemp seeds, paprika, and ½ **teaspoon salt** until finely ground. Transfer to a shallow bowl or plate.

❸ In another shallow bowl, stir together the mustard, mayonnaise, and ½ **teaspoon salt**.

❹ On a clean work surface, pat the chicken breasts dry with paper towels. Cut the breasts into 1-inch-thick strips on a diagonal against the grain. Working with a few at a time, coat the chicken strips in the mustard mixture, then dredge in the crispy rice mixture, pressing down and rolling the strips until coated fully. Arrange the chicken in an even layer on the prepared baking sheets.

❺ Bake until golden and crispy, about 15 minutes. Flip the fingers carefully with a spatula, then continue to bake for 5 minutes more. Let cool for 10 minutes on the baking sheets without moving.

❻ Arrange the crispy chicken on a platter and serve with the aioli.

GF   LF   DF   SF

Vgt   **V**   sub extra-firm sliced tofu for chicken; use plant-based yogurt or mayo

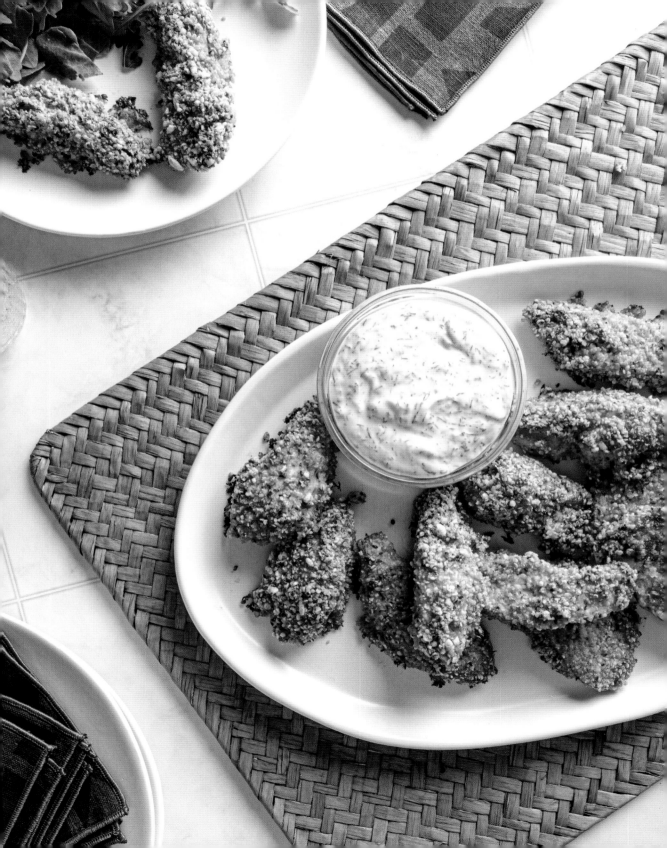

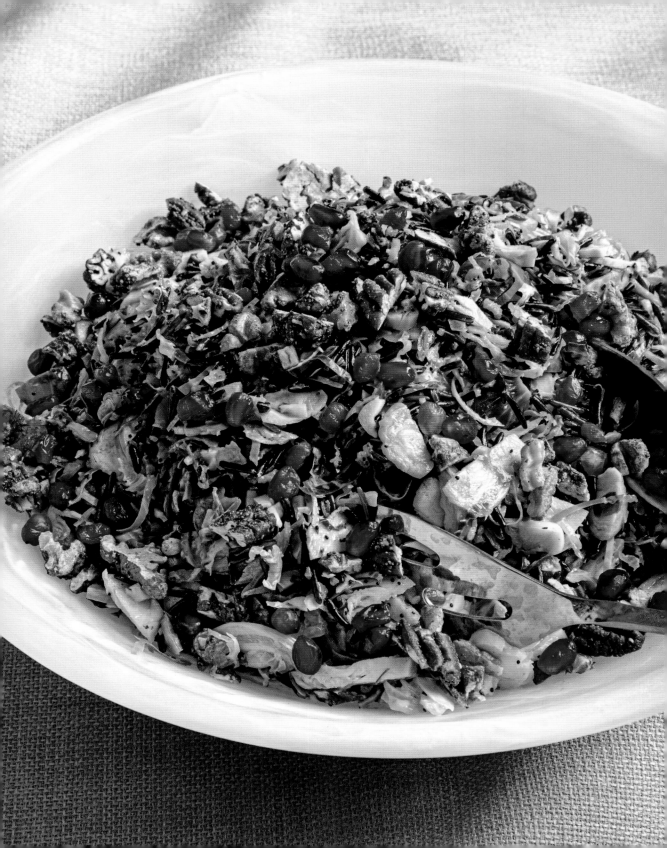

Brussels Sprouts & Wild Rice Salad with Maple Walnut–Pecan Spice Brittle

One of my favorite Carbivore sides to contribute to fall holiday meals is a wild rice salad. Unlike hulled rice, wild varieties hold their shape and texture. To add even more fiber and hardiness, I combine the rice with shredded Brussels sprouts and a bright lemon poppy dressing. If you want to save time, buy shredded Brussels sprouts or use a food processor to get them into little ribbons. The sprouts also let us get away with playing a little more with sweet additions to this savory salad. If you can't find pomegranate seeds, a scant amount (2 tablespoons) of dried cranberries or cherries will work. Like all good holiday dishes, every element can be made up to four days in advance and tossed together when ready to serve! If the lemon poppy dressing isn't your thing, this would also taste great with **Ginger-Walnut Sauce** (page 66) or **Basic Balsamic Vinaigrette** (page 60).

MAKES 6 SIDE SERVINGS

Sea salt

1 cup wild rice, rinsed

1 cup **Maple Walnut–Pecan Spice Brittle** (page 78) or chopped walnuts

1 pound Brussels sprouts, ends trimmed

½ cup **Lemon Poppy Vinaigrette** (page 64)

⅓ cup pomegranate seeds

❶ Bring a large pot of salted water (at least 2 quarts) to a boil over high heat. Add the rinsed rice to the boiling water and cook, uncovered, until al dente, about 45 minutes. About half the grains will burst open, but it's okay for the remaining rice to be chewy. Drain the wild rice and return it to the pot. Place a clean kitchen towel over the pot to catch the steam and let sit for 10 minutes.

❷ Meanwhile, make the **Maple Walnut–Pecan Spice Brittle.**

❸ Remove any tough outer leaves from the Brussels sprouts. Shred the sprouts using a food processor with the shredding disk, or by halving them and thinly slicing with a knife. Place the shredded sprouts in a large bowl.

❹ Add the cooked rice and the vinaigrette to the sprouts and toss to combine. Taste for seasoning, and add more salt as needed. Garnish with the brittle and pomegranate seeds.

GF DF Vgt V   LF sub 1 bunch shredded kale for sprouts

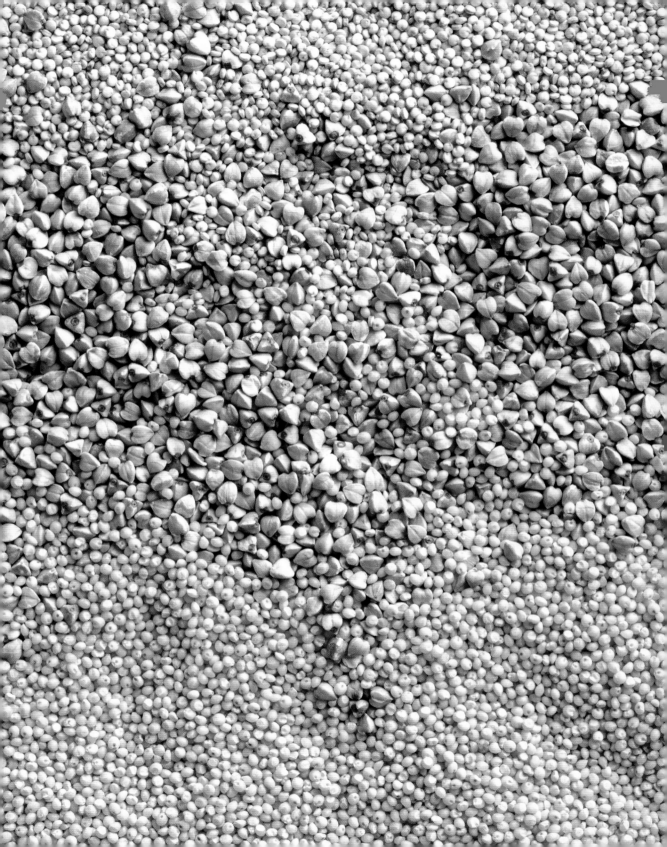

WHOLE GRAINS FROM AROUND THE WORLD

(Buckwheat, Millet, Quinoa)

. . .

Millet & Zucchini Cakes

Roasted Cauliflower Salad with Quinoa, Arugula
& Creamy Romesco Dressing

Buckwheat Crepes with Leek Confit, Salmon & Eggs

Quinoa Paella with Sausage & Shrimp

Chicken Satay Meatballs

Mom's Millet Flour Fish Fry with Tarragon-Chive Tartar Sauce

Turmeric-Pumpkin Fall Reset Soup

Kasha Pilaf with Mushrooms, Bacon & Greens

Ratatouille Quinoa Bake

Black Sesame–Buckwheat Banana Bread

PB & J Cups with Crunchy Quinoa

TYPES & PREPARATION TIPS

Beyond its blanket use as a marketing concept, the term "ancient grains" refers to crops that have maintained their genetic integrity, unaltered by modern agriculture, for centuries. Though we think of many of these as grains, some, like buckwheat, amaranth, and quinoa, are actually "pseudograins"—seeds from a bush rather than a field crop. In this chapter, I'm focusing on three types of whole grains that I cook with most—quinoa, millet, and buckwheat—but there are some recipes where the star carb could be easily swapped out for any of your favorites.

Buckwheat

Varieties: whole buckwheat groats or kasha; buckwheat flour
Popular preparation method: absorption
Ratio: 1 cup buckwheat groats to 2 cups liquid
Cook time: 15 to 25 minutes

Whole buckwheat groats are deeply tanned triangles that can be found in the same grocery section as most other grains. Kasha, whole groats that have been toasted, tends to have a slightly deeper flavor. The cooked groats maintain a lovely chew and can be used in grain salads and pilafs, whereas the uncooked grains can be used as a crunchy, nutty addition to any seed sprinkle or granola. Buckwheat flour is fine and dense, like the softest gray-sand beach. It works well in both savory (crepes, see page 149) and sweet (banana bread, see page 164) baked goods, but is best when offset by a more neutral flour (like white rice, oat, or all-purpose gluten-free flour) to give it some body and dull the intensity.

Millet

Varieties: whole millet, fonio, teff flour, millet flour
Popular preparation method: absorption
Ratio: 1 cup millet to 2 cups liquid
Cook time: 15 to 20 minutes

Millet becomes light and fluffy when cooked, making it a perfect gluten-free swap for couscous or bulgur wheat in tabbouleh. It is also one of my favorite grains to use in veggie burgers and fritters, like my **Millet & Zucchini Cakes** (page 145). But the most popular millet derivative in my kitchen is flour, which has a sandy texture that works well as a dredging for protein. **Mom's Millet Flour Fish Fry with Tarragon-Chive Tartar Sauce** (page 159) is one of my go-to recipes, but you can also use it for a chicken piccata or pan-fried veal cutlet.

Quinoa

Varieties: whole white, red, or black quinoa; quinoa flakes

Popular preparation method: absorption

Ratio: 1 cup quinoa to 1 $\frac{3}{4}$ cups liquid

Cook time: 15 minutes

Quinoa is quick cooking and forgiving, which makes it an easy swap for white rice in pilafs and casseroles, like my **Quinoa Paella with Sausage & Shrimp** (page 151) or **Ratatouille Quinoa Bake** (page 163). When cooked using the absorption method, quinoa plumps and reveals its germ, a small tail that winds around the grain. A good sign of overcooked quinoa is when this small hair detaches from the kernel or the grains become mushy. Most brands will tell you to use a ratio of 1:2 grain to water, but I find that quinoa is at its pearliest when you cook it in slightly less liquid, for slightly less time than called for.

Uncooked, the seeds can be toasted and used as a crunchy, fiber-rich topping (see **Seed Cracker Granola**, page 92, or **PB & J Cups with Crunchy Quinoa**, page 167) or commercially puffed as a breakfast cereal. You can also find cooked, flattened, and dried quinoa in the breakfast cereal aisle. Similar to rolled oats, quinoa flakes can be made into a quick porridge, or used as a whole-grain breadcrumb substitute as I do in my **Chicken Satay Meatballs** (page 155).

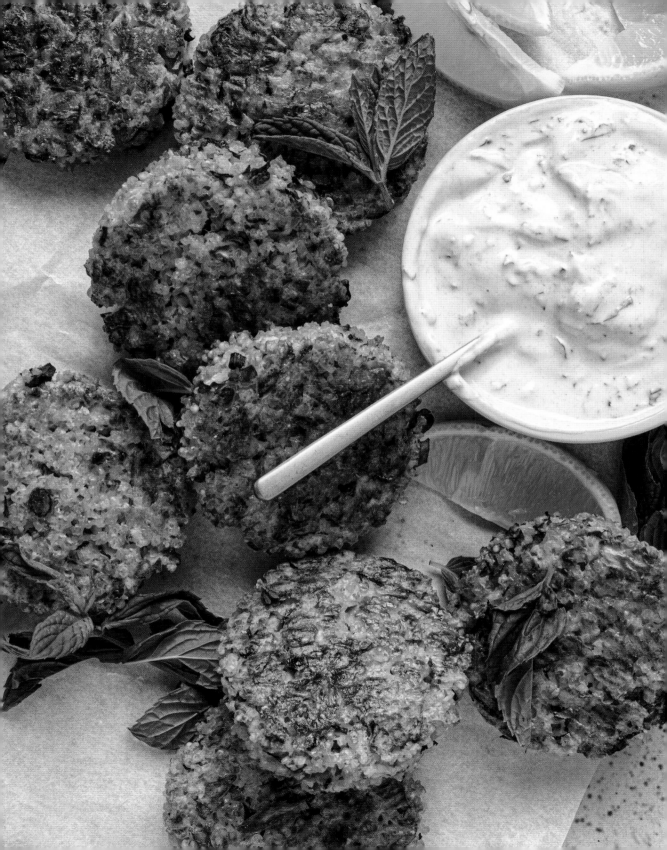

Millet & Zucchini Cakes

If you've previously thought of millet as a slightly lackluster grain, these crispy cakes will make you rethink those lukewarm feelings. Millet's craggy texture creates a layer of crunch after a trip to the oven—perfect for dipping in a fabulous sauce. Here yogurt gets jazzed up with harissa, a North African red pepper paste that can be mild or hot. These cakes, which make a great main course, snack, or appetizer, can be made ahead and re-crisped in a 400°F oven for 10 minutes.

MAKES 9

Extra-virgin olive oil

¾ cup millet

Sea salt

1 medium zucchini (8 ounces), coarsely grated

1 large egg

¼ cup full-fat plain Greek yogurt

¼ cup packed fresh mint, finely chopped

4 scallions, thinly sliced

1 teaspoon ground cumin

½ teaspoon Aleppo pepper, or ¼ teaspoon red pepper flakes

1 cup **Harissa Yogurt** (page 68)

❶ Preheat the oven to 400°F. Line a baking sheet with parchment paper and lightly brush it with oil.

❷ In a medium lidded saucepan, combine the millet, **1¼ cups water, ½ teaspoon salt**, and a drizzle of oil. Bring to a boil over high heat, then reduce to low and cover the pan. Cook the millet for about 15 minutes, or until all the liquid is absorbed and the grains are tender. Fluff with a fork, transfer to a large bowl, and set aside to cool. You can also refrigerate it to speed this up.

❸ Working over the sink, in a clean kitchen towel, gather the grated zucchini into a bundle and squeeze out all the water. You should have a baseball-size wad of zucchini as a result. Add the zucchini to the millet.

❹ Once the grains have cooled, add the egg, yogurt, mint, scallions, cumin, pepper, and **½ teaspoon salt**. Stir until well-incorporated.

❺ Grease a ⅓-cup measure lightly with oil and use it to portion the millet into 9 mounds on the prepared baking sheet. Shape the mounds into patties, 1 inch thick, patting them until compact. Brush the patties lightly with oil.

❻ Bake until the patties have dried out and formed a brown crust on the bottom, 20 minutes. Flip the patties and continue to bake for 10 to 15 minutes until crispy. Serve the cakes warm alongside the yogurt.

 GF **Vgt** **SF** **LF** **DF** omit sauce

Roasted Cauliflower Salad with Quinoa, Arugula & Creamy Romesco Dressing

There's a foolproof formula that I've used in dozens of ways: roasted veg + salad green + precooked grains + creamy dressing = Carbivore perfection. Spanish-inspired romesco sauce adds a punchy acidity that I love as a dressing. The vinegar is offset with sweetness from golden raisins, which we can get away with thanks to all the fiber-packed plants in this bowl. To add more protein, top the salad with grilled chicken breast or blackened shrimp and add crumbled feta, ricotta salata, or goat cheese as an additional delicious carb companion. Quinoa can easily be swapped with sorghum, millet, buckwheat groats, wild or brown rice, lentils, or non-gluten-free farro or barley.

MAKES 4 SERVINGS

1   medium head cauliflower, cut into 1-inch florets

Extra-virgin olive oil

1   teaspoon smoked paprika, divided

Sea salt

½   cup raw almonds, divided

One 16-ounce jar roasted red peppers (about 6 whole peppers), drained

1   tablespoon sherry vinegar or red wine vinegar

½   teaspoon red pepper flakes

5   ounces baby arugula

2   cups cooked quinoa (see headnote)

2   tablespoons golden raisins

❶ Preheat the oven to 425°F. Line a baking sheet with parchment paper.

❷ On the prepared baking sheet, toss together the cauliflower, **3 tablespoons oil, ½ teaspoon smoked paprika, and ½ teaspoon salt** until coated. Arrange in an even layer. Roast for about 25 minutes until lightly browned.

❸ Roughly chop **¼ cup almonds** and add them to the cauliflower. Continue to roast for 5 minutes more until the nuts are toasted. Remove and set aside.

❹ Meanwhile, make the romesco dressing: In a high-speed blender, combine the roasted peppers, remaining **¼ cup almonds,** the vinegar, red pepper flakes, **1 teaspoon salt,** remaining **½ teaspoon smoked paprika,** and **¼ cup oil.** Puree until smooth, adding more oil, as needed, to create a creamy consistency.

❺ In a large salad bowl, toss together the arugula, cooked quinoa, cauliflower, raisins, and **¼ cup romesco.** Serve with the remaining dressing on the side.

GF   DF   Vgt   V

LF   sub 1 pound carrots, sliced, for the cauliflower   **SF**   omit raisins

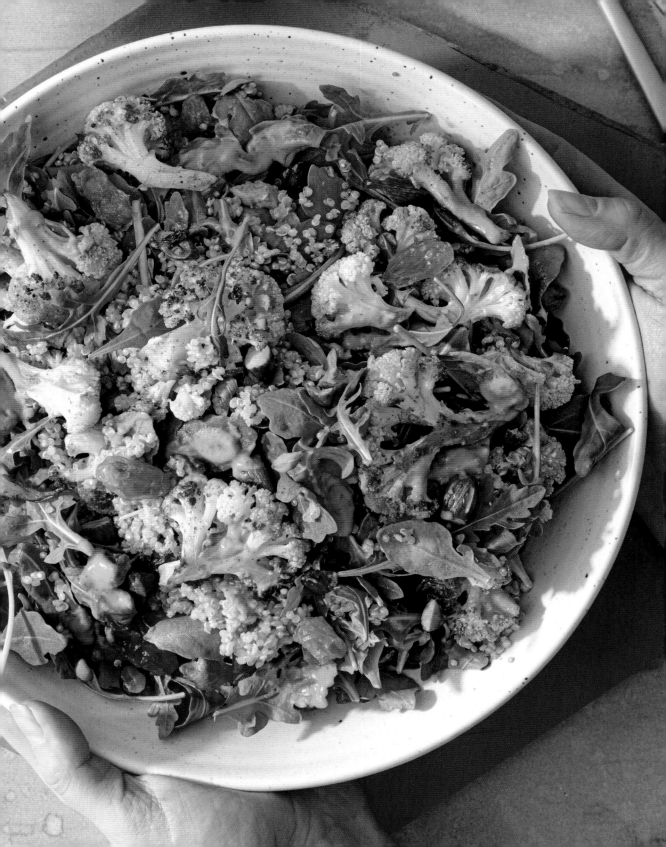

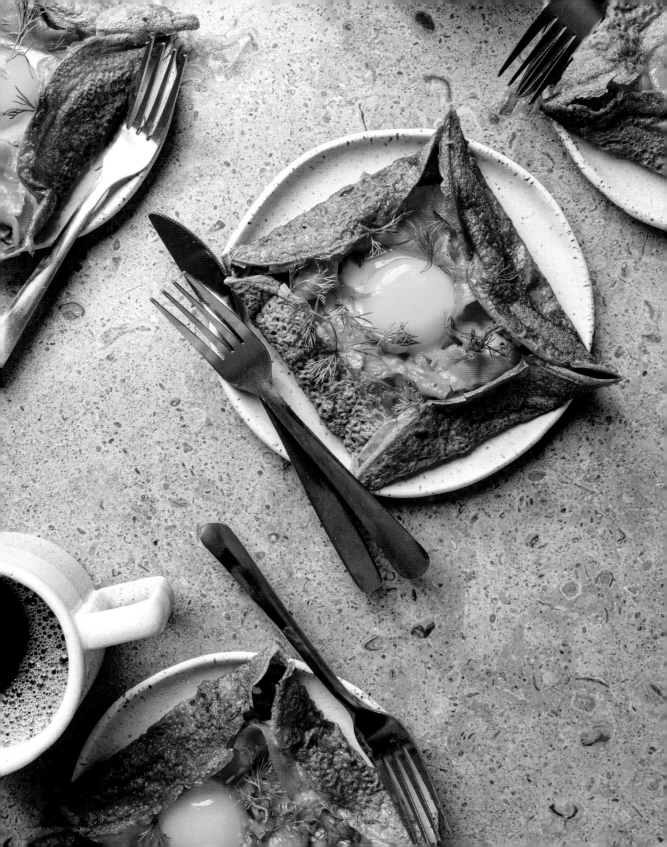

Buckwheat Crepes with Leek Confit, Salmon & Eggs

Buckwheat crepes (or *galettes bretonnes*) are one of the big gluten-free wins when in France, as they are traditionally made with 100 percent buckwheat flour. These crepes are loaded with savory local sundries and folded in on the sides to form a square with the fillings (often a fried egg) exposed in the middle like a partially wrapped present.

Though these galettes might sound intimidating, they are actually quite easy to make, whether for a crowd or individually throughout the week for breakfast. All the elements can be prepared in advance, and the crepes take only a few minutes to firm up on the stove. A cast-iron pan is heavier when it comes to tilting it to spread the batter, but it also helps produce a crunchy crepe instead of a flimsy one. If folding in the sides is challenging, feel free to serve the whole thing open-faced.

CHANGE OF SEASON: In summer, swap fresh tomatoes or shredded zucchini for the leeks, and top with shredded Gruyère instead of salmon.

MAKES 8 SERVINGS

Confit

- ¼ cup extra-virgin olive oil or unsalted butter
- 2 large leeks, halved, rinsed (see headnote, page 209), and thinly sliced
- ½ cup white wine
- ½ teaspoon sea salt

Crepes

- 1 large egg
- ½ cup whole milk or unsweetened nondairy milk
- ⅓ cup buckwheat flour
- ⅓ cup white rice flour or all-purpose gluten-free flour
- ¼ teaspoon sea salt

Unsalted butter or extra-virgin olive oil
- 8 ounces smoked salmon
- 8 large eggs
- 2 tablespoons roughly chopped fresh dill or tarragon

❶ **Make the confit:** In a medium saucepan, heat the oil over medium heat. Add the leeks and sauté until just beginning to brown, about 5 minutes. Add the wine and salt and cook for 1 minute more, then cover the pan and reduce the heat to low. Continue to cook, stirring occasionally, until the leeks are fully broken down and jammy, about 20 minutes. Taste for seasoning, and add more salt, as needed. Transfer to an airtight container until ready to use. The leek confit can be made up to 1 week in advance.

❷ **Make the crepe batter:** In a blender, combine the egg, milk, buckwheat flour, white rice flour, salt, and **1 cup lukewarm water.** Blend on medium speed until frothy and well combined. Give the batter one stir with a spoon to ensure the flour hasn't sunk to the bottom. The batter can be made up to a week in advance and kept chilled in the refrigerator (thin it with water if needed).

recipe continues →   149

❸ Cook the crepes: Heat a large (15-inch) cast-iron skillet over medium-high heat until just shy of smoking. Add **1 teaspoon butter** to melt and swirl the pan until fully coated, or use a brush to distribute.

❹ Ladle ⅓ cup batter into the skillet and quickly turn the pan to coat the whole bottom. It's easiest to do this in one quick motion, drizzling the batter while tipping the pan to coat. If you end up with a weird shape or don't have enough batter, simply drizzle in a little extra to fill in any holes. The crepe should be very thin and lacy with lots of air bubbles. If the batter doesn't cooperate, you may need to thin it slightly with a tablespoon or two of water.

❺ Cook the crepe until firm, crispy, and coming away from the sides, about 2 minutes. Adjust the heat if it starts to burn. Run your spatula along the perimeter of the crepe, then flip it in one swift motion. Cook the second side for another minute until the batter is set. Transfer to a plate, crispy-side down, and repeat with the remaining batter.

❻ Assemble the crepes: Working one at a time, return the crepe to the skillet over medium-low heat, crispy-side down (the first side you cooked it on). Crack an egg in the center and use the back of a spoon to spread the white evenly over the surface. Don't be afraid to separate the white from the yolk—treat it like a condiment and cover the center of the crepe. Cook until the white has partially set, then spoon a few dollops of leek confit over the egg and arrange a slice or two of salmon around the yolk, tearing it into pieces, if needed. Cook until the white has completely set, about 2 minutes.

❼ Fold in the sides of the crepe to create a square galette with the egg yolk exposed in the center. Alternatively, slide the crepe onto a plate. Season the egg with a little salt and garnish with dill.

❽ Repeat with the remaining crepes, leek confit, and filling, or cook your next galette to order at a later date!

GF DF SF   Vgt omit salmon

Quinoa Paella with Sausage & Shrimp

In Spain, paella is traditionally flexible in terms of proteins used, often incorporating a mix of chicken, sausage, and seafood. The authenticity comes down to technique, which I have to warn you, in case the quinoa wasn't a tip-off, this recipe does not religiously abide by! While we lose the traditional crispy rice bits by using quinoa, we make up for it in fiber and other benefits. The quinoa maintains its pearly texture, and yes, also gets a little crunchy around the edges, especially if you use a heavy-bottomed cast-iron pan to cook it. For this version, I combine shrimp with precooked sausage from the deli aisle—two proteins I usually keep stocked in my freezer. Choose something smoky, like kielbasa, bratwurst, or chorizo (not the dried kind). A no-nitrate hot dog also won't disappoint!

CARB SWAP: For a traditional paella, sub Bomba or Arborio rice for the quinoa.

MAKES 4 SERVINGS

- 2 tablespoons extra-virgin olive oil
- 12 ounces precooked sausage links (see headnote), sliced
- 1 pound large shrimp, peeled and deveined
- Sea salt
- 1 medium Spanish or Vidalia onion, diced
- 1 red bell pepper, diced
- 1 cup uncooked white quinoa
- 2 garlic cloves, minced
- 1 teaspoon smoked paprika
- 1 teaspoon ground turmeric
- ¼ teaspoon red pepper flakes
- 1 bunch leafy greens (chard, kale, or collards), thinly sliced
- 2 cups diced or crushed tomatoes (fresh or from one 15-ounce can)
- 2 cups chicken, fish, or vegetable stock
- 2 tablespoons chopped fresh parsley
- 1 lemon, halved

1 In a large heavy-bottomed skillet (preferably cast iron), heat the olive oil over a medium-high flame. Sauté the sausage until browned, about 4 minutes. With a slotted spatula, leaving as much oil behind as possible, transfer the sausage to a bowl and set aside.

2 Add the shrimp to the skillet, season lightly with salt, and sauté until just barely cooked—they will be pink and curled—about 2 minutes. Transfer to a separate bowl.

3 Add the onion and bell pepper to the skillet, along with more oil, as needed. Cook, stirring occasionally, until soft, about 5 minutes. Stir in the quinoa, garlic, smoked paprika, turmeric, red pepper flakes, and **1 teaspoon salt**. Sauté until the spices are fragrant and the quinoa is coated well, 2 minutes. Fold in the greens and cook until they are wilted, about 3 minutes.

recipe continues →

4 Stir in the tomatoes with their juices, scraping up any browned bits from the bottom of the skillet. Spread the quinoa mixture into an even layer. Arrange the sausage on top and cover with the stock. Bring to a boil over high heat, then reduce the heat to medium-low and simmer, uncovered, for 15 minutes. Give the top layer of grains a quick stir to redistribute, then spread into an even layer again. Cook for 10 minutes, undisturbed, until the quinoa is pearly and the edges have crisped.

5 Arrange the shrimp on top of the paella and continue to cook, uncovered, until most of the liquid has evaporated, the grains are al dente, and the shrimp are heated through, about 3 minutes.

6 Off the heat, squeeze a lemon half over the shrimp. I like to do this over my opposite hand, letting the juice slip through my fingers, but catching the seeds. Taste for seasoning, and add more salt, as needed.

7 Cut the remaining lemon half into 4 wedges. Garnish with parsley, and serve with the lemon wedges on the side.

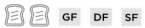

GF   DF   SF

LF omit sausage, onion, and garlic; use LF stock   **Vgt** **V** omit sausage and shrimp

Carbivore

152

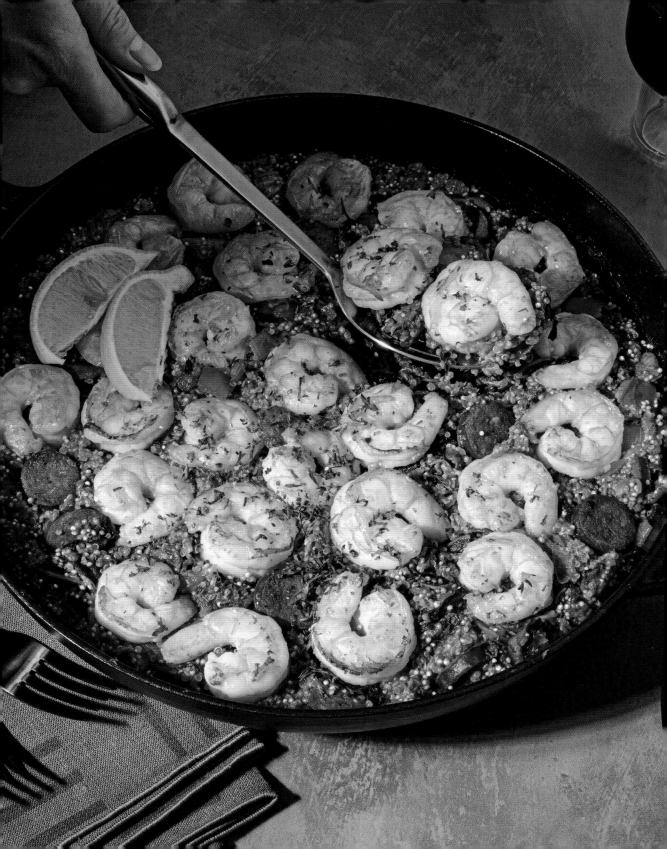

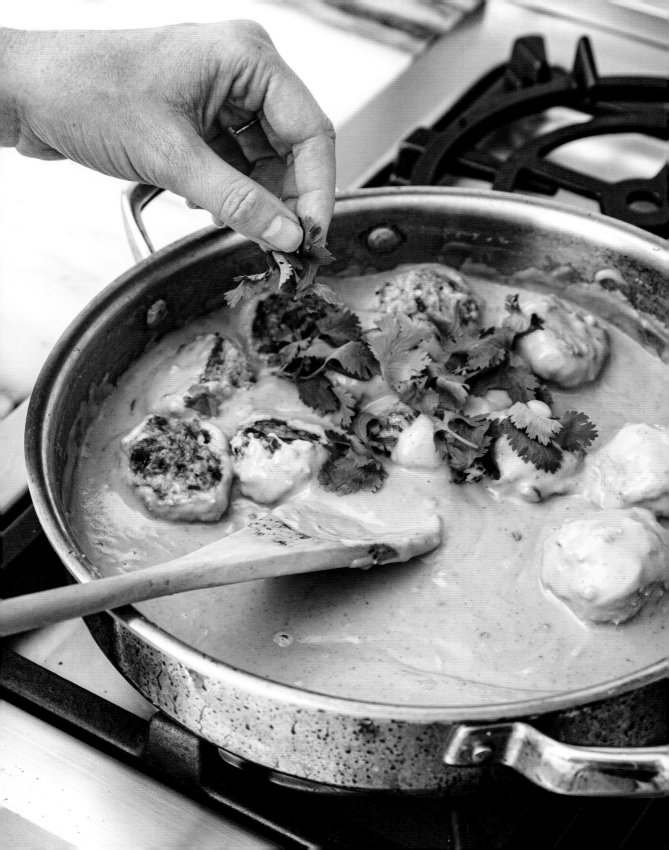

Chicken Satay Meatballs

Satay (or sate, depending on where you are) is a ubiquitous street food in Southeast Asia, particularly Indonesia, Singapore, and Thailand. It usually consists of sliced or cubed meat strung onto skewers, marinated in turmeric, and served with peanut sauce. In this recipe, we skip the skewers and, instead, pack all those signature flavors into chicken meatballs. My binder of choice here is quinoa flakes, which you can find in the breakfast aisle of the supermarket near the oatmeal. They melt into the background more quickly than oats and are healthier on the carb front than breadcrumbs, but you could substitute either in a pinch. I usually serve these balls as a main course but you can roll them smaller for a party appetizer with the sauce on the side for dipping, if your goal is no skewer left behind.

*MAKE IT A MEAL: Serve alongside **Braised Coconut-Lime Sweet Potatoes & Bok Choy** (page 226) or **Minty Green Rice Pilaf with Chiles & Peanuts** (page 134), or **Peanut & Lime Slaw** (page 83).*

MAKES 4 SERVINGS

Meatballs

1 ½ pounds ground chicken (preferably dark meat)

¾ cup quinoa flakes (see headnote)

½ cup finely chopped fresh cilantro leaves, plus more for garnish

2 garlic cloves, minced

1 large egg, beaten

1 teaspoon sea salt

1 teaspoon ground coriander

1 teaspoon ground turmeric

½ teaspoon ground ginger

¼ teaspoon cayenne pepper

Sauce

Avocado oil

2 tablespoons finely chopped fresh ginger

1 serrano chile, thinly sliced

One 13.5-ounce can full-fat coconut milk

½ cup chicken stock or water

½ cup creamy peanut butter

2 tablespoons fish sauce

2 tablespoons fresh lime juice

1 tablespoon maple syrup

½ teaspoon sea salt

① Preheat the oven to 400°F. Line a baking sheet with parchment paper.

② **Make the meatballs:** In a large bowl, combine the ground chicken, quinoa flakes, cilantro, garlic, egg, salt, coriander, turmeric, ground ginger, and cayenne. With clean hands (wet or grease them, as the mixture is sticky!), mix the ingredients until loosely combined. You don't want to overly break up the meat. Form the mixture into 2-inch balls (an ice-cream scoop works well for portioning), and roll in your hands until round and smooth. You should have about 16 balls. Arrange the balls on the prepared baking sheet. Bake for about 20 minutes until the bottoms are lightly browned but the tops aren't overly crispy.

recipe continues →

③ **Make the sauce:** While the balls bake, place a large heavy skillet over medium-high heat and coat it with a thin layer (about ⅛ inch) of oil. Add the fresh ginger and chile to the pan. Sauté for 1 minute until fragrant. Pour in the coconut milk and stock and bring to a simmer, scraping up any browned bits from the bottom of the skillet. Whisk in the peanut butter, fish sauce, lime juice, maple syrup, and salt until smooth. Simmer gently for about 5 minutes until the sauce has reduced enough to coat the back of a spoon.

④ Transfer the baked meatballs to the sauce and toss to coat. Cook for 2 minutes in the sauce, until the balls are heated through.

⑤ Garnish with a handful of torn cilantro leaves and enjoy warm.

GF   DF

LF omit garlic; reduce coconut milk to 1 cup   SF omit maple syrup

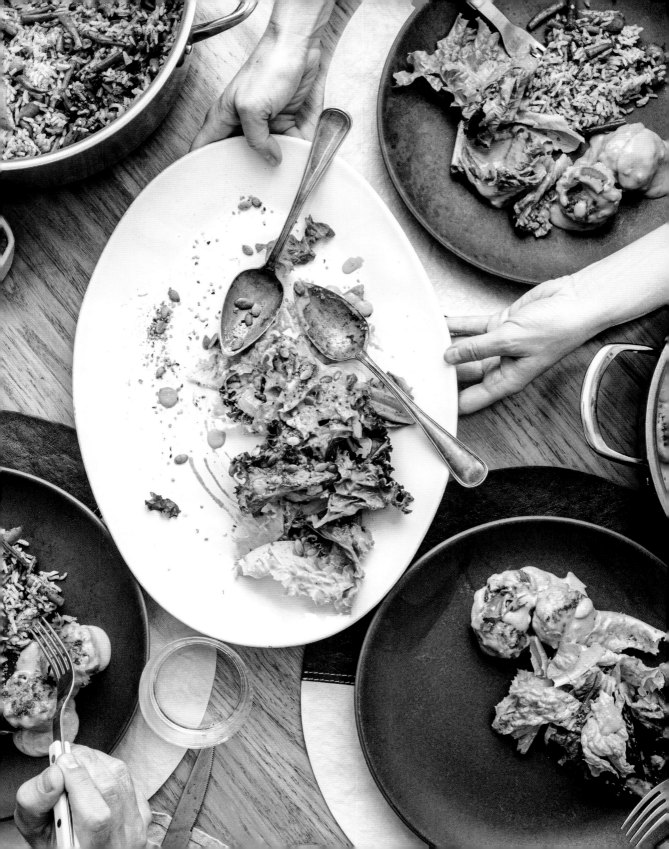

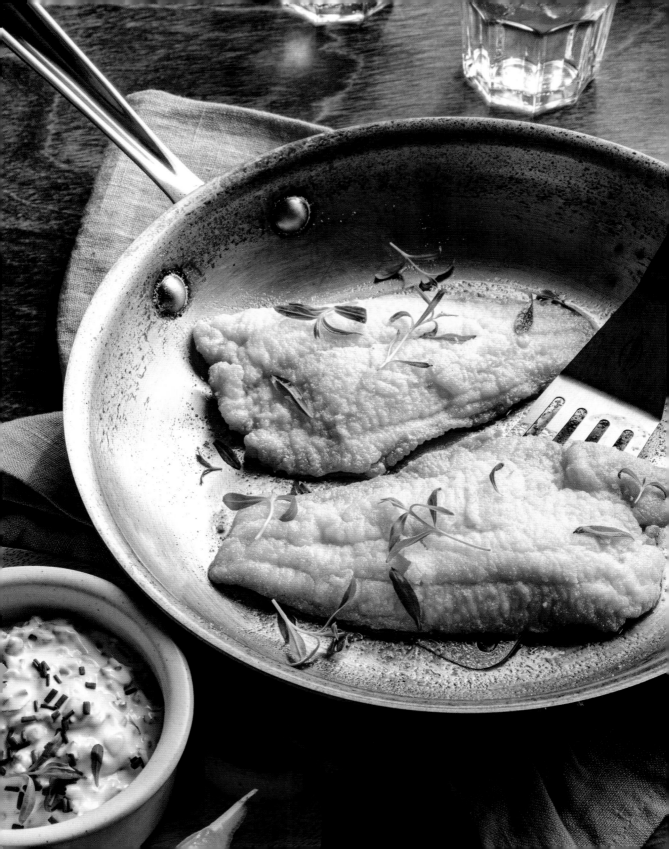

Mom's Millet Flour Fish Fry with Tarragon-Chive Tartar Sauce

One of the dishes I grew up eating every summer is pan-fried yellowtail flounder. My mother, who was gluten-free long before it was cool or even a well-known dietary restriction, discovered that millet flour's sandy texture is perfect for dredging fish and crisping it until golden brown and begging for tartar sauce. The secret here is using the thinnest, smallest fish fillets possible. The little yellowtail flounder found in most fish shops across New England is particularly cut out for the job, as the fillets maximize the crispy-coating-to-tender-fish ratio and cook in a matter of seconds. If you can't find them, go with whatever looks thin and delicate at the fish market, like sole, catfish, or fluke (tilapia is too meaty). If your fish is thicker and has a higher water content, you might end up with slightly soggier results—but nothing that a giant dollop of herby tartar sauce can't fix.

MAKES 4 SERVINGS

1 ½ cups millet flour

2 pounds flounder, sole, or the smallest, thinnest white fish fillets you can find

Avocado oil

Sea salt

1 lemon, cut into wedges

Tarragon-Chive Tartar Sauce (page 69)

❶ Put the millet flour on a large plate. Rinse the fish and place the clean fillets on a second plate. Line a third plate with paper towels and set aside.

❷ Place a large heavy-bottomed skillet over medium-high heat until just shy of smoking, then add a thin layer (about ⅛ inch) of oil.

❸ Working in batches, dredge the fillets in the flour until well coated, shaking off any excess, and place the fish in the hot oil, making sure not to crowd the pan. Pan-fry until golden brown, about 2 minutes per side. It's easiest to flip the fish with two flat spatulas. Transfer the cooked fish to the paper towel–lined plate and repeat with the remaining fillets, adding more oil, as needed.

❹ Season the crispy fish with salt (if you do this before frying, the salt will draw out the fish's moisture and the fish will become soggy!). Serve with the lemon wedges and **Tarragon-Chive Tartar Sauce.**

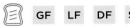

GF LF DF SF

Turmeric-Pumpkin Fall Reset Soup

One of the hardest lines to walk for Carbivores with gut issues is making sure you get your fiber without it wreaking havoc on your digestive system. I started creating these "reset soups" as a solution for days when your gut needs a little downtime. This version has lots of finely chopped low-FODMAP vegetables (carrots, parsnips, broccoli) and hearty quinoa, cooked until soft and easier to assimilate. There's no garlic or onion, but you are welcome to add them along with hot sauce or red pepper flakes if your gut can handle it. You can also swap in any fall veggies you like—turnips and butternut squash work well—and frozen chopped kale or leafy greens can stand in for the broccoli. Finally, toss in some shredded rotisserie chicken if you want more protein. Thanks to the anti-inflammatory turmeric and ginger, this soups get tastier after a day or two in the fridge (and it freezes well).

CARB SWAP: Sub white rice for quinoa if that's easier on your digestion, or chickpeas for more fiber.

MAKES 6 APPETIZER SERVINGS

- 2 tablespoons coconut oil or grass-fed ghee
- 4 medium carrots (8 ounces), unpeeled, finely diced
- 2 medium parsnips (8 ounces), peeled, finely diced
- ½ cup uncooked quinoa
- 2 tablespoons minced fresh ginger
- 2 teaspoons ground turmeric
- 1 teaspoon sea salt
- ¼ teaspoon freshly ground black pepper
- 6 cups vegetable or chicken stock
- One 13.5-ounce can full-fat coconut milk
- 1 ½ cups unsweetened pumpkin puree (from one 15-ounce can)
- 3 cups finely chopped broccoli florets (from 1 medium crown)
- 2 tablespoons fresh lime juice
- ¼ cup roughly chopped fresh cilantro

❶ In a large stockpot or Dutch oven, heat the coconut oil over a medium flame. Sauté the carrots and parsnips until they begin to lightly brown, about 5 minutes. Stir in the quinoa, ginger, turmeric, salt, and pepper. Cook, stirring, until the quinoa is coated well in the spice mixture and the ginger is quite fragrant, about 2 minutes. Add the stock, coconut milk, and pumpkin puree to the pot; stir until smooth. Bring to a boil over high heat, then reduce the heat to medium-low and simmer, uncovered, until the quinoa is pearly and plump, about 15 minutes. Stir in the broccoli and simmer for 3 minutes, or until al dente.

❷ Off the heat, stir in the lime juice and taste for seasoning, adding more salt, as needed. Ladle the soup into bowls and garnish with cilantro to serve.

GF DF Vgt V SF

LF reduce coconut milk to 1 cup **P** omit quinoa

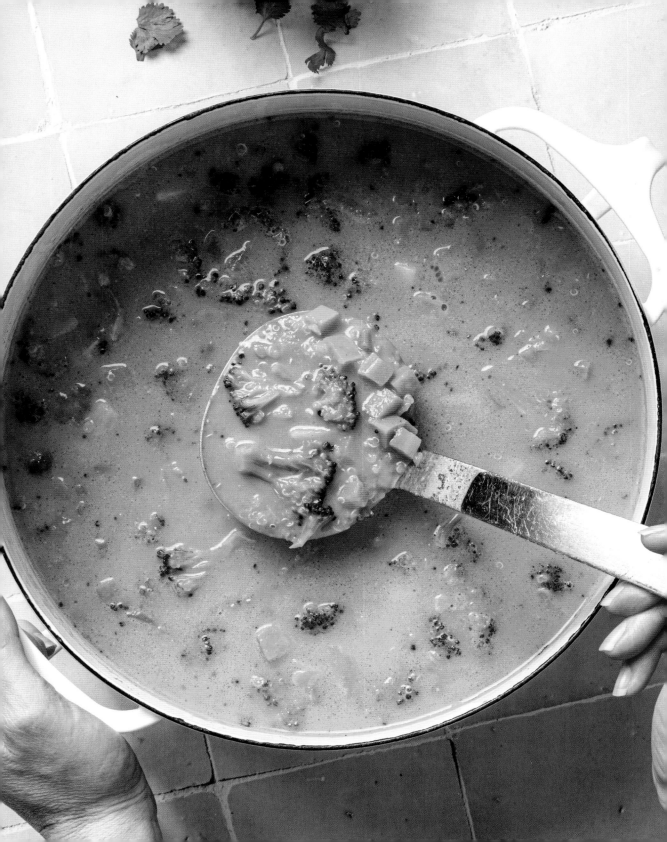

Kasha Pilaf with Mushrooms, Bacon & Greens

Buckwheat groats (or kasha, as it's called when roasted) are one of the most underrated pseudograins—trust me on this! In pilafs, the grains maintain their chewiness after being cooked low and slow with mushrooms and greens. Kasha is widely eaten for breakfast in many Eastern European countries, but it also works for a side dish or cozy dinner.

CARB COMPANIONS: Add a fried egg on top and/or some plain full-fat yogurt.

MAKES 4 SERVINGS

1	cup kasha (roasted buckwheat groats)
4	sugar- and nitrate-free uncured bacon slices
1	shallot, thinly sliced
12	ounces cremini mushrooms, stemmed and sliced
1	bunch Swiss chard, stems and leaves separated, thinly sliced
1	tablespoon extra-virgin olive oil
1	teaspoon sea salt
2	tablespoons chopped fresh dill

1 In a dry medium Dutch oven or lidded saucepan, toast the kasha over medium heat until slightly darker in hue and nutty smelling, 3 to 5 minutes. Transfer to a bowl and set aside. Wipe out the pot if there's any residue.

2 Return the pot to the heat and add the bacon. Cook until the fat has rendered and the bacon is crispy on both sides, about 4 minutes. Using tongs, transfer the bacon to a paper towel–lined plate. When cool enough to touch, roughly chop or crumble the bacon into bite-size pieces.

3 Pour out all but 2 tablespoons of the bacon fat from the pot. Add the shallot, mushrooms, and chard stems. Sauté until the mushrooms are glossy and browned, 5 minutes. Fold in the chard leaves and cook for 1 minute more, until wilted.

4 Stir in the toasted kasha, oil, and salt, stirring until the grains are coated well in the vegetable mixture. Add **2 cups water**, scraping up any browned bits from the bottom of the pan, and bring to a boil. Reduce the heat to low and cook, covered, for about 20 minutes, until the liquid is absorbed and the kasha is tender. Remove from the heat and let rest for 10 minutes.

5 To serve, divide the kasha among four bowls and garnish with the crispy bacon and dill.

 GF **DF** **SF**

LF omit mushrooms and shallot   **Vgt** **V** omit bacon

Ratatouille Quinoa Bake

In case your Pixar trivia is a little rusty, ratatouille is a French dish made from summer vegetables like zucchini, eggplant, bell peppers, and tomatoes. These luscious vegetables simmer together until they nearly fall apart and brim with caramelized flavor. In this quinoa bake, we start the ratatouille on the stovetop and, good news for your knife work: the vegetables get added sequentially so you can chop as you go, even without the help of a small furry sous chef. After that, the vegetables stew with the quinoa, releasing lots of wonderful juices that are absorbed by the grains. Quinoa bakes are most delicious with melted cheese on top. I've opted for a scant amount, but you can double or omit it, depending on how the healthy hedonism scales are falling.

CARB SWAP: Sub Arborio rice for quinoa—it works great in most casseroles.

MAKES 4 SERVINGS

¼ cup extra-virgin olive oil

2 medium shallots, thinly sliced

1 red or orange bell pepper, finely diced

1 small eggplant (8 ounces), diced

1 medium zucchini (8 ounces), diced

1 medium summer squash (8 ounces), diced

2 garlic cloves, minced

1 teaspoon sea salt

½ teaspoon red pepper flakes

1 cup uncooked quinoa

2 cups diced plum or Roma tomatoes, or one 15-ounce can diced tomatoes

2 cups vegetable stock or water

¼ cup roughly chopped fresh basil leaves, divided

1 cup shredded mozzarella or Gruyère cheese

1 Preheat the oven to 400°F.

2 In a large ovenproof skillet, heat the oil over a medium-high flame. Sauté the shallots and bell pepper until soft, about 5 minutes. Stir in the eggplant and continue to cook, stirring occasionally, until glossy and no longer opaque, 5 minutes. Stir in the zucchini, summer squash, garlic, salt, and red pepper flakes. Cook until the garlic is quite fragrant, 2 minutes. Fold in the quinoa and the tomatoes with their juices, pour in the stock, and bring to a simmer over high heat. Once the casserole is bubbling, sprinkle in half the basil and transfer to the oven.

3 Bake the casserole for 25 minutes until most of the liquid is absorbed. Remove from the oven and fluff the quinoa with a fork so some of the crispy grains on top are reincorporated. Smooth into an even layer and sprinkle the cheese on top. Continue to bake until the cheese is lightly browned and the sides develop a crust, 5 to 10 minutes.

4 Garnish with the remaining basil and serve directly from the skillet.

   GF   Vgt   SF

LF omit shallot and garlic; reduce cheese to ½ cup   **DF**   **V** omit cheese

Black Sesame–Buckwheat Banana Bread

I learned from Ashlae Warner of the blog *Oh, Lady Cakes* that the trick to the best banana bread is to use completely blackened (borderline rotten) bananas. This maximizes the natural sugars and ensures that the banana almost becomes a puree upon mashing. Both buckwheat flour and black sesame seeds are wonderfully earthy. This bread gets double-duty sesame from the tahini, while the seeds spread throughout help keep the fiber content high. (If you can't find black sesame seeds, white will work fine, as will poppy seeds in a pinch!) For more of a dessert bread, add chocolate chunks to the finished batter and flaky sea salt on top. Since it's such a moist quick bread, refrigerate any leftovers in an airtight container to help it keep for up to a week.

CARB COMPANIONS: Enjoy a slice toasted with a slather of nut butter, coconut butter, or more tahini.

MAKES 1 LOAF

1 ¾ cups mashed banana (from 4 large, very ripe bananas)

3 large eggs, at room temperature

¼ cup tahini

¼ cup extra-virgin olive, avocado oil, or melted coconut oil

3 tablespoons maple syrup or honey

2 teaspoons vanilla extract

½ cup oat flour or other neutral gluten-free flour

⅓ cup buckwheat flour

¼ cup black sesame seeds, plus 1 teaspoon, divided

1 teaspoon baking soda

1 teaspoon ground cinnamon

½ teaspoon sea salt

❶ Preheat the oven to 350°F. Line a loaf pan with two strips of parchment paper, one widthwise and one lengthwise.

❷ In a large bowl, combine the banana, eggs, tahini, oil, maple syrup, and vanilla and mix by hand until smooth. Stir in the oat flour, buckwheat flour, **¼ cup sesame seeds**, baking soda, cinnamon, and salt until the flour is just incorporated (a few swirls of flour is better than overmixing the batter). Transfer to the prepared pan and smooth the top. Sprinkle the loaf with the remaining **1 teaspoon sesame seeds**.

❸ Bake for 45 minutes to 1 hour until the top is nicely browned and cracked like a brownie and a toothpick or knife inserted into the center comes out clean.

❹ Let rest in the pan until cool enough to touch, about 15 minutes, then slice and enjoy.

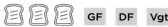

GF DF Vgt

LF use maple syrup; safe serving is 1 slice (about one-ninth of the loaf)

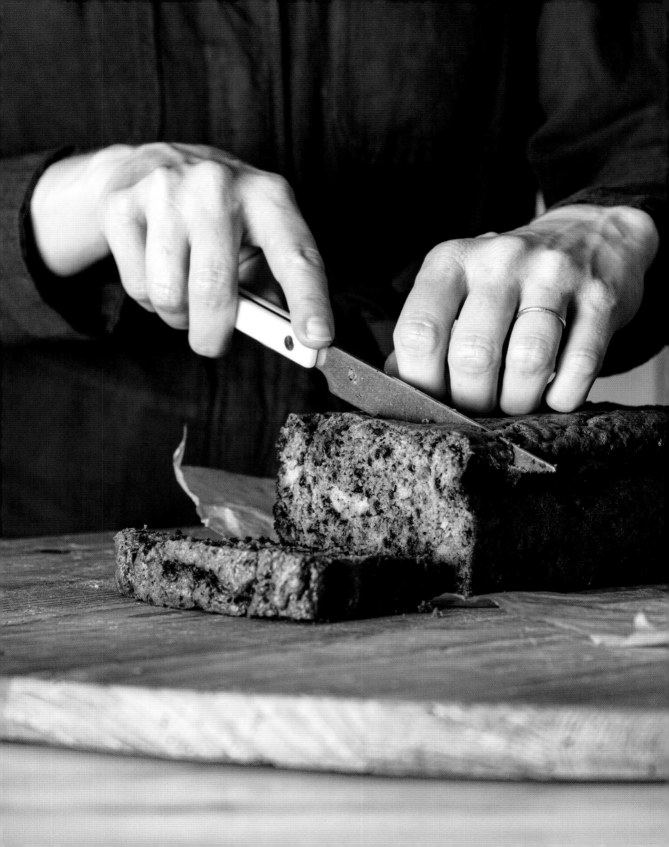

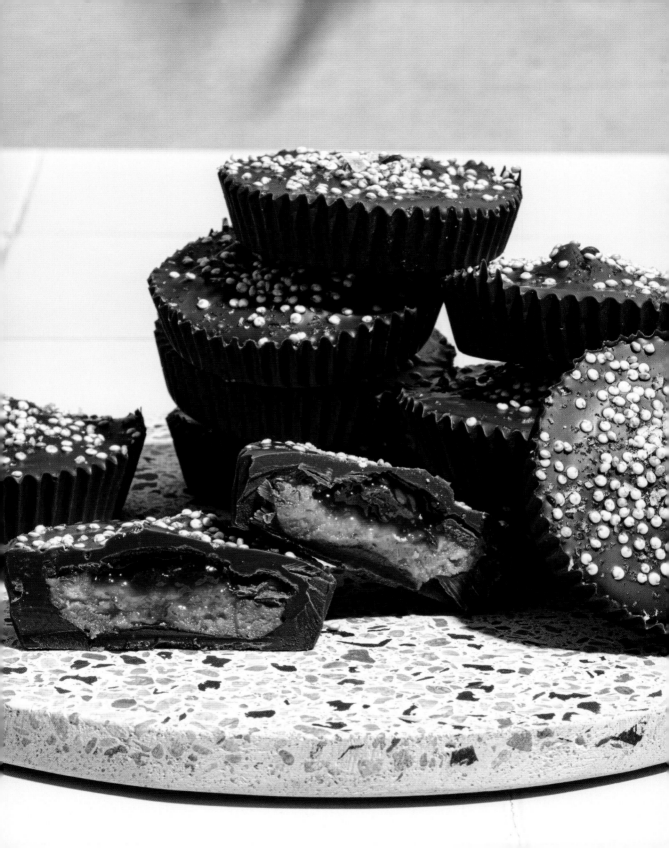

PB & J Cups with Crunchy Quinoa

My husband and I have a bit of an obsession with Hu Kitchen chocolate, particularly their cashew butter and raspberry bar. It is second only to our love of Justin's almond butter cups with puffed quinoa—which is how this candy aisle love child was born. Making chocolates at home can be equal parts fun and messy, but the pros outweigh the cons, especially when you get to control exactly what goes into them. I recommend starting with a good quality dark chocolate (at least 70 percent cacao) that's low in sugar. To add extra fiber, I use my **Raspberry-Chia Jam** (page 73). You can always cut a corner with store-bought, but be aware of the amount of sugar that will be added to your treats. Lastly, the "puffed" quinoa is a wonderful way to add texture and an extra carb companion to your candy. Just FYI, the quinoa will be toastier and crunchier than store-bought "puffed" options when using the at-home method.

MAKES 12 CUPS

⅓ cup **Raspberry-Chia Jam** (page 73) or store-bought raspberry jam

¼ cup uncooked quinoa

9 ounces dark chocolate chips (about 1 ½ cups) or roughly chopped baking chocolate (see headnote)

⅓ cup smooth peanut butter

3 tablespoons unsweetened nondairy milk

½ teaspoon coarse sea salt

❶ Make the **Raspberry-Chia Jam**, if not using store-bought. Set aside in the fridge to cool.

❷ Line a standard cupcake or muffin tin with paper liners. Clear enough space in the refrigerator to fit the pan.

❸ Place a large shallow saucepan over medium heat. Once quite hot (water droplets should sizzle), add the quinoa to the hot pan in an even layer. It should start to pop immediately, like popcorn. Cook, shaking the pan every 30 seconds to redistribute, and adjusting the heat if the quinoa begins to darken too quickly, until the popping slows, about 3 minutes. Transfer the quinoa to a bowl.

❹ In a heatproof microwave-safe bowl, melt the chocolate in a microwave in 30-second intervals, or place the bowl over a gently simmering pot of water on the stove, stirring occasionally.

❺ Place a scant 1 tablespoon of chocolate in the center of each liner. Using a spoon, in a swirling motion from the center, encourage the chocolate to spread evenly across the bottom, trying to get it as thin as possible. Then, with the side of your spoon, push the chocolate

recipe continues →

¼ inch up the sides of the liners. You want to have a hollow chocolate cup to hold the filling. Refrigerate the tin for at least 10 minutes, or until the chocolate is firm. Reserve the remaining chocolate.

6 In a small bowl, whisk the peanut butter and nondairy milk until completely smooth and pliable.

7 Remove the tin from the refrigerator. Place 1 heaping teaspoon of the peanut butter mixture in the center of the chocolate cups, flattening it as best you can, followed by 1 scant teaspoon of jam, keeping it in the center.

8 Reheat the remaining melted chocolate for 15 seconds if it's firmed up (you want it very runny), and add another tablespoon to the center of each cup so it completely covers the filling. Use your spoon to nudge the chocolate to spill into the corners, being careful not to expose the jam beneath the surface (if you do, don't worry, you'll cover any mistakes in the next step).

9 Top the cups with a sprinkle of puffed quinoa and coarse sea salt. It will look almost like a quinoa nonpareil!

10 Return the tin to the refrigerator until firm, about 10 minutes more. Remove the PB & J cups from the pan, in their liners, and refrigerate in an airtight container for up to 2 weeks.

GF LF DF Vgt V   P omit quinoa

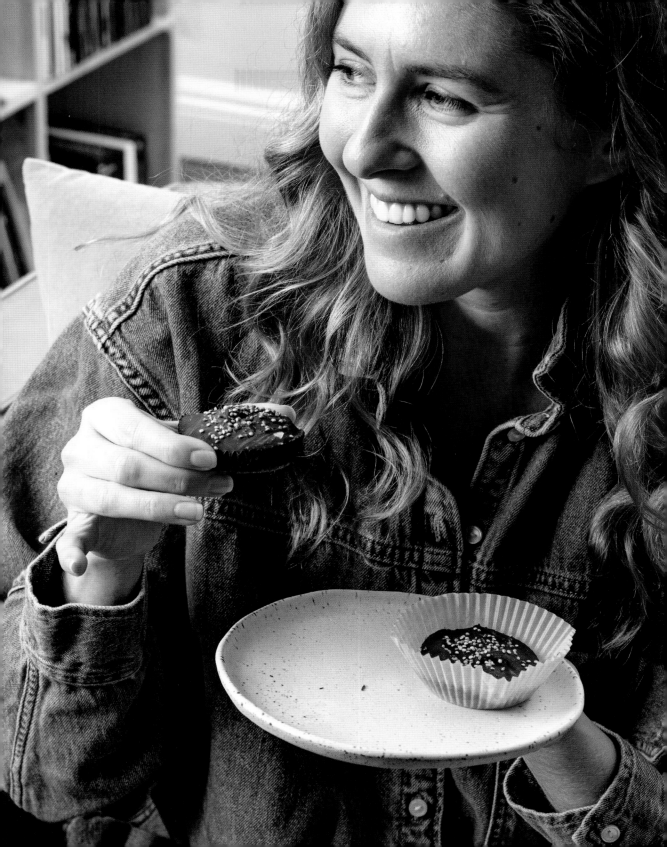

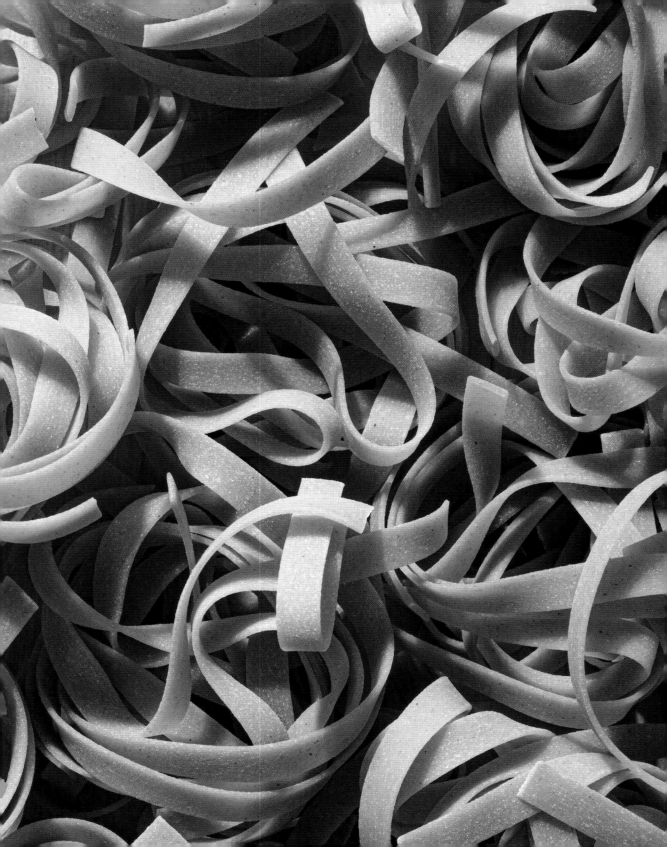

NOODLES

· · ·

Spinach-Artichoke Dip Mac & Cheese

Inside-Out Egg Roll Noodles

Cod & Orzo Arrabbiata

Green Curry Ramen with Eggplant & Green Beans

Creamy Sesame Noodle Salad with Smashed Cucumbers

Spaghetti with Harissa Bolognese & Mint-Almond Gremolata

Salmon & Broccoli Noodle Casserole

Eggs Mimosa Pasta Salad with Crispy Prosciutto,
Asparagus & Piles of Herbs

Linguine with Chorizo, Clams & Kale

Ginger-Scallion Chicken Soba Noodle Soup

Grilled Skirt Steak & Vermicelli Bowls with Nuoc Cham

Spanakopita Lasagna

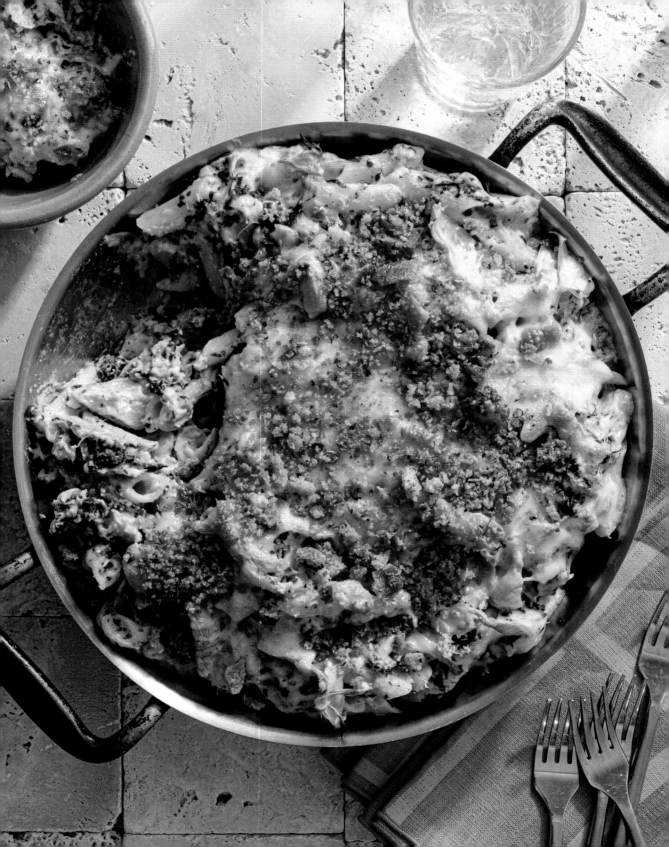

Spinach-Artichoke Dip Mac & Cheese

My upbringing was heavy on the millet, light on the fast food. Being an East Coast kid, California Pizza Kitchen was among the most mythic of these forbidden establishments. When I finally went as an adult, I fell hard and fast for the thick and creamy spinach-artichoke dip. Here, I've used it as inspiration for a mac and cheese, going heavier on the veggies. Artichokes are one of the most fiber-rich plants around, as evidenced by their stringy, woody leaves. If you'd rather not chew your way through that in a baked pasta, puree the artichokes like you would in a dip. To streamline prep, start by pulsing the parmesan, then the breadcrumbs, and finally the artichokes. Feel free to use more cheese than I've called for, or substitute a plant-based alternative to make this vegan.

MAKES 6 SERVINGS

Sea salt

12 ounces gluten-free penne, fusilli, or elbow pasta

1 pound frozen chopped spinach (about 6 cups), thawed

4 tablespoons extra-virgin olive oil or unsalted butter

1 medium shallot, sliced

2 garlic cloves, minced

2 teaspoons paprika

¼ teaspoon cayenne pepper (optional)

¼ cup all-purpose gluten-free or white rice flour

4 cups whole milk or unsweetened almond milk

Two 14-ounce cans artichoke hearts, rinsed, drained, and finely chopped

1 ½ cups (6 ounces) shredded sharp white cheddar cheese, divided

⅓ cup finely grated parmesan cheese, divided

¾ cup fresh gluten-free breadcrumbs

❶ Preheat the oven to 400°F.

❷ Bring a large pot of salted water to a boil over high heat. Add the pasta and cook for half the time specified on the package directions. The noodles should still have a bite to them and not be fully edible yet. Drain thoroughly and set aside.

❸ Working over the sink, gather the thawed spinach in a clean kitchen towel and squeeze until all the moisture is released. You should be left with a baseball-size wad of dry spinach. Set aside.

❹ In a large (15-inch) ovenproof skillet, heat the oil over a medium-high flame. Sauté the shallot, garlic, paprika, and cayenne pepper (if using) until soft, 3 minutes. Sprinkle in the flour and stir to coat. Cook for 1 minute, then whisk in the milk until smooth. Bring to a simmer and cook, whisking frequently, until thickened enough to coat the back of a spoon, about 4 minutes.

Noodles

5 Off the heat, whisk in **1 ½ teaspoons salt,** spinach, and artichokes. Fold in the cooked pasta, **1 cup cheddar,** and half the parmesan. (Alternatively, if you don't have a big enough skillet to hold everything, transfer the ingredients to a 9 × 13-inch casserole dish.) Spread the pasta mixture in an even layer and top with the remaining cheddar and parmesan. In a small bowl, toss the breadcrumbs with a drizzle of oil and scatter over the cheese.

6 Bake until lightly browned and bubbling, about 15 minutes. Let stand in the skillet for a few minutes until solidified, then serve.

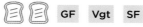

GF   **Vgt**   **SF**

LF   use nondairy milk; omit artichokes, garlic, and shallot

DF   **V**   use nondairy milk and cheese

Inside-Out Egg Roll Noodles

Some of my best recipes have been a product of my first failed idea (see: *SIBO Made Simple* Beef Negimaki Stir-Fry). In this case, I was hard at work on an egg roll recipe, when I realized my gluten-free work-around was not cutting it. So, I threw the filling into a pan and stir-fried it with the dipping sauce and some noodles. The result was double the deliciousness without all the trouble. To save even more time, use a food processor to shred the vegetables. Though pork is most traditional, these noodles also taste terrific with ground chicken or turkey—or even chopped shrimp, smoked tofu, or mushrooms, for the veg heads.

CARB COMPANIONS: Instead of raw cashews, use the **Tangy Peanut-Cashew Crunch** *(76) for garnish and skip step 4.*

MAKES 4 SERVINGS

Sea salt

2 medium carrots

1 red bell pepper

½ small head (8 ounces) green or napa cabbage

2 tablespoons minced or grated fresh ginger

6 scallions, thinly sliced, white and green parts separated

¼ cup gluten-free tamari or soy sauce

2 tablespoons rice vinegar

1 tablespoon toasted sesame oil

2 teaspoons sesame seeds

1 teaspoon maple syrup or honey

1 teaspoon sriracha or ½ teaspoon red pepper flakes

Avocado oil or coconut oil

½ cup raw cashews, roughly chopped

1 pound ground pork, chicken, or dark-meat turkey

8 to 10 ounces flat stir-fry or pad Thai rice noodles

① Bring a large pot of salted water to a boil over high heat.

② Meanwhile, finely chop the carrots, bell pepper, and cabbage—or pulse in a food processor until shredded (this is more efficient!). Set aside with the minced ginger and white scallions.

③ In a small bowl, whisk together the tamari, vinegar, sesame oil, sesame seeds, maple syrup, and sriracha.

④ In a large nonstick or cast-iron skillet, heat **1 tablespoon avocado oil** over medium heat. Add the cashews and toast, stirring occasionally, until lightly browned and very fragrant, about 3 minutes. Transfer to a bowl and season lightly with salt.

recipe continues →

175

Noodles

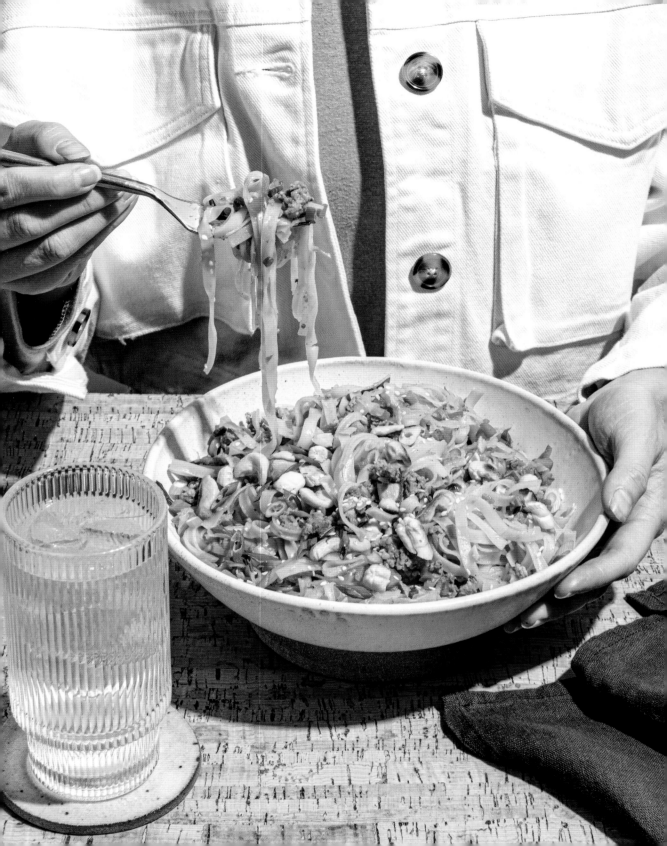

⑤ Raise the heat to medium-high and add the carrots, bell pepper, cabbage, ginger, white scallions, and another **1 tablespoon avocado oil** to the skillet. Sauté until the vegetables are soft and beginning to caramelize, about 7 minutes.

⑥ Push the veggies to the side of the skillet and add the ground pork. Press the meat down into a thin layer and season with salt. Cook, undisturbed, until a brown crust forms on the bottom, about 5 minutes. Break the meat into chunks with a spatula and stir to incorporate with the veggies. Continue cooking, stirring occasionally, until the pork is cooked through, about 2 minutes more.

⑦ While the meat cooks, prepare the noodles according to the package directions. Drain and add to the skillet with the meat and veggies.

⑧ Drizzle the sauce over the noodles and add half the green scallions. Toss everything together a few times until incorporated.

⑨ Garnish with the remaining green scallions and the cashews.

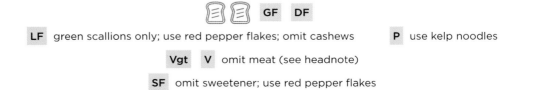

GF   DF

LF   green scallions only; use red pepper flakes; omit cashews   P   use kelp noodles

Vgt   V   omit meat (see headnote)

SF   omit sweetener; use red pepper flakes

Noodles

Cod & Orzo Arrabbiata

I have a bit of an obsession with Rao's jarred arrabbiata sauce. It's loaded with just enough red pepper flakes to make the tomato sauce feel angry, per its Italian name, but not so many that my tummy is too. Here, my homemade version works together with orzo, sturdy chard leaves, and flaky cod loin to create an ultra-flavorful Italian-ish one-pan meal. Cod, like most white fish, is on the mild side, but this makes it a perfect canvas for "big sauces." If you can't find cod, hake, haddock, or halibut will work. You want thicker fillets so they can nestle in the tomato sauce without taking up the entire surface area of the pan. Chard is the fiber all-star here, but you can use any leafy green (kale, collards, spinach, etc.). Broccoli rabe or broccolini, cut into 1-inch pieces, would also pair nicely with the fiery sauce. Lastly, if you need a carb swap, use long-grain white rice instead of the orzo.

MAKES 4 SERVINGS

- 2 tablespoons extra-virgin olive oil
- ½ medium yellow onion, finely diced
- 1 bunch Swiss chard, stems and leaves separated, thinly sliced
- 2 garlic cloves, minced
- ½ teaspoon red pepper flakes
- One 28-ounce can crushed tomatoes
- 1¼ cups gluten-free orzo
  Sea salt
- 2 cups fish or vegetable stock, or water
- 1½ pounds cod loin, skin removed, cut into 4 equal fillets
- ½ lemon
- ⅓ cup loosely packed fresh basil leaves, torn

1 Preheat the oven to 425°F.

2 In a large ovenproof skillet or saucepan, heat the oil over a medium-high flame. Add the onion, chard stems, garlic, and red pepper flakes to the skillet. Sauté until the onion is translucent, about 7 minutes. Fold in the chard leaves and cook for 2 minutes until wilted.

3 Carefully stir in the tomatoes, followed by the orzo and ¾ teaspoon salt. Once combined, pour in the stock, raise the heat to high, and bring to a boil. Reduce the heat to maintain a simmer and cook, uncovered, stirring frequently to keep the orzo from sticking, until the pasta has plumped but isn't fully cooked through, about 7 minutes. Off the heat, nestle the fillets into the orzo so they are partially submerged. Season the fish generously with salt.

4 Transfer the pan to the oven and bake until the fish is fork-tender and the orzo is al dente, about 10 minutes. Remove from the oven and squeeze the lemon half over the fish, using your opposite hand to catch any seeds.

5 Serve directly in the skillet, garnished with the torn basil and more red pepper flakes, if desired.

GF DF SF

LF sub 2 diced carrots for onion; omit garlic; use water   Vgt V omit fish

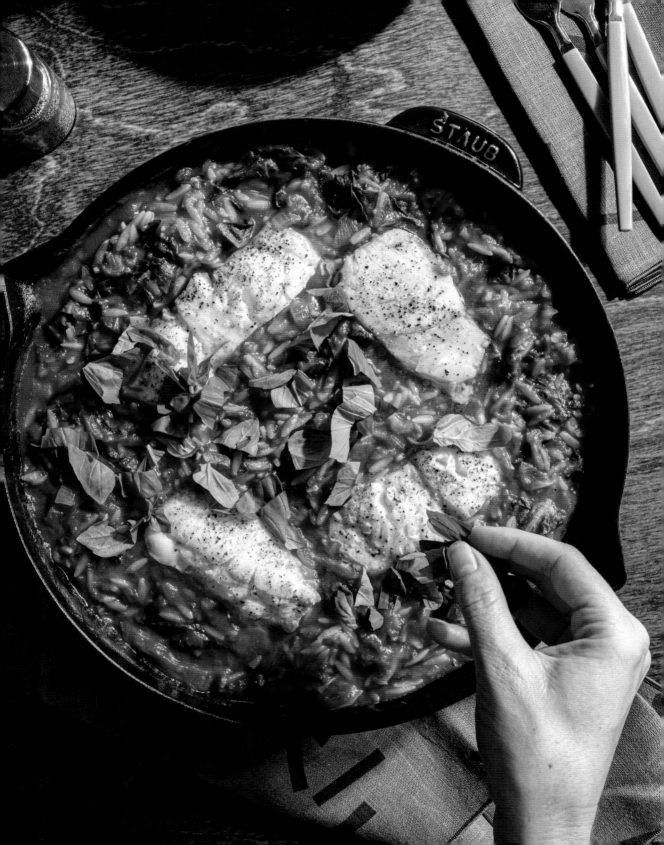

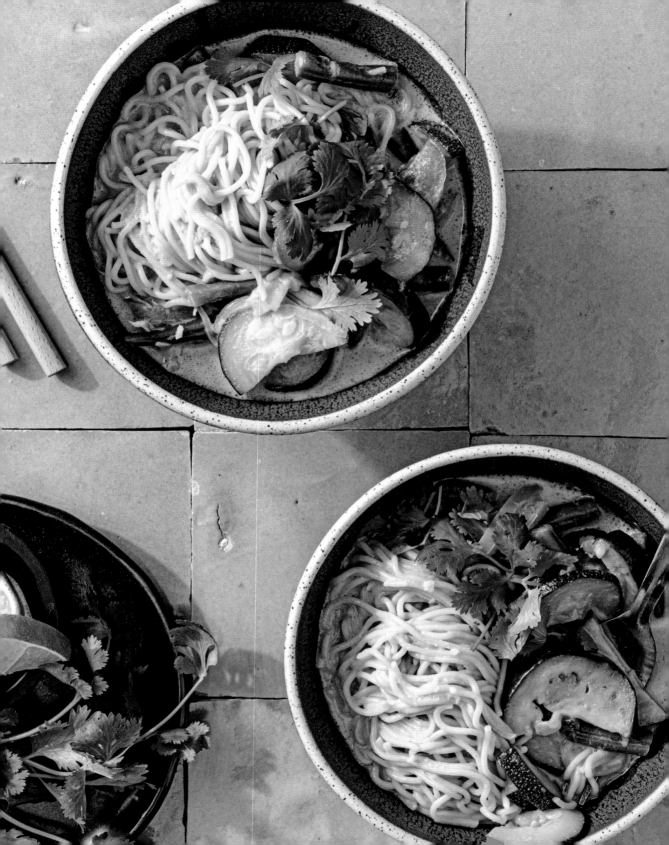

Green Curry Ramen with Eggplant & Green Beans

During COVID lockdown, when we'd be at the end of our grocery haul and out of fresh produce, we'd reach for this weeknight dish. All you need for the base is pantry items—brown rice ramen noodles, coconut milk, curry paste, and frozen vegetables. It became such a comfort staple that we still have it in our rotation. To keep with the current times, this recipe has been altered to use fresh vegetables typically found in a Thai green curry: eggplant, green beans, and bell peppers. To save on dishes, the noodles cook directly in the liquid, helping thicken the sauce to the consistency of a creamy curry—less brothy than a noodle soup, but still something that can be eaten with both chopsticks and a spoon. The most important element of this recipe is to use a pasta that cooks fairly quickly (under 5 minutes). I love Lotus Foods Millet & Brown Rice Ramen for this.

CARB COMPANIONS: For additional veg, fresh or frozen broccoli, cabbage, and kale all work well.

MAKES 4 SERVINGS

2   tablespoons avocado oil or coconut oil

1   large shallot, thinly sliced

1   green bell pepper, thinly sliced

2   tablespoons minced fresh ginger

3   tablespoons green curry paste

1   small eggplant (8 ounces), halved lengthwise and thinly sliced into half-moons

1   medium zucchini (8 ounces), halved lengthwise and thinly sliced into half-moons

8   ounces green beans, cut into 1-inch pieces

One 13.5-ounce can full-fat coconut milk

3   cups vegetable or chicken stock

1   teaspoon sea salt

5 to 6 ounces brown rice ramen or pad Thai noodles (see headnote)

2   tablespoons fresh lime juice (from 1 or 2 limes)

¼   cup chopped fresh cilantro leaves

❶ In a large Dutch oven or stockpot, heat the oil over medium heat. Add the shallot, bell pepper, and ginger. Sauté until the shallot is soft, about 5 minutes. Stir in the green curry and add the eggplant. Stir-fry until the eggplant softens slightly, about 3 minutes.

❷ Add the zucchini and green beans. Stir in the coconut milk, stock, and salt, scraping up any browned bits from the pan. Raise the heat to high and bring to a boil.

recipe continues →

3 Add the noodles, pushing them under the vegetables so they are submerged in the broth. Continue to simmer, over medium heat, stirring occasionally so the noodles don't cling together, until the strands are pliable, about 3 minutes, depending on the brand.

4 Remove the pot from the heat and let stand for 5 minutes—the noodles will plump more and the broth will continue to thicken as it cools. Stir in the lime juice and taste for seasoning, adding more salt, as needed, especially if using low-sodium stock. Garnish with the cilantro leaves, ladle into bowls, and serve.

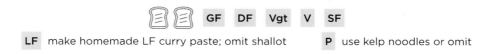

GF   DF   Vgt   V   SF

LF   make homemade LF curry paste; omit shallot   P   use kelp noodles or omit

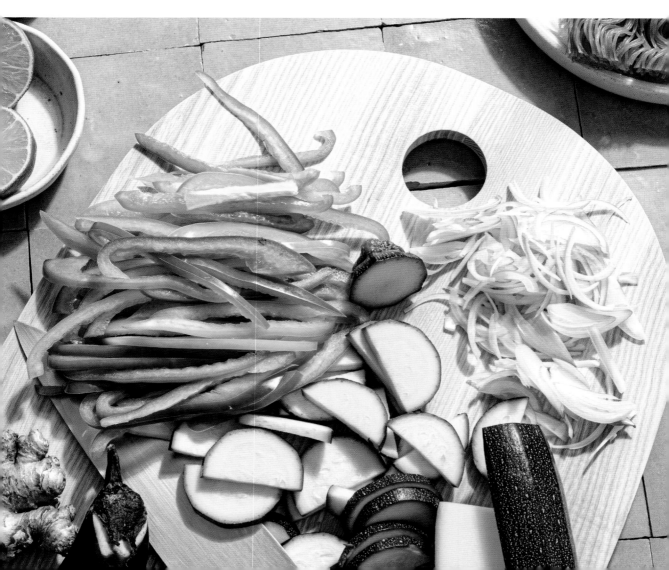

Creamy Sesame Noodle Salad with Smashed Cucumbers

I first learned the technique for smashing cucumbers with the back of a knife from Hetty McKinnon's book *To Asia, with Love*, which is a must-buy for Chinese-influenced vegetarian cooking. The watery, crunchy cukes get all the more jagged, allowing a creamy sauce to cling to all the rough edges. In Hetty's version (and this one), that dressing is a creamy combination of tahini, sesame oil, and mild Korean chili flakes. Once her cucumber salad became a constant companion to our weeknight meals, I started tossing it with rice noodles to make a complete dinner. It's similarly easy to peanut noodles, but this version is nut-free thanks to the sesame.

MAKES 4 SIDE SERVINGS

Sea salt

8 ounces rice noodles (pad Thai–style, vermicelli, or spaghetti in a pinch)

1 tablespoon avocado oil

4 small Persian or Kirby cucumbers (about 12 ounces)

⅓ cup **Spicy Sesame Dressing** (page 60)

2 scallions, thinly sliced

1 tablespoon sesame seeds

Chili crisp (optional)

Optional toppings: chopped kimchi, sliced radishes, sliced snap peas, shredded purple cabbage, smoked tofu, or shredded rotisserie chicken

❶ Bring a large pot of salted water to a boil over high heat. Add the noodles and cook according to the package directions. Drain, then run the noodles under cold water until cooled to room temperature. Transfer to a large bowl and toss with the oil to coat.

❷ Meanwhile, on a clean work surface, trim off the ends from the cucumbers and halve them lengthwise. Turn each half cut-side down and place a large knife flat against the cucumber. Using your hand, smash the knife so the cucumber cracks open through the center into two pieces. Using the back of your knife, whack the cucumber logs at a 45-degree angle into bite-size pieces. Alternatively, slice them or break apart into pieces with your hands. Transfer to a medium bowl and toss the cucumbers with **½ teaspoon salt**.

❸ Make the **Spicy Sesame Dressing**, if you haven't already.

❹ Add half the dressing to the noodles and toss to coat. Arrange the noodles on a platter and top with the cucumbers, scallions, sesame seeds, chili crisp (if using), and any optional toppings you like. Serve with the remaining dressing on the side.

 GF **DF** **Vgt** **V** **SF** **LF** green scallions only **P** use kelp noodles

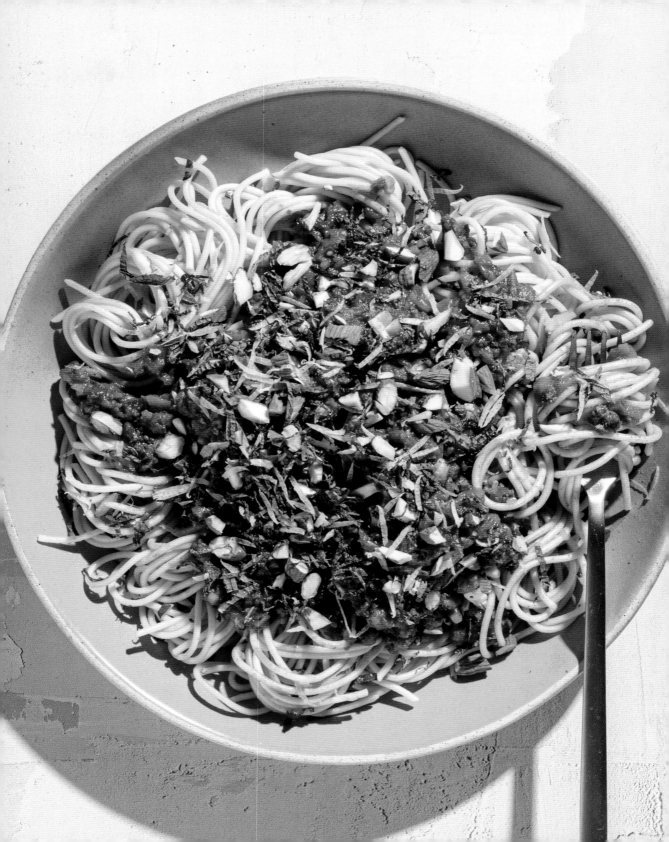

Spaghetti with Harissa Bolognese & Mint-Almond Gremolata

Though Bolognese is usually a hearty winter recipe, the spicy harissa and zippy gremolata brighten up this version. The sauce is fairly hands-off once it gets going, but is one of those ragus that tastes better the longer it simmers (keep reading for alternative methods using a slow cooker).

Gremolata—a mixture of nuts, herbs, and lemon zest—is this pasta's built-in carb companion. Though this topping is easy to execute by hand, you can pulse the ingredients in a food processor or grind them in a mortar and pestle for a finer texture. The vegetables in the mirepoix also can be finely chopped in a food processor. Mina is the brand of harissa available at most supermarkets and it comes in a mild and a spicy version. If using the milder condiment, you may want to double the quantity. Finally, even though we've taken the Bolognese slightly out of Italy, you can't ever take Italy out of the Bolognese...which is to say that if you love parmesan on your pasta, it will still work here.

---

*MAKE IT A MEAL: Serve alongside **Smoky Cauliflower Wedges** (page 250), **Braised Chickpeas & Broccolini** (page 323), or **Stuffed Artichokes with Italian Stallion Breadcrumbs** (page 261).*

MAKES 4 SERVINGS

Extra-virgin olive oil

1 large onion, finely chopped

2 medium carrots, finely chopped

1 red bell pepper, finely chopped

1 pound ground beef or lamb

2 medium garlic cloves, minced

½ teaspoon ground cumin

½ teaspoon paprika

½ cup tomato paste (from one 6-ounce can)

2 tablespoons harissa paste

Sea salt

1 cup dry red wine

12 ounces brown rice spaghetti or quinoa spaghetti

½ cup packed fresh mint leaves, finely chopped

½ cup raw almonds, finely chopped

Grated zest of 1 lemon

❶ In a large skillet or saucepan, heat **2 tablespoons olive oil** over medium-high heat. Sauté the onion, carrots, and bell pepper until soft and beginning to caramelize, 8 to 10 minutes. Push the vegetables to the side of the pan and add the ground beef in an even layer. Sprinkle the garlic, cumin, and paprika over the meat. Let the meat sear, undisturbed, for about 3 minutes, until a slight crust forms on the bottom. Continue to cook, breaking apart the meat with a spatula, until it is deeply browned and in pebble-size chunks, about 10 minutes. Don't stress about any browned bits on the bottom of the pan—they will come up later!

Noodles

recipe continues →

② Add the tomato paste, harissa, and **1 ½ teaspoons salt**. Toss to coat the meat. Continue to cook until the tomato paste begins to caramelize, about 5 minutes. Pour in the wine and stir, scraping up any browned bits from the bottom. Once the liquid has mostly cooked off, add **3 cups water**. Bring to a rapid simmer, then reduce the heat to low.

③ Let the meat simmer, uncovered, until the sauce is thick and dark and most of the liquid has evaporated, at least 45 minutes to 1 hour. If the sauce gets too dry and is no longer bubbling freely, add another **½ cup water**. The longer you cook the sauce, the more complex the flavors—you can keep going, adding more water as needed, for up to 3 hours. Taste for seasoning and add more salt or harissa as needed. The Bolognese can be made 3 days ahead, or even longer and frozen.

④ When you're ready to eat, bring a large pot of salted water to a boil over high heat. Add the pasta and cook according to the package directions, reserving **½ cup pasta water**. Drain the pasta and toss it to coat in the harissa Bolognese, incorporating the reserved pasta water as needed to loosen the sauce.

⑤ In a small bowl, stir together the mint, almonds, and lemon zest.

⑥ Divide the pasta among bowls and garnish each serving with a heaping tablespoon of the gremolata.

Slow Cooker Instructions: **At the beginning of step 3, transfer to a slow cooker. Cook for 2 to 4 hours on high, or 4 to 6 hours on low.**

Electric Pressure Cooker Instructions: **At the beginning of step 3, cook on high pressure for 20 minutes. Let the pressure release naturally.**

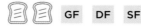

GF **DF** **SF**

LF omit onions, garlic, and harissa; sub 2 teaspoons Aleppo pepper

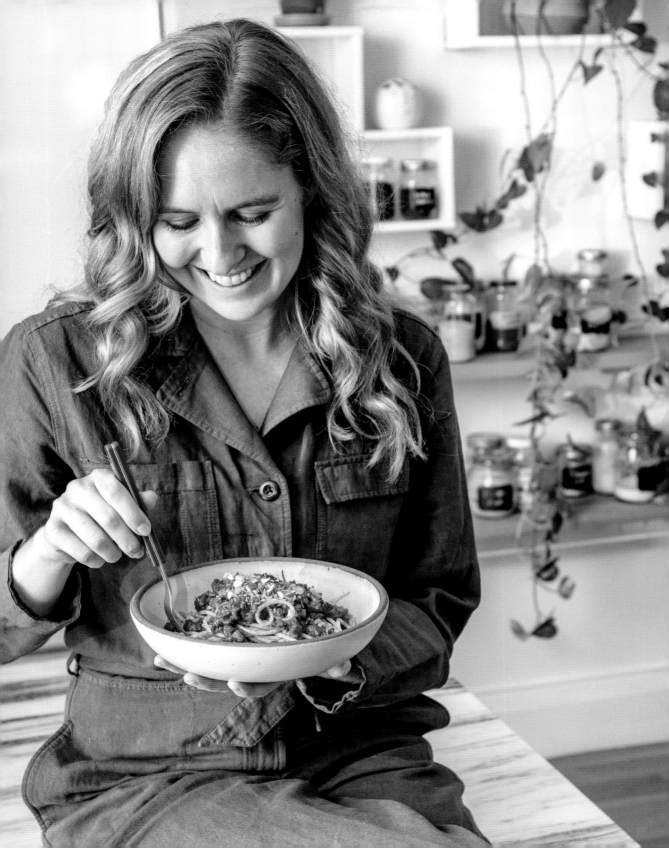

Salmon & Broccoli Noodle Casserole

My modern take on tuna noodle casserole is a cult favorite on my blog. What its supporters lack in numbers, they make up for in *passion*. The problem with expanding membership to this noodle casserole fan club is that I often lose people at "tuna." So this is my appeal to the skeptics, using canned salmon as the base and broccoli, leeks, and shiitakes as the carb companions. Instead of the usual canned "cream of whatever" soup, this casserole uses a quick coconut milk béchamel. But what makes it a staple for both '50s housewives and this girl right here is that you can make the whole pan a few days in advance (up until the crumb topping). Although I love the extra carb crunch, if you don't have breadcrumbs on hand, just skip them.

CHANGE OF SEASON: In summer, swap broccoli and mushrooms for 1 small zucchini, grated, and 2 cups fresh corn kernels.

MAKES 4 SERVINGS

Sea salt

12 ounces gluten-free fusilli or penne

2 tablespoons extra-virgin olive oil

1 medium leek, white and light green parts only, halved, rinsed (see headnote, page 209), and thinly sliced (about 2 cups)

1 cup thinly sliced shiitake mushrooms (about 2 ounces)

1 medium head broccoli, cut into very small florets (about 3 cups)

¾ cup dry white wine

2 tablespoons grass-fed ghee, unsalted butter, or plant-based butter

3 tablespoons white or brown rice flour

One 13.5-ounce can full-fat coconut milk

Grated zest of 1 lemon

2 tablespoons fresh lemon juice

1 tablespoon Dijon mustard

½ teaspoon red pepper flakes

5 ounces canned salmon

½ cup gluten-free breadcrumbs or **Plain Jane Breadcrumbs** (page 237)

❶ Preheat the oven to 375°F.

❷ Bring a large pot of salted water to a boil over high heat. Add the pasta and cook according to the package directions until just shy of al dente, about 8 minutes. Drain and set aside.

❸ Meanwhile, in a large cast-iron skillet or casserole dish, heat the oil over a medium flame. Add the leek and cook until translucent and flimsy, stirring occasionally, about 5 minutes. Add the mushrooms and cook until they release their moisture, 2 minutes.

Fold in the broccoli and season generously with salt. Continue to cook until the broccoli turns a more vibrant green but isn't fully cooked through, about 3 minutes. Pour in the wine and cook until the liquid is mostly absorbed, 2 minutes. Turn off the heat and scrape the broccoli mixture into a bowl. Set aside.

④ Place the skillet over low heat and add the ghee. Once melted, sprinkle the flour evenly over the ghee and stir to create a paste. Pour in the coconut milk and bring to a simmer over medium-high heat. Reduce the heat to medium-low and stir until the sauce is thick enough to coat the back of your spoon, smoothing out any lumps during the process.

⑤ Off the heat, stir the lemon zest, lemon juice, mustard, **½ teaspoon salt,** and red pepper flakes into the sauce until combined. Gently fold in the cooked pasta, broccoli mixture, and salmon, flaking it with a fork, until fully distributed. Top evenly with the breadcrumbs.

⑥ Bake for 15 minutes until bubbling and browned. Serve immediately.

GF **DF** **SF**

P use cassava pasta   **Vgt** **V** omit salmon

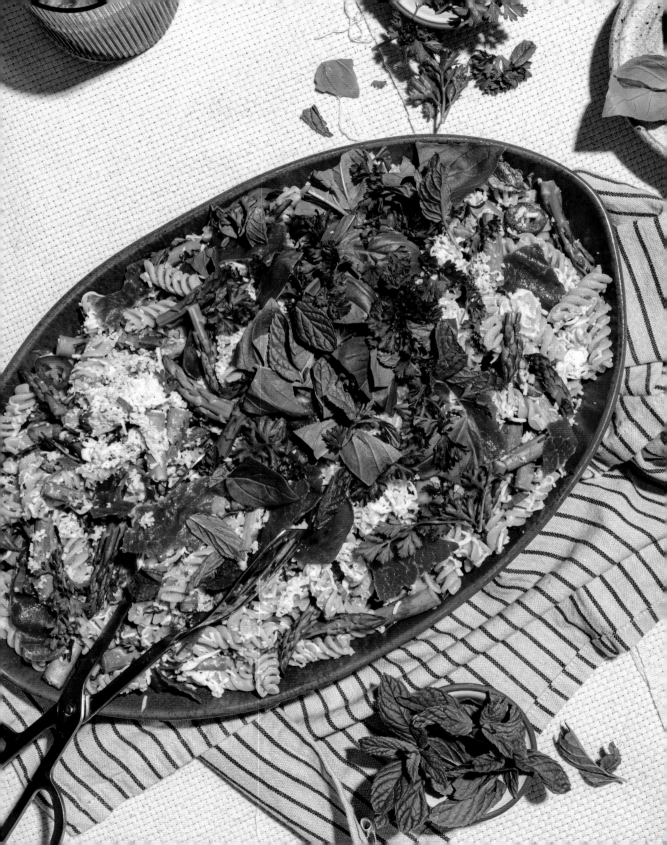

Eggs Mimosa Pasta Salad with Crispy Prosciutto, Asparagus & Piles of Herbs

There are few things in this world I wouldn't put mayo on, but pasta is a bridge too far. Especially when pasta salad can be so delicious with just olive oil, lemon, and herbs. Here we take an all-of-the-above approach, but swap the mayo for pillowy grated hard-boiled egg. The beauty of this recipe is that you can boil everything together sequentially in the same pot!

I like this pasta with a little added heat in the form of a fresh red chile. If you can't find one, a green serrano works, or ½ teaspoon red pepper flakes or chili crisp. Truly, any combination of fresh herbs will be terrific, but if you need some suggested duos, try dill and chives, or mint and basil. I like serving this pasta as a spring or summer side dish with grilled chicken and a green salad. If you don't manage to clean the platter, any leftovers keep well for the week ahead.

CARB SWAP: Sub 1 pound baby or fingerling potatoes, halved, for the pasta (set your timer for 15 minutes)—you'll have a perfect mayo-free potato salad!

MAKES 6 SIDE SERVINGS

6	slices prosciutto	1	small shallot, minced	¼	cup extra-virgin olive oil
	Sea salt	1	garlic clove, minced		
12	ounces gluten-free short shape pasta (I like fusilli or shells)	1	fresh red chile, thinly sliced (see headnote)	1	cup roughly chopped fresh herbs (chives, dill, parsley, mint, and/or basil)
			Grated zest of 1 lemon		
3	large eggs				
1	bunch asparagus, trimmed, cut into 2-inch pieces	2	tablespoons fresh lemon juice (from 1 lemon)		

1 Preheat the oven to 375°F. Line a baking sheet with parchment paper.

2 Arrange the prosciutto slices on the prepared sheet pan and bake until dark and crispy, about 10 minutes. Let cool on the sheet pan, then break apart into large pieces.

3 While the prosciutto cooks, bring a large pot of salted water to a boil over high heat. Add the pasta and cook according to the package directions until al dente. When you have 8 minutes left on the timer, using a slotted spoon, carefully lower the eggs into the boiling water. When the timer hits the 3-minute mark, add the asparagus. (Note: if your pasta takes less than 8 minutes to cook, add it after the eggs so the cook time matches the package instructions).

recipe continues →

4 While the pasta cooks, in a large bowl, stir together the shallot, garlic, chile, lemon zest, lemon juice, oil, and **½ teaspoon salt.**

5 Drain the pasta, eggs, and asparagus. Fish out the eggs, run them under cold water, and set aside until they are cool enough to handle. Transfer the pasta and asparagus to the bowl with the dressing.

6 Peel the eggs. Using the fine holes of a box grater, grate the eggs into the pasta bowl.

7 Add the herbs and toss to combine. Taste for seasoning, and add more salt or lemon juice, as needed.

8 Serve the pasta warm or at room temperature (as more of a pasta salad) with the crispy prosciutto crumbled on top.

GF **DF** **P** **SF**   **Vgt** omit prosciutto

Linguine with Chorizo, Clams & Kale

This pasta is a hybrid of two of my favorite dishes: linguine alle vongole, the iconic Italian clam pasta, and caldo verde, a Portuguese kale and sausage soup. The briny seafood only makes the smoky, fatty chorizo, bright cherry tomatoes, and spicy red pepper flakes better. I prefer this recipe with a hard, cured sausage. If you can't find red-tinged chorizo, any Italian hard salami will do. Alternatively, use a cooked sausage from the deli aisle, ideally linguica to stick with the caldo verde theme. But as a general rule, bacon or pancetta would not be terrible either. If you can't find clams in your area, mussels or shrimp work too. For the latter, just sauté, uncovered, with the kale. Finally, I always recommend cooking with a wine you'd want to drink: anything on the dry side from Portugal (Vinho Verde), Italy (Vermentino, Verdicchio, Pinot Grigio), or Spain (Albariño).

CARB SWAP: Omit the pasta and add 1 pound finely diced potatoes to the pan with the chorizo.

MAKES 2 TO 4 SERVINGS

2 pounds cockles, Manila clams, or littlenecks (the smaller the better)

Sea salt

2 tablespoons extra-virgin olive oil

4 ounces Spanish or Portuguese chorizo (hard, cured), finely diced

1 shallot, thinly sliced

1 pint cherry tomatoes, halved

1 garlic clove, minced

¼ to ½ teaspoon red pepper flakes (optional)

1 cup dry white wine

2 cups finely chopped kale leaves

12 ounces gluten-free linguine

¼ cup finely chopped fresh parsley

❶ Rinse the clams well and place them in a large bowl. Cover with cold water and let soak while prepping the remaining ingredients.

❷ Bring a large pot of salted water to a boil over high heat.

❸ In a large Dutch oven or lidded saucepan, heat the oil over medium-high heat. Add the chorizo and shallot and sauté until the shallot is soft, 5 minutes. If browned bits form on the bottom of the pan, don't worry.

❹ Add the cherry tomatoes, garlic, and red pepper flakes (if using) and cook for 5 minutes until the tomatoes soften and release their juices. Stir in the wine, scraping

recipe continues →

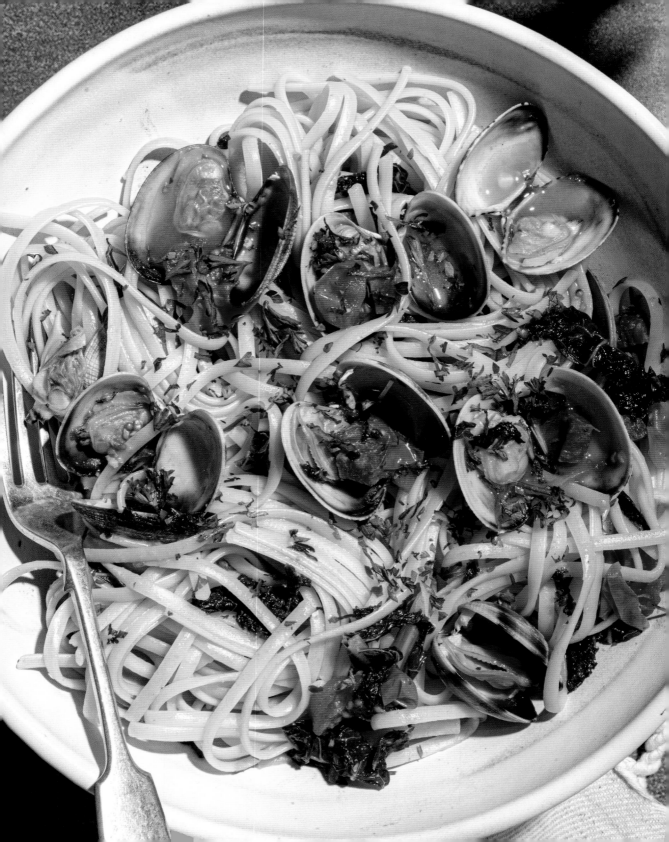

up any browned bits from the bottom of the pan, and season with **½ teaspoon salt**. Simmer until the liquid has reduced by about half, around 2 minutes.

⑤ Stir in the kale and arrange the clams on top, pulling them directly from the bowl of water and leaving any grit behind (don't drain through a colander). Bring the remaining liquid in the pan to a simmer over medium heat, cover the pan, and steam for 5 minutes, or until all the clams have opened. Discard any clams that do not open.

⑥ Meanwhile, add the linguine to the boiling water and cook according to the package directions. Drain and add directly to the pan with the clams. Toss until the pasta is fully coated in the chorizo and its starch has thickened the sauce.

⑦ Garnish the pasta with the parsley and enjoy immediately.

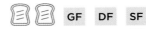

GF   DF   SF

LF omit chorizo, garlic, and shallot   **P** use cassava pasta

Ginger-Scallion Chicken Soba Noodle Soup

You've heard of knife-and-fork salads? Well, this is a knife-and-fork soup! Rather than your traditional chicken noodle soup where you get everything in one bite, this soba bowl is made of just a few ingredients in their simplest form: noodles, bok choy, and sliced chicken breast. The soba noodles thicken the soup as they cook, resulting in a texture closer to a hot-and-sour soup or noodle congee than a brothy ramen. You can make the noodles separately if you prefer a consommé to something heartier. This is an ideal one-pot meal for a bad gut day thanks to the ginger, low-FODMAP veggies, and lean poultry.

CARB SWAP: Swap 1 cup white rice for the noodles. Chop the bok choy and cooked chicken for a more traditional chicken and rice soup.

MAKES 4 SERVINGS

2 tablespoons avocado oil or coconut oil	2 boneless, skinless chicken breasts (about 1 pound)	3 baby bok choy, quartered
1 shallot, thinly sliced	8 cups chicken stock	1 tablespoon rice vinegar
4 scallions, thinly sliced, white and green parts separated	1 tablespoon gluten-free tamari or soy sauce	2 teaspoons toasted sesame oil
1 tablespoon minced fresh ginger	1 teaspoon sea salt	1 tablespoon sesame seeds or **Salty Sesame-Sunflower Gomasio** (page 75)
1 garlic clove, minced	8 ounces soba noodles (100 percent buckwheat, if gluten-free)	Sriracha or chili crisp (optional)

❶ In a large heavy-bottomed Dutch oven or stockpot, heat the oil over a medium flame. Add the shallot, white scallions, and ginger to the pot. Sauté until soft, about 3 minutes. Add the garlic and cook for 1 minute. Arrange the chicken in the pot in an even layer. Pour in the stock and tamari and add the salt. Bring to a simmer, then turn the heat to medium-low and continue to simmer gently until the chicken is cooked through, 10 to 15 minutes. Transfer the chicken to a plate and set aside to rest for 10 minutes, then thinly slice it.

❷ Return the liquid in the pot to a boil. Add the noodles and simmer rapidly until they are 2 minutes shy of the package directions (they will continue to cook in the hot liquid once you remove the pot from the heat). Add the bok choy to the noodles during the last minute of cooking.

❸ Off the heat, stir in the vinegar and sesame oil.

❹ Divide the noodles among four bowls, followed by the bok choy and chicken slices—I like each element to have its own real estate in the bowl. Ladle some broth over the noodles and garnish with the green scallions and sesame seeds. Feel free to hit your bowl with sriracha or chili crisp, if you like heat.

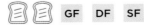 **GF** **DF** **SF**

LF omit garlic, shallots, white scallions, sriracha; use LF stock

Vgt **V** omit chicken; use veg stock

Grilled Skirt Steak & Vermicelli Bowls with Nuoc Cham

Vietnamese cuisine treats fresh herbs like their own food group. Where there are noodles, there are usually also piles of fresh mint, cilantro, or basil. This is one of the reasons the region makes for such great healthy hedonist inspiration, especially cold noodle salads like *bun bo xao*, which is, essentially, a bowl of various carb companions: thinly sliced marinated beef, pickled vegetables, fresh lettuces, ground peanuts, and those aforementioned herb piles. The whole dish comes together in less than 30 minutes and can hang out at room temperature until you're ready to eat.

Skirt steak is one of my favorite cuts of meat, but you can substitute flank steak (skirt's slightly thicker cousin) or chicken thighs, or go surf and turf by adding a pound of shrimp strung onto skewers. If you don't feel like breaking out the grill, use a cast-iron skillet. I like to keep my lettuce leaves whole so the bowls can be eaten as lettuce wraps for those who feel inclined to get handsy.

CARB COMPANIONS: *Other toppings include julienned cucumber, bean sprouts, or spiralized zucchini.*

MAKES 4 SERVINGS

Nuoc cham sauce

- ½ cup fresh lime juice (from 6 to 8 limes)
- ½ cup fish sauce
- 3 tablespoons honey or maple syrup
- 2 garlic cloves, minced or pushed through a press
- 2 tablespoons minced fresh ginger
- 1 small red Fresno chile or jalapeño, seeded and thinly sliced

Bowls

- 1 pound skirt steak
- Avocado oil or other neutral oil
- Sea salt
- 12 ounces rice vermicelli noodles
- 1 medium daikon radish, or 6 red radishes, julienned
- 2 medium carrots, julienned
- 2 tablespoons rice vinegar

- 1 head butter or Little Gem lettuce, leaves separated
- 2 cups fresh mint or cilantro leaves (or a mix)
- ¼ cup finely chopped peanuts or **Tangy Peanut-Cashew Crunch** (page 76)

1 Make the nuoc cham: In a medium bowl or 2-cup liquid measuring cup, whisk together the lime juice, fish sauce, honey, garlic, ginger, and chile until blended.

2 **Make the bowls:** Place the steak in a shallow bowl and add **¼ cup nuoc cham sauce** and **1 tablespoon oil**. Using clean hands, swish the meat around until it's fully covered. Set aside to marinate while you prep the remaining ingredients.

3 Meanwhile, bring a large pot of salted water to a boil over high heat. Add the noodles and cook according to the package directions. Drain and rinse the noodles with cold water. Set aside.

4 In a large bowl, combine the radish, carrots, vinegar, **2 tablespoons nuoc cham sauce**, and **⅛ teaspoon salt**. Toss to combine and set aside to pickle, stirring occasionally to redistribute.

5 Preheat an outdoor gas or charcoal grill or place a grill pan over high heat on the stovetop. Remove the steak from the marinade and shake off any excess. Season the meat lightly with salt, then place it on the grill. Cook until nicely charred on both sides, about 3 minutes per side for medium-rare. Set aside on a cutting board to rest for at least 5 minutes, then thinly slice the steak against the grain.

6 Divide the noodles among four bowls (alternatively, arrange the components on one large platter), along with a few lettuce leaves, the pickled radish and carrots, sliced steak, and herb leaves. Garnish with the peanuts and drizzle with a few tablespoons of nuoc cham sauce. Serve the remaining sauce on the side.

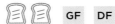 **GF** **DF**

LF omit garlic; use maple syrup   **P** sub spiralized zucchini for rice noodles

SF omit sweetener

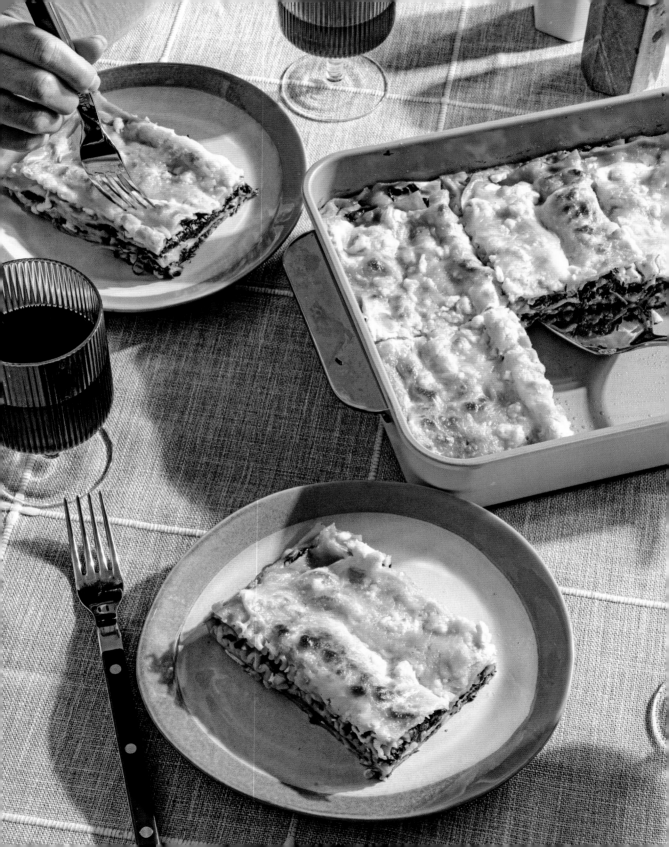

Spanakopita Lasagna

Spanakopita, the Greek phyllo stuffed with spinach, feta, and herbs, is one of those dishes that doesn't need much tweaking to be a Carbivore winner. However, I did it anyway, by turning it into a filling for lasagna. The amount of herbs and greens in this dish may seem like a lot, but they wilt as you toss them together, and then even more once they hit the oven. This recipe uses one of my time-saving lasagna hacks: Greek yogurt instead of a béchamel. It melts away along with the scant amount of cheese and stock to create a creamy base. If feta isn't your thing, omit it—the pasta will still end up tasting like white pizza.

MAKES 4 TO 6 SERVINGS

- 1   pound baby spinach
- 1   small red onion, finely diced
- 1   bunch scallions, thinly sliced
- 1   bunch fresh dill, finely chopped
- 1   bunch fresh flat-leaf parsley, finely chopped
- 1   bunch fresh mint, finely chopped
- 2   large eggs
-     Sea salt
- 4   ounces feta cheese (optional)
- 1   cup chicken or vegetable stock, divided
- 9   ounces gluten-free no-boil lasagna noodles
- 1   cup full-fat plain Greek yogurt, divided
- 1   cup shredded mozzarella cheese, divided

❶ Preheat the oven to 375°F.

❷ In a large bowl, combine the spinach, red onion, scallions, dill, parsley, mint, eggs, and **1 ½ teaspoons salt**. Mix vigorously with clean hands, massaging the spinach until it is completely wilted and combined with the other ingredients. Crumble in all but a few tablespoons of feta (if using). Mix everything again—the cheese should be broken down into small crumbs and well incorporated.

❸ Pour **½ cup stock** into a 9 × 13-inch casserole dish. Arrange a layer of noodles, overlapping them slightly. Slather the noodles with **⅓ cup yogurt** and season lightly with salt. Top with half the spinach mixture and **⅓ cup mozzarella**. Repeat with another layer of noodles, yogurt, salt, spinach, and mozzarella. Finish the lasagna with a final layer of noodles, yogurt, mozzarella, and the reserved feta (if using). Pour the remaining **½ cup stock** around the edges of the lasagna. Cover the pan with aluminum foil.

❹ Bake for 30 to 40 minutes, or until the noodles are tender. Remove the foil and bake for 10 minutes more until the cheese is nicely browned on top. If the top layer of noodles puffs up, don't stress. Push it down when checking for doneness. Let the lasagna rest for 10 minutes, then cut it into slabs and serve.

 GF **SF** **Vgt** use veg stock

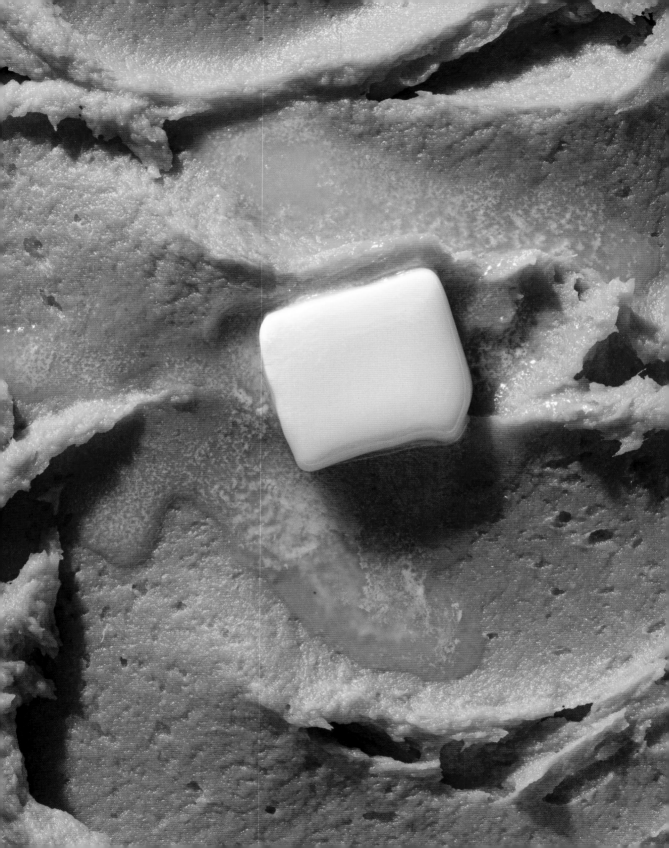

SPUDS

· · ·

One-Pan Provençal Chicken Thighs & Slivered Potatoes

Spring Potato-Leek Soup with Asparagus

Brussels Sprouts & Sweet Potato Hash with Eggs & Leftover Salsa

Braised Lemony Colcannon

Seared Tuna Niçoise-ish Salad with Creamy Caper Dressing

Chili con Carne Shepherd's Pie with Sweet Potato Mash

Spicy Beef Tagine with Apricots & Rosemary

Crab Cake Twice-Baked Potatoes

Parsnip-Potato Latkes

Braised Coconut-Lime Sweet Potatoes & Bok Choy

Gnocchi Primavera with Peas & Lemon "Cream" Sauce

Sweet Potato & Cabbage Rosti with Kimchi Aioli

Russet

Popular preparation methods: baking, frying, thickening soups

Russets are one of the most versatile potatoes on the block. Known for its coarse, craggy brown skin and sturdy, starchy flesh, the russet is a perfect vessel for baking and stuffing, like in my **Crab Cake Twice-Baked Potatoes** (page 223). The high starch content also makes them ideal for french fries or shredded fritters, like **Parsnip-Potato Latkes** (page 225). And since they are often on the larger side, in preparations where you do need to peel your potatoes, they are often the easiest to work with. The starchy flesh is particularly useful for thickening pureed soups, like **Spring Potato-Leek Soup with Asparagus** (page 209), or making dumplings, not that you need to start from scratch with my **Gnocchi Primavera with Peas & Lemon "Cream" Sauce** (page 229).

Yukon Gold

Popular preparation methods: mashing, scalloping

The yellow, rich flesh of these potatoes is extra luscious for mashing, or using in any dish where you want the flavor of the potato to take center stage, like **Braised Lemony Colcannon** (page 213). Because their skin is thin, tender, and papery, these potatoes are also great for preparations that don't require peeling, like the thinly sliced galette in my **One-Pan Provençal Chicken Thighs & Slivered Potatoes** (page 207).

Red Potatoes

Popular preparation methods: boiling, roasting, smashing

Thanks to their vibrant red skin and small size, these potatoes are ideally left unpeeled. They can form a classy, simple side if halved and roasted at a high temperature in the oven, like the crispy potatoes in my **Seared Tuna Niçoise-ish Salad with Creamy Caper Dressing** (page 215), or boiled and smashed into a coarser mashed potato. Their skins also add texture and color to a mayo-based potato salad.

Sweet Potatoes (Also Called Yams)

Popular preparation methods: braising, mashing, roasting, stewing

In America, the terms "yam" and "sweet potato" are used interchangeably. However, most American supermarkets are selling you sweet potatoes, even if the label says "yam." Sweet potatoes, with their classic orange flesh, are what come to mind for most people. But the interiors can also be purple or white, as with Japanese sweet potatoes. True yams, on the other hand, are much larger, have a similar texture and flavor to yuca (not sweet), and rough brown skins (like russets). They are most commonly grown in Latin America, West Africa, the Caribbean, and Asia.

Because the flesh tends to be true to its name, sweet potatoes are one of my favorite ingredients to add sweetness to a complex dish without any added sugar. They offset the heat in **Spicy Beef Tagine with Apricots & Rosemary** (page 220) or **Brussels Sprouts & Sweet Potato Hash with Eggs & Leftover Salsa** (page 212). You can leave the skin on and cut them into wedges, like in **Braised Coconut-Lime Sweet Potatoes & Bok Choy** (page 226), or leave them whole since their tough skin, like russets, can double as a vessel in **Roasted Sweet Potatoes with Beans & Greens** (page 311). Finally, they are equally delicious mashed as a sweet topping for **Chili con Carne Shepherd's Pie** (page 217). No, you will not find a marshmallow in this book.

Purple & Blue Potatoes

Popular preparation methods: steamed, roasted

Like their orange cousins, the vibrant colors of purple and blue potatoes are natural indicators of their nutrient value. But in purely aesthetic terms, they are also a fun way to change the palette of your tablescape. I like boiling them to maintain their vibrancy and using them in non-mayo-based potato salads.

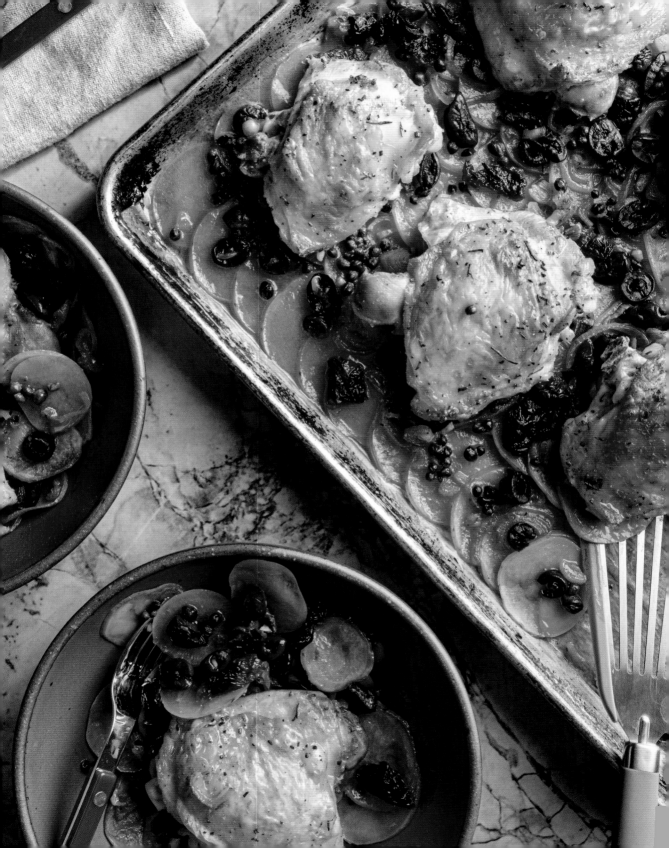

One-Pan Provençal Chicken Thighs & Slivered Potatoes

Keeping olives, capers, and sun-dried tomatoes in my fridge at all times is my strategy for packing tons of flavor into my dishes without a trip to the grocery store. In this case, they turn an ordinary weeknight sheet pan meal into something special enough for company. The potatoes are thinly sliced (use a mandoline, if you have one!) and arranged galette-style into an elegant overlapping base for the chicken to rest on. The preserved vegetables get fanned on top and release their brine as they cook, which your potatoes gladly soak up. This dish can be made an hour ahead and reheated in the oven right before you eat. A large cod loin would also work instead of the poultry—just add it to the pan during the last 10 minutes of cooking. Because there aren't green vegetables in this recipe, it's a good time to add a starter salad (see page 81)!

MAKES 4 TO 6 SERVINGS

Extra-virgin olive oil

Grated zest of 1 lemon

2 tablespoons fresh lemon juice

2 teaspoons chopped fresh rosemary

1 teaspoon Dijon mustard

Sea salt and freshly ground black pepper

8 bone-in, skin-on chicken thighs

1 ¾ pounds Yukon Gold potatoes (4 large), unpeeled

1 cup pitted kalamata olives, chopped

10 oil-packed sun-dried tomatoes, chopped

⅓ cup capers (from one 3-ounce jar)

2 garlic cloves, minced

2 shallots, thinly sliced

❶ Preheat the oven to 425°F. Line a rimmed sheet pan with parchment paper and lightly grease it with oil.

❷ In a large bowl, whisk together the lemon zest, lemon juice, rosemary, mustard, **2 tablespoons oil, 1 teaspoon salt,** and **¼ teaspoon pepper.** Add the chicken and toss until well-coated. Set aside to marinate.

❸ On a clean work surface, thinly slice each potato into ⅛-inch-thick slivers using a sharp knife or a mandoline. Keep the sliced potatoes more or less together as you go, then fan the slices on the prepared sheet pan in rows lengthwise, overlapping slightly. Season lightly with salt.

❹ In a medium bowl, combine the olives, sun-dried tomatoes, capers, garlic, shallots, and **1 tablespoon oil.** Toss to coat. Spread the antipasti mixture evenly over the potatoes. Arrange the chicken, skin-side up, on the potatoes.

❺ Bake for about 50 minutes, or until the potatoes are tender with nicely browned edges, and the chicken is cooked through with crispy skin. Remove from the oven and serve directly from the pan.

GF DF P SF   LF omit shallots and garlic

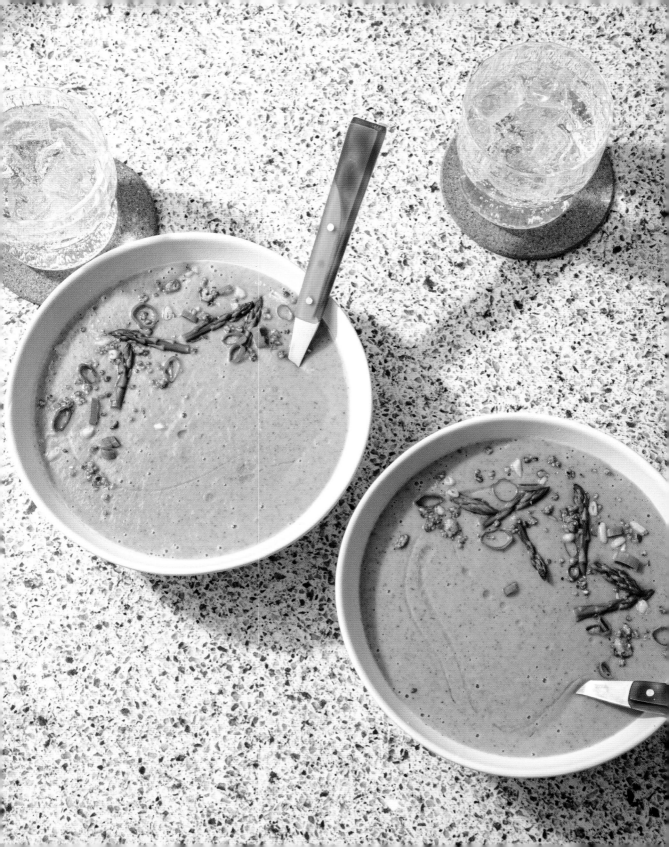

Spring Potato-Leek Soup with Asparagus

Confession: I've always found potato-leek soup to be a little on the gluey side. So, when I make it at home, I try to add a green element, especially in spring months. Asparagus becomes quite subtle in this soup and pairs well with the anise-y fennel and peppery arugula in the background. Any manner of peas (sweet, sugar snap, snow) could be swapped for the asparagus. Because we are pulverizing much of the fiber in this recipe, I garnish the soup with a few raw asparagus spears as a carb companion.

Leeks can be quite gritty. To wash them, cut off the stringy base and the dark-green top (right above where the outermost leaf separates from the layers below). Halve the leek lengthwise and then rinse each half under the running water, fanning the outer layers so any grit is washed away. Then, thinly slice each half into half moons.

MAKES 4 SERVINGS

¼ cup extra-virgin olive oil

1 fennel bulb, sliced

1 large leek, thinly sliced (see headnote)

1 bunch scallions, thinly sliced, white and light green parts separated

2 garlic cloves, minced

1 pound russet potatoes (about 2 medium), unpeeled, cut into 1-inch cubes

6 cups vegetable or chicken stock

1 teaspoon sea salt

1 pound asparagus

2 cups packed baby arugula or watercress

1 tablespoon fresh lemon juice

¼ cup **Anise-y Pine Nut–Almond Crunch** (page 77; optional)

❶ In a large stockpot or Dutch oven, heat the olive oil over a medium-high flame. Add the fennel, leek, and white scallions. Cook, stirring occasionally, until soft and starting to lightly brown, about 7 minutes. Add the garlic and cook for another few minutes until becoming golden.

❷ Add the potatoes, stock, and salt. Bring to a boil, then reduce the heat to medium-low and simmer, uncovered, until the potatoes are soft enough to pierce with a fork, about 15 minutes.

❸ Meanwhile, trim the asparagus by removing the tough bottom inch, or any section that is thick, white, and hard to cut through, and discard. Roughly chop all but 4 asparagus spears. Finely chop the remaining spears and set aside for garnish.

❹ Once the potatoes are tender, stir in the roughly chopped asparagus and all but 2 tablespoons of the green scallions. Cook for 2 minutes until the asparagus is al dente and vibrant green.

Spuds

5 Off the heat, stir in the arugula and lemon juice, stirring until the greens wilt. Carefully transfer the soup to a high-speed blender, or use an immersion blender, to puree until smooth. Taste for seasoning, and add more salt, as needed.

6 Ladle the soup into bowls and garnish with the reserved scallions, raw asparagus pieces, a drizzle of oil, and the pine nut crunch (if using).

GF   DF   P   Vgt   V   SF

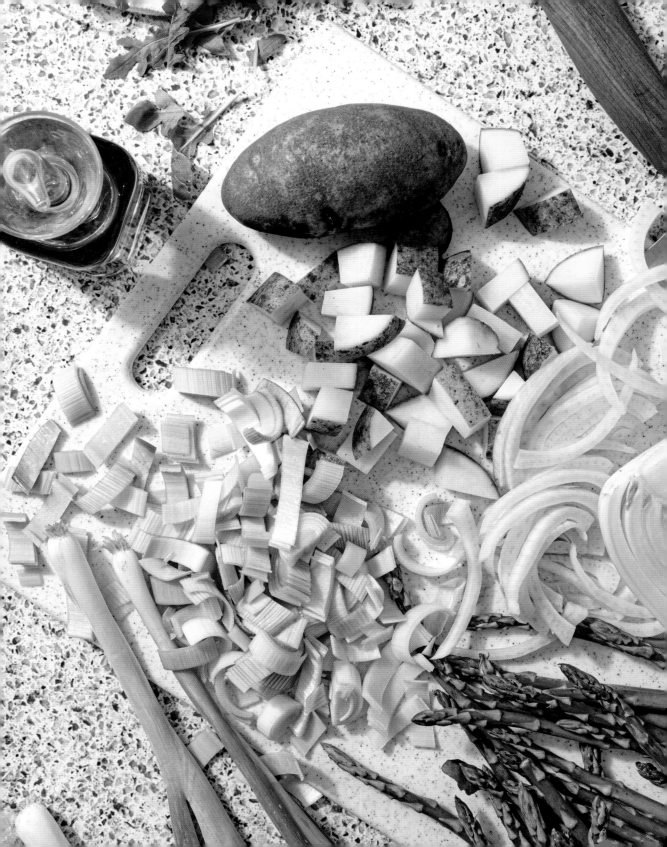

Brussels Sprouts & Sweet Potato Hash with Eggs & Leftover Salsa

We are not big snackers in my household but I often buy store-bought salsa as an easy appetizer when entertaining, especially if making cantina fare, like **Baked Fish Tacos with Ginger-Mango Slaw** (page 291). Inevitably, only half the container gets consumed. Somewhere over the years, I started to get more proactive and use the extra salsa to make our weekend brunch potatoes more exciting. Although not the crispiest roasted potato out there, the spicy, smoky tomato coating makes up for it in the flavor department. Even mediocre salsa only gets better the longer it's cooked. I use the technique here as a one-pan breakfast with equal parts sweet potatoes and shredded Brussels sprouts.

CHANGE OF SEASON: Sub fingerling potatoes and 4 ears sweet corn, kernels removed, for the sweet potatoes and Brussels sprouts. Add the corn at the beginning of step 4.

MAKES 4 SERVINGS

- 1 pound sweet potatoes, unpeeled, cut into ½-inch cubes
- 1 pound Brussels sprouts, trimmed, thinly sliced or shredded
- 4 scallions, thinly sliced, white and green parts separated
- ½ teaspoon ground cumin
- ½ teaspoon sea salt
- 2 tablespoons extra-virgin olive oil
- ¾ cup store-bought salsa
- 4 large eggs
- Fresh cilantro leaves (optional)
- 1 lime, cut into wedges

❶ Preheat the oven to 425°F. Line a rimmed sheet pan with parchment paper.

❷ On the prepared sheet pan, toss together the sweet potatoes, Brussels sprouts, white scallions, cumin, salt, and oil until coated. Arrange in an even layer.

❸ Bake for 15 minutes. Toss the potato mixture to redistribute, then bake for 10 minutes more, or until the sweet potatoes and sprouts have begun to brown and crisp.

❹ Remove the pan from the oven, add the salsa, and toss to coat. Spread in an even layer. Using a spoon or spatula, create 4 wells in the vegetable mixture for the eggs. Crack 1 egg into each well. Return to the oven until the egg whites are set but the yolks are still runny, 5 to 7 minutes.

❺ Garnish with the green scallions and cilantro (if using). Divide among plates and serve with the lime wedges on the side, along with any additional leftover salsa!

GF DF P Vgt SF   V omit eggs

Braised Lemony Colcannon

If I had to choose my desert island potato (and french fries were not an option), it would be a tie between lemony Greek potatoes and my mother's colcannon, which combines mashed potatoes with cooked greens or cabbage. Carbivore fiber considerations aside, I love the way the veggies lighten up the spuds, and if using green cabbage, it often melts away so much that you can't even tell it's there. This dish is my perfect mash-up (see what I did there?), cooking the cabbage and potatoes in pungent lemon juice, then smashing it into a coarse puree. This is one of those fabulous all-purpose sides that can be the carb quadrant of any blue plate special, and is a sneaky way to get picky eaters to offset their carbs with vegetables without even knowing it.

---

*MAKE IT A MEAL: Serve alongside **Dijon Turkey Meat Loaf with Spinach** (page 101), roast chicken, pork chops, or steamed fish with a simple salad or vegetable side—green beans, Brussels sprouts, or sweet peas.*

MAKES 4 SERVINGS

¼ cup extra-virgin olive oil

½ medium yellow onion, diced

3 cups finely chopped green cabbage

2 ½ pounds Yukon Gold potatoes, unpeeled, cut into 2-inch chunks

3 cups chicken or vegetable stock

⅓ cup fresh lemon juice (from 2 or 3 lemons)

1 teaspoon sea salt

1 tablespoon finely chopped fresh dill or parsley

❶ In a large lidded saucepan or Dutch oven, heat the olive oil over medium heat. Add the onion and cabbage and cook, stirring occasionally, until soft and just beginning to brown, about 5 minutes. Stir in the potatoes and cover with the stock, lemon juice, and salt. Bring to a boil, then reduce the heat to medium-low. Cover the pot and cook, stirring to redistribute once or twice, for 15 minutes, or until the potatoes are tender but not falling apart.

❷ Remove the lid and continue simmering, stirring occasionally, until most (but not all) of the liquid has evaporated and the potatoes are falling apart, about 10 minutes more.

❸ Off the heat, mash the potatoes directly in the pot until almost smooth.

❹ Garnish with the dill and a drizzle of olive oil, if desired.

GF   DF   P   Vgt   V   SF   LF   omit onion

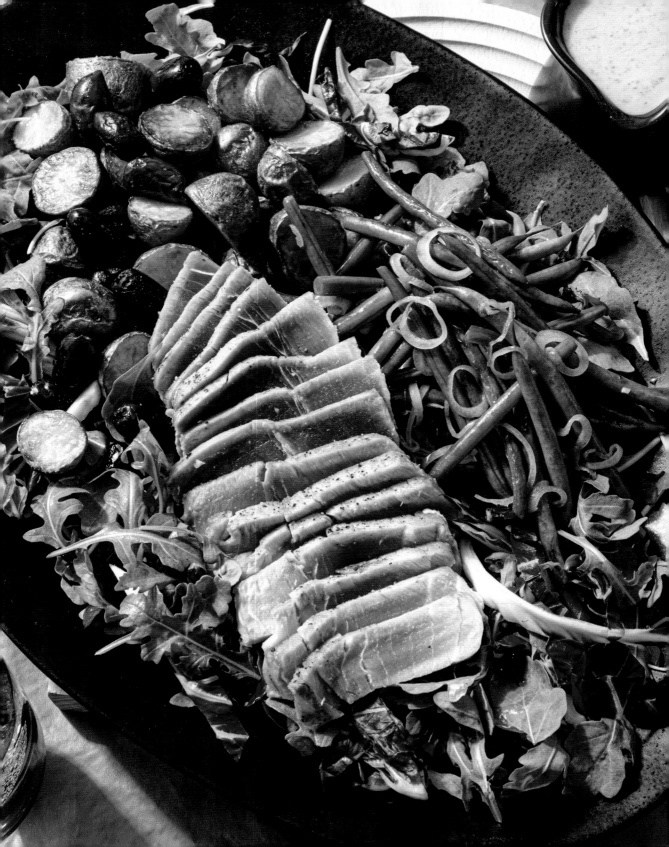

Seared Tuna Niçoise-ish Salad with Creamy Caper Dressing

A French *salade niçoise* is an ideal easy-breezy meal to prepare on a hot day. The toppings are all raw or steamed and can be made in advance. In this version, I cut back on the ingredient list (no hard-boiled egg or tomato here!) and, instead, make each component the best it can be for year-round dining. The potatoes get crisped in the oven, the olives warmed, the green beans sautéed with shallots. The tuna is a gorgeous yellowfin steak that gets seared until medium-rare. To take this salad over the top, the dressing is a salty, herby, biting combination of Dijon, capers, parsley, and lemon juice. It's a salad that's chic enough for company (it's French, after all), but not so labor-intensive that you can't get it together in under an hour for a weeknight meal.

MAKES 4 SERVINGS

1   pound baby red potatoes or fingerlings, halved

    Extra-virgin olive oil

    Sea salt

1   cup pitted kalamata olives

1 ½   pounds tuna steaks (about 2)

2   garlic cloves, smashed

4   thyme sprigs, or ½ teaspoon dried leaves

    Grated zest of 1 lemon

8   ounces haricots verts or green beans, trimmed

1   large shallot, sliced

5   ounces baby arugula (4 cups, packed)

2   cups roughly chopped radicchio (from ½ small head)

1   cup **Creamy Caper Dressing** (page 61)

❶   Preheat the oven to 425°F. Line a rimmed sheet pan with parchment paper.

❷   On the prepared pan, toss together the potatoes, **2 tablespoons oil**, and **¼ teaspoon salt** to coat. Arrange the potatoes cut-side down. Roast until browned on the bottom and the skin is puckered on top, 20 to 25 minutes. Add the olives to the pan and bake for 3 minutes more, or until the olives are heated through and juicy. Set aside.

❸   While the potatoes roast, place the tuna steaks in a medium bowl with **2 tablespoons oil**, the garlic, thyme, and lemon zest. Season lightly with salt and slosh the steaks around until coated well, rubbing the garlic and thyme onto the steaks. Set aside at room temperature.

❹   In a large heavy-bottomed skillet (I like cast iron), heat a thin layer (about ⅛ inch) of oil over medium-high heat. Add the green beans and shallot. Sauté until the beans are al dente, about 5 minutes. If your beans are charring but not getting cooked through, add a few tablespoons of water and they will steam. Season with salt and transfer to a plate.

Spuds

recipe continues →

⑤ Wipe out any remnants of shallot from the skillet and add another thin layer (about ⅛ inch) of oil. Raise the heat to high. Once the oil is just shy of smoking, add the tuna steaks (leaving behind the garlic and thyme sprigs). Sear until the bottom is browned, but the fish isn't opaque all the way up the sides, about 2 minutes. Flip the steaks and repeat on the opposite side for 1 minute for medium-rare, or longer if you want it cooked through. Transfer the tuna to a work surface and let rest for a few minutes before slicing.

⑥ Assemble the salad: On a large serving platter, scatter the arugula and radicchio. Pile the crispy potatoes and olives, sautéed green beans, and tuna slices in sections. Drizzle with half the dressing and serve the remainder on the side.

GF   DF   P   SF   LF   omit garlic and shallot   Vgt   V   omit tuna

Chili con Carne Shepherd's Pie with Sweet Potato Mash

If you couldn't tell by now, I love taking my favorite dishes and smashing them together. In this recipe, the usual savory ground lamb or beef mixture that forms the base of Irish shepherd's pie is revamped à la Texas chili con carne. What the pie lacks in peas and carrots, it makes up for in beans and chilies. Instead of regular potatoes for the mash, I've gone with sweet potatoes, both for their health benefits and because they balance the heat so nicely. You can substitute regular potatoes to make it look more like a traditional shepherd's pie, but I love the way the orange flesh stands out. If you're a cheese lover, sprinkle ½ cup shredded cheddar over the pie before baking. Feel free to crisp up the leftover roasted sweet potato skins to munch on while the meal cooks. Fiber is fiber!

CARB SWAP: Swap the sweet potatoes for regular russets or, for an avant-garde shepherd's pie, sub creamy grits (see page 268) for the mash.

MAKES 6 SERVINGS

2 ½ pounds sweet potatoes (about 3 medium)

Extra-virgin olive oil

Sea salt

1 small yellow onion, finely diced

1 pound ground beef (chicken or turkey work too)

2 garlic cloves, minced

1 tablespoon chili powder

1 teaspoon ground cumin

1 teaspoon paprika

One 15-ounce can crushed tomatoes

One 4-ounce can diced mild green chilies

2 cups cooked pinto, kidney, or black beans (from one 15-ounce can, rinsed and drained)

½ cup fresh cilantro leaves, divided

Dash ground cinnamon

Optional garnishes: sour cream or full-fat plain Greek yogurt, sliced jalapeños, shredded white cheddar cheese

❶ Preheat the oven to 425°F. Line a baking sheet with parchment paper.

❷ Halve the potatoes lengthwise. Brush the flesh with oil and season lightly with salt. Place the potato halves, cut-side down, on the prepared baking sheet. Roast until fork-tender, about 25 minutes. Set aside to cool.

❸ While the potatoes cook, in a large ovenproof skillet, heat **2 tablespoons oil** over medium-high heat. Sauté the onion until soft, about 5 minutes. Push the onion to the sides of the pan and add the ground beef. Cook the meat, breaking it apart with a spatula, until nicely browned, crumbled, and cooked through, 5 minutes.

recipe continues →

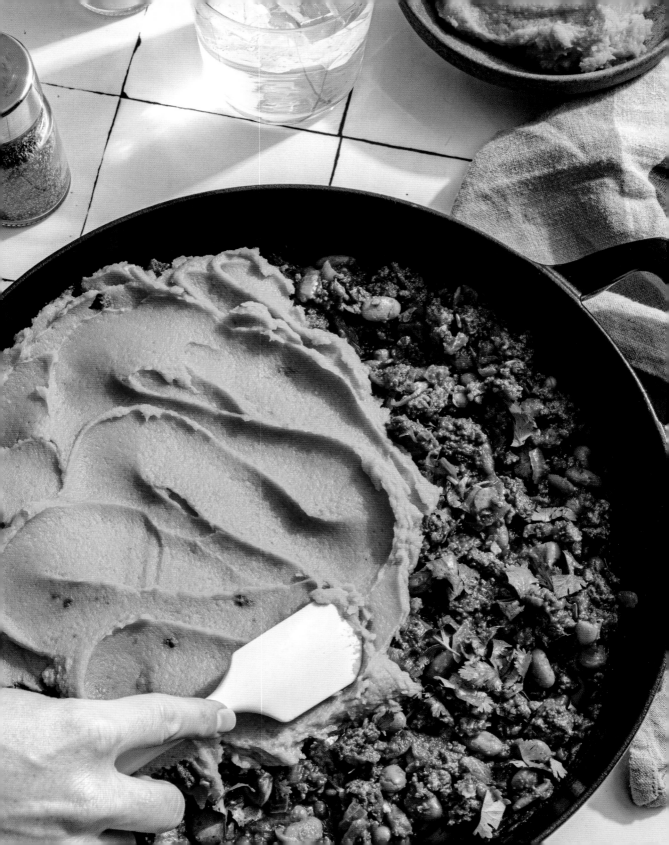

Stir in the garlic, chili powder, cumin, paprika, and **1 teaspoon salt**. Cook for 2 minutes, or until the spices are fragrant. Carefully pour in the tomatoes, green chilies, and beans. Bring to a simmer and cook over medium-high heat, scraping up any browned bits from the bottom of the skillet, until the liquid has reduced and the chili is thick, 5 to 10 minutes. Smash some of the beans with the back of a spoon or a spatula to make the chili even thicker as it cooks.

④ Off the heat, stir in half the cilantro. Taste for seasoning, and add more salt, as needed.

⑤ When the sweet potatoes are no longer too hot to handle, remove the skins and place the flesh in a medium bowl. Add **1 tablespoon oil**, the cinnamon, and **¼ teaspoon salt** and mash until smooth. Taste for seasoning and adjust as needed. Spoon the sweet potato mash evenly over the chili, making sure it covers the whole pie. Smooth the potatoes with a spoon or spatula so there are no gaps where filling can leak through. It doesn't have to be perfect—the craggy bits will form crispy edges in the oven.

⑥ Bake for 15 minutes, or until piping hot and bubbling around the sides.

⑦ Garnish with the remaining cilantro and any optional toppings you like.

GF   **DF**   **SF**   **LF** omit garlic, onion, and beans   **P** omit beans

Spicy Beef Tagine with Apricots & Rosemary

The summer after I graduated college, my mother and I took a trip to Morocco. It was a formative experience for a few reasons, the most unfortunate being the parasite I acquired that eventually (I suspect) catalyzed my autoimmune disease. But on the other side of that coin, it opened up a whole new world of healthy cooking. I fell in love with Moroccan stews, cooked in a cone-like terracotta dish called a tagine, which were always packed with digestive spices, fork-tender meats, vegetables, and dried fruit. This version is deeply warming, spicy, and slightly sweet thanks to the cinnamon sticks, dried apricots, and sweet potatoes. Harissa, the North African red pepper paste, is what helps light this stew on fire. Because I've found that the spice level varies by brand (I use Mina's spicy jar), it's better to err on the side of caution if you're sensitive, tasting the broth as it cooks. You can always add more harissa toward the end.

CARB COMPANIONS: For more fiber, add diced parsnips, butternut squash, kale, or fresh or canned pumpkin to this stew.

MAKES 4 SERVINGS

- 2 tablespoons grass-fed ghee or avocado oil
- 1 ½ pounds beef chuck, cut into 1-inch cubes
- Sea salt and freshly ground black pepper
- 1 small yellow onion, diced
- 4 carrots, unpeeled, thinly sliced on a diagonal
- 3 tablespoons minced or grated fresh ginger

- 2 tablespoons chopped fresh rosemary (from 3 or 4 sprigs)
- 2 to 3 tablespoons harissa paste (see headnote)
- 1 teaspoon Aleppo pepper, or ¼ teaspoon cayenne pepper
- 2 cinnamon sticks, or ½ teaspoon ground cinnamon
- 2 cups diced or crushed tomatoes (from one 15-ounce can or jar, undrained)

- 8 dried apricots, halved
- 1 pound sweet potatoes, unpeeled, cut into 1-inch cubes
- 1 tablespoon fresh lemon juice
- 2 tablespoons chopped toasted pistachios
- 2 tablespoons chopped fresh cilantro

❶ In a large Dutch oven, heat the ghee over medium-high heat. Season the beef with salt and pepper and add it to the pot in an even layer, working in batches, if needed, so as not to crowd the pot. Brown the beef until nicely seared on all sides, about 10 minutes total. Transfer to a plate.

2 Reduce the heat to medium and add the onion and carrots to the pot, plus more ghee, as needed. Sauté until the onion is translucent, about 5 minutes. Stir in the ginger, rosemary, harissa, Aleppo pepper, cinnamon sticks, and **1 teaspoon salt**. Cook for several minutes until a fragrant paste forms.

3 Return the beef to the pot and toss to coat in the spice mixture. Add the tomatoes and their juices and simmer for a few minutes to get rid of their acidity. Stir in the apricots and cover with **3 cups water**, or enough to submerge the beef.

4 Bring to a simmer, then turn the heat to low, cover the pot, and cook for about 1 hour 30 minutes until the beef can be broken easily into smaller pieces with a spatula, but isn't yet fork-tender or falling apart.

5 Fold in the sweet potatoes, trying to submerge them under the remaining liquid (add more water, as needed). Simmer over medium heat, uncovered, for 30 minutes until the sweet potatoes are very tender and the broth has reduced.

6 Off the heat, stir in the lemon juice. Taste for seasoning, and add more salt or harissa, as needed.

7 Ladle the tagine into bowls and garnish with the pistachios and cilantro.

Slow-Cooker Instructions: At the end of step 3, transfer the ingredients to a slow cooker and, instead of bringing to a simmer, cook for 3 hours on high. Add the sweet potatoes and continue to cook for 1 to 2 hours until tender.

Electric Pressure Cooker Instructions: After step 3, cook the beef on high pressure for 20 minutes. Let the pressure release naturally. Add the sweet potatoes and cook for 15 minutes on high pressure. Let the pressure release naturally.

GF DF P

LF omit onion, harissa, apricots, and pistachios   **SF** omit apricots

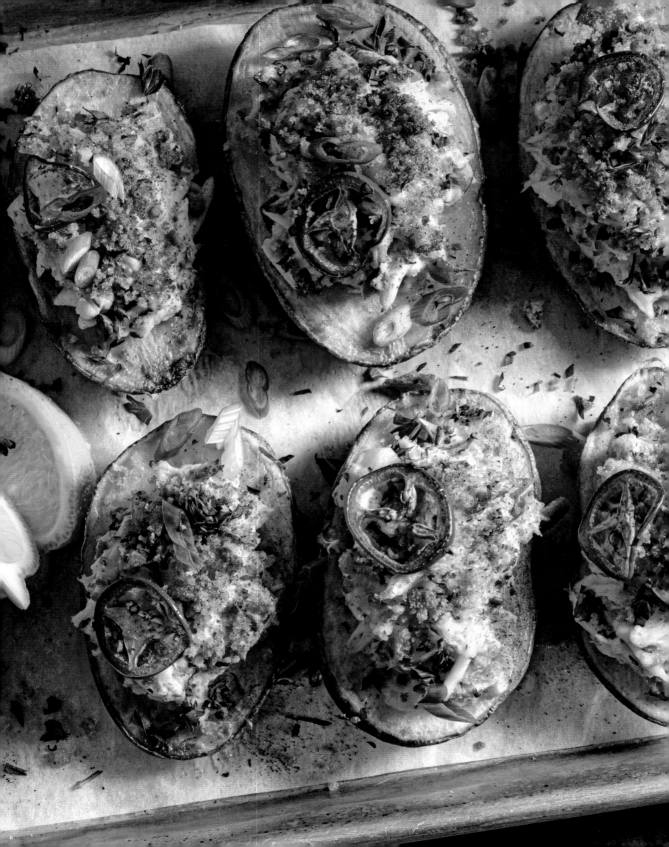

Crab Cake Twice-Baked Potatoes

About once a summer, Charlie and I treat ourselves to a decadent tin of lump crabmeat. Because it is a luxury that should be savored, I'm always looking for ways to stretch the crab while still doing it justice. Somewhere along the way, I started making crab cakes on top of baked potatoes. This not only eliminates the need for frying, but also allows you to use some of the cooked mash as a binder for the crab instead of a mass of breadcrumbs. I love serving these potatoes as a dinner party main course (each person gets a half) alongside an impressive salad like **Big Leaf Lettuces with Summer Tomato-Cashew Dressing** (page 81). If crabmeat is too rich for your blood, a smoked fish fillet like trout or bluefish could also be flaked as a substitute.

MAKES 8 SERVINGS

4 medium russet potatoes (1 ½ pounds)	2 medium jalapeños	2 tablespoons chopped fresh flat-leaf parsley
Extra-virgin olive oil	8 ounces fresh lump crabmeat	1 tablespoon fresh lemon juice
Sea salt	¼ cup mayonnaise	Old Bay seasoning or paprika
½ cup **Zesty Old Bay Breadcrumbs** (page 238) or regular dried breadcrumbs, divided	1 tablespoon Dijon mustard	Lemon wedges
	2 scallions, finely chopped	

❶ Preheat the oven to 425°F. Line a baking sheet with parchment paper.

❷ Halve the potatoes lengthwise. Brush with oil and season with salt. Place, cut-side down, on the prepared baking sheet.

❸ Bake until fork-tender, 25 to 30 minutes. Remove from the oven and set aside until cool enough to handle. (You can also refrigerate them for 20 minutes to help develop the resistant starch.) Leave the oven on.

❹ Meanwhile, **make the Zesty Old Bay Breadcrumbs** (page 238), if not using store-bought crumbs.

❺ **Make the crab cake filling:** Finely mince 1 jalapeño and transfer to a medium bowl. Thinly slice the remaining jalapeño and set aside. Add the crabmeat, mayo, mustard, **2 tablespoons breadcrumbs**, the scallions, parsley, lemon juice, and ¼ **teaspoon salt** to the minced jalapeño and mix until combined.

Spuds

recipe continues →

6 When the potatoes are no longer too hot to handle, scoop out some of the flesh from the center of each potato, leaving ⅓-inch shell around the skin, into a medium bowl. Using a fork, mash the potato until smooth. Add ¾ cup of the mashed potato to the crab mixture and stir to incorporate. Taste the crab filling for seasoning, and add more salt or lemon juice, as needed.

7 Return the potato skins to the parchment-lined baking sheet, hollow-side up. Scoop a generous amount of the crab mixture into each shell (there should be a heaping dome). Sprinkle each with some of the remaining breadcrumbs, then top with a jalapeño slice and a sprinkle of Old Bay. Bake until the tops of the cakes are set and the breadcrumbs are golden, about 10 minutes.

8 Serve with lemon wedges as a main course or side dish for a summer BBQ.

GF   DF   SF   LF green scallions only

P omit breadcrumbs

Parsnip-Potato Latkes

Latkes are a labor of love, and also a labor of labor. Grating potatoes and onions—or anything for that matter—might be one of my most dreaded kitchen tasks. But I'm pretty sure that having scabby knuckles by the end of Hanukkah season is an important cultural part of being Jewish. And it is usually worth it for the crispy, frayed potato edges and a good condiment to dip them in. Because there's so little flour, latkes are easy to make gluten-free, and also a great opportunity to cut half the spuds with a vegetable that packs more fiber—in this case, sweet, woody parsnips and leeks. You can serve the latkes alongside **Sugar-Free Ginger Applesauce** (page 72), **Dill Aioli** (page 69), full-fat plain Greek yogurt, or crème fraîche. If you're feeling flush, a bump of caviar never hurt. They also work well as a breakfast side.

MAKES 6 SERVINGS

1   large leek, white and green parts only, halved lengthwise, rinsed (see headnote, page 209), and thinly sliced

1   medium parsnip (8 ounces), peeled and coarsely grated

1   small russet potato (8 ounces), peeled and coarsely grated

4   large eggs, beaten

½   cup white rice flour or all-purpose gluten-free flour

1   teaspoon sea salt

    Avocado oil

1   In a large bowl, combine the leek, parsnip, potato, eggs, flour, and salt and stir until incorporated.

2   Line a plate with paper towels and set aside.

3   In a large heavy-bottomed skillet (preferably cast iron), heat a thin layer (about ⅛ inch) of oil over high heat. Working in batches, place 1-tablespoon portions of the latke mixture in the skillet and fry until lightly browned on both sides, about 2 minutes per side. Transfer to the prepared plate and repeat with the remaining batter, adding more oil, as needed (about four batches total, depending on the size of your pan).

4   Serve the latkes immediately, or save for later and reheat on a baking sheet in a 425°F oven until sizzling, about 10 minutes.

GF   DF   Vgt   SF   LF   omit leek

Braised Coconut-Lime Sweet Potatoes & Bok Choy

Braising is one of my go-to techniques for spuds. Cover the wedges with a potent broth and more oil than you'd usually cook with, and you have a completely hands-off method to set and forget. In this case, scallions and ginger infuse the coconut-lime broth, and the dish is rounded out by an equal portion of baby bok choy, which are quartered to mimic the potato spears. It's equally fitting for an easy weeknight hybrid side or a holiday table. This dish is on the mild side, but you can add a dash of sriracha or a tablespoon of red curry paste if you prefer a little heat.

*MAKE IT A MEAL: Serve as a side with **Chicken Satay Meatballs** (page 155) and **Peanut & Lime Slaw** (page 83), or as a vegetarian main over **Minty Green Rice Pilaf with Chiles & Peanuts** (page 134).*

MAKES 6 SIDE SERVINGS

1 ½   pounds small sweet potatoes (about 3)

4   garlic cloves, crushed

One 13.5-ounce can full-fat coconut milk

¼   cup extra-virgin olive oil

¼   cup fresh lime juice (from 2 or 3 limes)

1   tablespoon minced fresh ginger

1   teaspoon sea salt

2   scallions, thinly sliced, white and green parts separated

3   baby bok choy, quartered

¼   cup chopped salted peanuts, cashews, or **Tangy Peanut-Cashew Crunch** (page 76)

1 Preheat the oven to 375°F.

2 On a clean work surface, halve the sweet potatoes lengthwise. Cut each half into ½-inch wedges. They should look like (slightly larger) steak fries. Arrange the sweet potatoes in a 9 × 13-inch baking dish, in an even layer, and scatter the garlic over the top.

3 In a medium bowl or 4-cup liquid measuring cup, whisk together the coconut milk, oil, lime juice, ginger, salt, and white scallions until smooth (some coconut chunks are fine—they will melt). Pour the coconut mixture over the sweet potatoes. They should be submerged halfway.

4 Bake, undisturbed, for about 30 minutes, or until the potatoes are al dente but not falling apart.

5 Add the bok choy and toss gently to redistribute. Bake for 15 minutes until most of the liquid has evaporated. Serve directly in the pan, garnished with the nuts and green scallions.

GF   DF   P   Vgt   V   SF

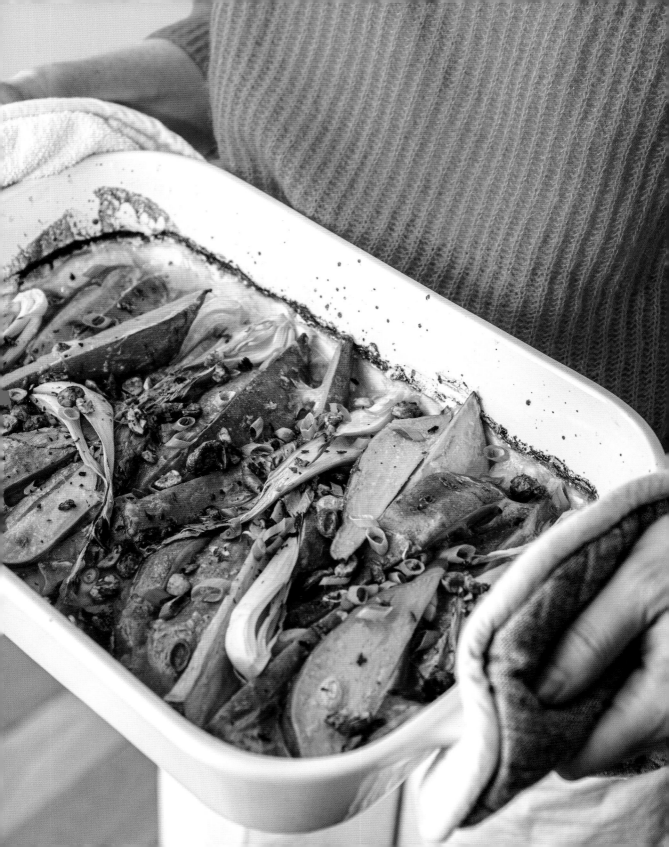

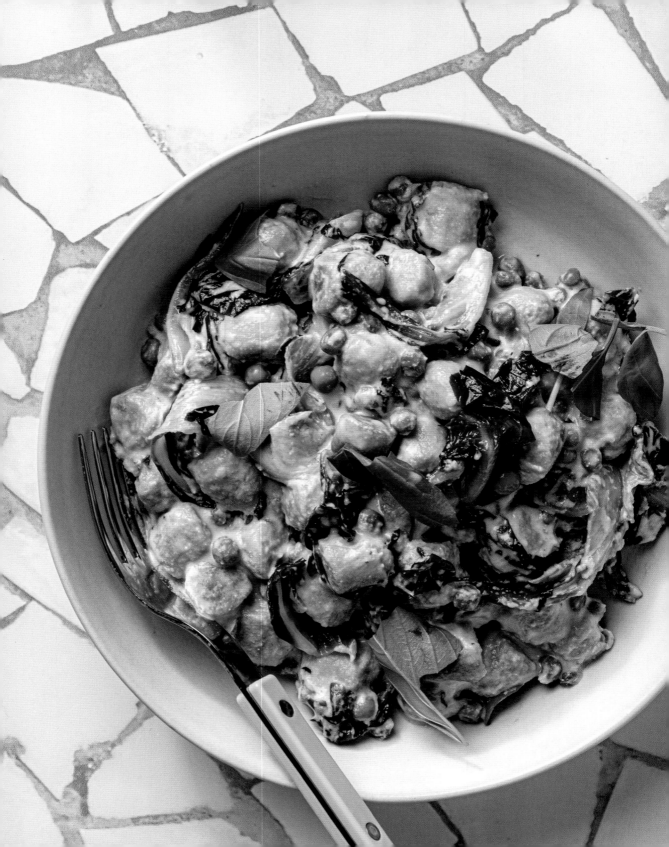

Gnocchi Primavera with Peas & Lemon "Cream" Sauce

Cashews get all the attention in the plant-based world as a trick for creating thick, luscious sauces without cream. But you can accomplish this with many ingredients. Sunflower seeds, which are used here, are relatively neutral and take little time to soften in boiling water. This lemony, rich sauce is truly the star of our gnocchi, and one I encourage you to double for future weeknight pastas. For the vegetables in my primavera, I use sweet peas and bitter greens—radicchio, arugula, or a mix—which wilt, and have their bitter, peppery notes offset by the sharp lemon in the sauce. You can use kale, fennel, or asparagus for even more spring vibes. Though this recipe is vegan, if you want more protein, hot Italian sausage adds richness to the greens.

CARB SWAP: Sub 12 ounces gluten-free pasta for the gnocchi.

MAKES 2 TO 4 SERVINGS

⅓ cup raw sunflower seeds

Extra-virgin olive oil

2 shallots, thinly sliced

2 garlic cloves, thinly sliced

¾ cup unsweetened plant-based milk

3 tablespoons fresh lemon juice (from 1 or 2 lemons)

Grated zest of 1 lemon

¼ teaspoon red pepper flakes

Sea salt

12 ounces gluten-free sweet potato or regular gnocchi

2 cups roughly chopped arugula, escarole, or radicchio (or a mix)

½ cup fresh or frozen sweet peas

½ cup roughly torn fresh basil leaves

❶ Bring a kettle filled with at least **1 cup of water** to a boil.

❷ Place the sunflower seeds in a medium heatproof bowl and cover with boiling water. Allow to sit for 10 minutes, then drain.

❸ Meanwhile, in a large nonstick or stainless-steel skillet, heat **2 tablespoons oil** over a medium-high flame. Cook the shallots and garlic until soft and beginning to lightly brown, about 4 minutes. Scrape the garlic and shallots into a blender. Reserve the skillet.

❹ To the blender, add the milk, lemon juice and zest, red pepper flakes, **½ teaspoon salt,** and the drained soaked sunflower seeds. Puree until smooth. Taste for seasoning, adding more salt or lemon juice, as needed. Set aside.

Spuds

⑤ Bring a large pot of salted water to a boil. Add the gnocchi and cook according to the package directions until al dente. Reserve ¼ cup cooking water, then drain.

⑥ Meanwhile, in the same skillet, add another **1 tablespoon oil** and sauté the arugula over medium heat until very wilted, about 3 minutes. Add the peas and cook for 1 minute until warmed or thawed (if frozen). Season lightly with salt and scrape the veggies into a bowl.

⑦ Add another **1 tablespoon oil** to the skillet and place it over medium-high heat. Arrange the gnocchi in an even layer and cook until nicely crisped on one side, 1 to 2 minutes—be careful not to move them before a crust forms.

⑧ Off the heat, carefully fold the veggies and **1 cup cream sauce** into the gnocchi. Add a splash of the reserved pasta water if it's too thick (the potato starch will thicken it further). Add more cream sauce, as needed.

⑨ Garnish with the basil leaves and serve immediately.

 GF   DF   Vgt   V   SF

Sweet Potato & Cabbage Rosti with Kimchi Aioli

Rosti is, essentially, Swiss hash browns made from coarsely grated raw potato, pan-fried until crispy on the outside and pillow-y soft on the inside. Okonomiyaki is a Japanese savory pancake usually made with shredded cabbage and other vegetables in a light batter. This recipe borrows from both, combining shredded sweet potatoes, green cabbage, and scallions to create a blood sugar–friendly hash, which is then topped with a sesame-infused, probiotic-rich kimchi aioli. The most labor-intensive part is shredding the sweet potato, but once you've paid those culinary dues, the pancake cooks in under 10 minutes.

---

*MAKE IT A MEAL: The rosti can be eaten at breakfast alongside fried or scrambled eggs, or as an easy dinner side for **Ginger-Salmon Burgers** (page 249) or roast chicken.*

MAKES TWO 10-INCH PANCAKES

1	medium sweet potato (about 12 ounces), coarsely grated (2 cups, packed)
2	cups very thinly sliced green cabbage (from about ¼ medium head)
4	scallions, thinly sliced on a diagonal, divided
½	cup white or brown rice flour
¼	cup potato starch or cornstarch
½	teaspoon sea salt
2	large eggs
	Avocado oil
¼	cup finely chopped kimchi, drained
⅓	cup mayonnaise
1	tablespoon sesame seeds
½	teaspoon toasted sesame oil

1 In a large bowl, combine the sweet potato, cabbage, and half the scallions. Using clean hands, massage the veggies until the sweet potato releases some of its starch and the cabbage releases a bit of its water. Things will start to feel damp—when you clench a fistful of veggies, they'll mostly hold together.

2 Add the flour, potato starch, and salt and toss to combine. Add the eggs and, using a spoon, stir to combine thoroughly.

3 Heat a 12-inch cast-iron or nonstick skillet over medium heat. Once the skillet is hot, add a thin layer (about ⅛ inch) of avocado oil to fully coat the skillet. Add half the sweet potato mixture and spread it into an even layer, packing it down with a spatula. Keep it relatively thick, about 1 inch. Cook until the sides are crispy and beginning to come away from the sides of the pan, about 5 minutes. If the pan smokes, turn down the heat.

④ Flip the pancake using a spatula. If you feel nervous about getting a clean flip, use a second spatula in your nondominant hand to add support, or invert the pancake onto a plate that's larger than your skillet. If it breaks, don't stress. It will still be crispy and delicious.

⑤ Cook the second side for 5 minutes over medium heat until firm and crispy. Use your spatula(s) to transfer the pancake to a plate. Repeat this process once more with the remaining sweet potato mixture.

⑥ While the pancakes cook, in a small bowl, stir together the kimchi, mayonnaise, sesame seeds, sesame oil, and remaining scallions. Taste for seasoning, and add salt, as needed.

⑦ Cut each pancake into four wedges and serve immediately with the kimchi aioli. If you want to save one pancake for later, you can re-crisp the rosti in a 425°F oven for 5 to 10 minutes.

GF DF Vgt SF   LF green scallions only; omit kimchi

P sub ¼ cup coconut flour for rice flour

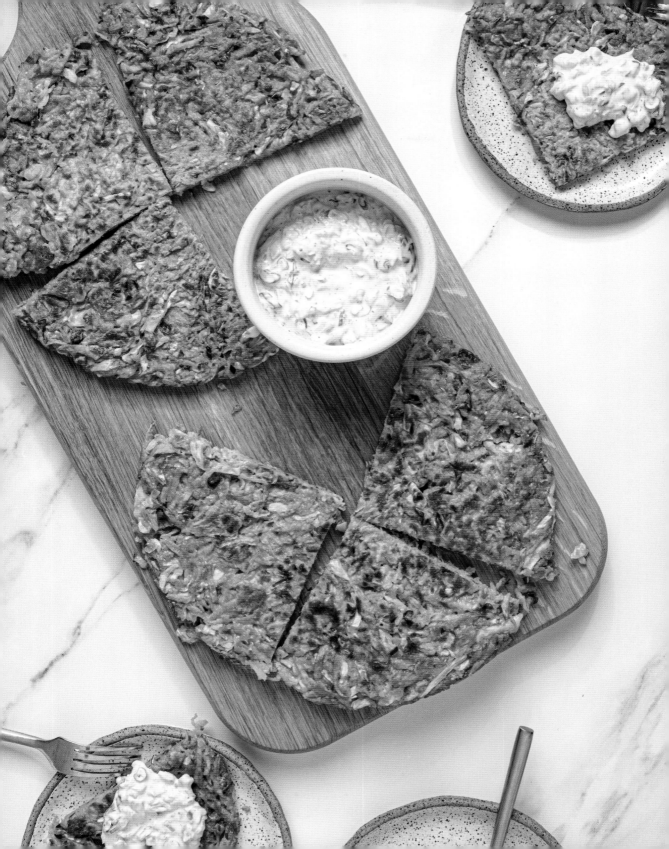

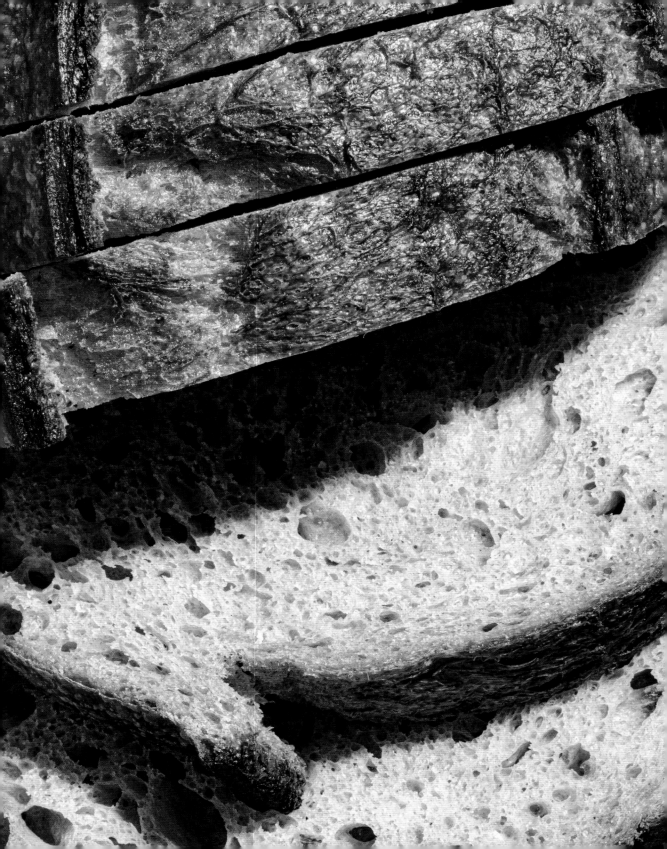

LOAVES & CRUSTS

. . .

Better-Than-the-Box Breadcrumbs, 3 Ways

Fancy Croutons, 3 Ways

Sheet Pan Chicken BLT Panzanella with Vinegared Tomatoes

Muhammara Roasted Red Pepper Dip

Ginger-Salmon Burgers

Smoky Cauliflower Wedges with Zesty Old Bay Breadcrumbs

Grilled Balsamic Mushroom Melts

Grilled Romaine with Parmesan Pangritata & Caesar-ish Dressing

Greenhouse Gazpacho

Basque Tuna Salad Tartines

Butternut Squash & Leek Stuffing

Stuffed Artichokes with Italian Stallion Breadcrumbs

Pepperoni Pizza with Okra, Collards & Hot Honey

Apple-Cinnamon Baked French Toast

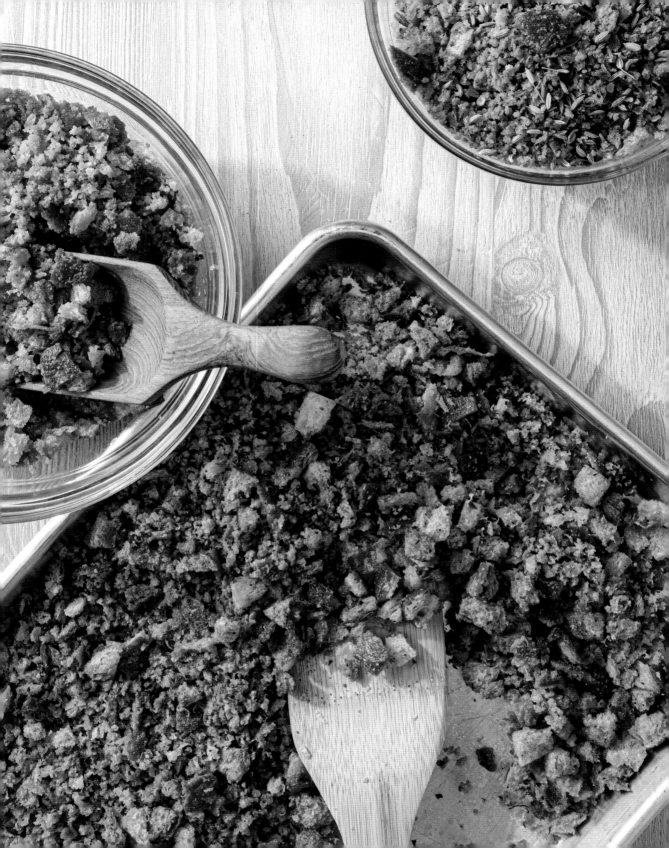

Better-Than-the-Box Breadcrumbs, 3 Ways

When a recipe calls for *fresh* breadcrumbs, you can simply take whatever loaf (especially the butts!) you have lying around and pulse it in a food processor to create pillow-y soft clumps. Dried breadcrumbs, on the other hand, like these better-than-the-box recipes, are precrisped. You can substitute any store-bought unseasoned dried breadcrumbs (panko or traditional), but I gotta say, these crumbs live up to their name. If you can make these to keep on hand, they will definitely add to your dish. Premade, these crumbs last for months on the counter but can also be frozen for later. Fresh or dried breadcrumbs defrost in under an hour at room temperature. If you're adding them directly to a casserole, they can be sprinkled on frozen and ushered directly into the oven.

Plain Jane Breadcrumbs

MAKES 2 CUPS

4   cups cubed or torn gluten-free or regular sourdough bread

¼   cup extra-virgin olive oil

¼   teaspoon sea salt

❶ Preheat the oven to 400°F. Line a baking sheet with parchment paper.

❷ Place the bread cubes in a food processor and pulse until coarse crumbs form. You can continue pulsing for a finer consistency, but I prefer chunky crumbs. Transfer the crumbs to a medium bowl and toss with the oil and salt to coat. Spread the crumbs evenly on the prepared baking sheet.

❸ Bake for about 10 minutes until the crumbs are golden brown and crisp. Let cool completely on the baking sheet, then transfer to an airtight container.

LF   DF   Vgt   V   SF   GF   use GF bread

Loaves & Crusts

Zesty Old Bay Breadcrumbs

These are the breadcrumbs I keep on hand to use indiscriminately in seafood recipes. They liven up any weekday fish when sprinkled on top before a trip to the oven. Or you can use them in the following dishes: **Crab Cake Twice-Baked Potatoes** (page 223), **Smoky Cauliflower Wedges with Zesty Old Bay Breadcrumbs** (page 250), or **Linguine with Chorizo, Clams & Kale** (page 193).

MAKES 2 CUPS

4   cups cubed or torn gluten-free or regular sourdough bread

¼   cup extra-virgin olive oil

     Finely grated zest of 2 lemons

2   tablespoons finely chopped fresh parsley, or 1 teaspoon dried

1   teaspoon Old Bay seasoning

¼   teaspoon sea salt

❶ Preheat the oven to 400°F. Line a baking sheet with parchment paper.

❷ Place the bread cubes in a food processor and pulse until coarse crumbs form. You can continue pulsing for a finer consistency, but I prefer chunky crumbs. Transfer the crumbs to a medium bowl and toss with the oil, lemon zest, parsley, Old Bay, and salt to coat. Spread the crumbs evenly on the prepared baking sheet.

❸ Bake for about 10 minutes until the crumbs are golden brown and crisp. Let cool completely on the baking sheet, then transfer to an airtight container.

LF   DF   Vgt   V   SF   GF   use GF bread

Italian Stallion Breadcrumbs

With crushed fennel seed, basil, oregano, and red pepper flakes, I designed these breadcrumbs with Italian American red sauce recipes in mind—the cacciatores, parmesans, and baked zitis of this world. They taste fabulous with most proteins, especially chicken, pork, and sausage, and elevate any simple vegetable, like **Stuffed Artichokes** (page 261).

MAKES 2 CUPS

2   teaspoons fennel seeds

4   cups cubed or torn gluten-free or regular sourdough bread

¼   cup extra-virgin olive oil

2   tablespoons finely chopped fresh basil

2   tablespoons finely chopped fresh oregano leaves

1   garlic clove, minced, or ½ teaspoon garlic powder (optional)

¼   teaspoon red pepper flakes

¼   teaspoon sea salt

❶ Preheat the oven to 400°F. Line a baking sheet with parchment paper.

❷ In a small food processor, pulse the fennel seeds until broken down into smaller grains.

❸ Add the bread cubes to the processor and continue pulsing until coarse crumbs form. You can continue pulsing for a finer consistency, but I prefer chunky crumbs. Transfer the fennel crumbs to a medium bowl and toss with the oil, basil, oregano, garlic (if using), red pepper flakes, and salt to coat. Spread the crumbs evenly on the prepared baking sheet.

❹ Bake for about 10 minutes until the crumbs are golden brown and crisp. Let cool completely on the baking sheet, then transfer to an airtight container.

    DF **Vgt** **V** **SF**   **GF** use GF bread   **LF** omit garlic

Fancy Croutons, 3 Ways

If you're going to add bread to your salad, you might as well make it count. Start with a good quality bread—but it doesn't necessarily need to be in its prime. Making croutons is an excellent way to recycle loaves that have gone south, as stale bread is perfect for soaking up other flavors and getting crispy in the oven quickly. There's a lot of controversy in the crouton community about tearing versus cubing. I am a cube girl, but feel free to exercise your personal preference. The same goes for how long you bake them. I prefer my croutons to have a little give to them and to avoid the fossilized state that give my molars too much action. Like homemade breadcrumbs, you can store them on the counter for a few months, or freeze leftovers and thaw in a 375°F oven for 5 to 10 minutes until crispy again.

Simple Sourdough Croutons

MAKES 4 CUPS

4   cups cubed gluten-
     free or regular
     sourdough bread
     (from 6 to 8 slices)

¼   cup extra-virgin
     olive oil

½   teaspoon sea salt

1 Preheat the oven to 375°F. Line a baking sheet with parchment paper.

2 In a medium bowl, combine the bread cubes, oil, and salt and toss to coat. Spread the bread evenly on the prepared baking sheet.

3 Bake until the croutons are golden brown but not hard to the touch, about 15 minutes. Remove from the oven, toss once to redistribute, and continue to bake for 5 minutes more until the bread dries out further and the croutons are firm. The fresher the bread, the longer the croutons will take to dry out. Let the croutons cool completely on the baking sheet, then transfer to an airtight container (see headnote).

 GF LF DF Vgt V SF   GF use GF bread

Rosemary-Shallot Focaccia-Style Croutons

Although I sometimes miss the crispy, yet pillow-y texture of focaccia, if I'm being honest, I was mostly in it for the toppings. Luckily, that means it's been fairly easy to feed that gluten-free craving in crouton form. If you want the shallot, sun-dried tomatoes, and rosemary to become one with your bread, pulse them with half the olive oil in a small food processor to create a paste. This is always an option to avoid chopping, too!

MAKES 4 CUPS

4	cups cubed gluten-free or regular bread (from 6 to 8 slices)
1	large shallot, minced
4	sun-dried tomatoes, minced
2	teaspoons chopped fresh rosemary leaves, or 1 teaspoon dried
¼	cup extra-virgin olive oil
¼	teaspoon sea salt

❶ Preheat the oven to 375°F. Line a baking sheet with parchment paper.

❷ In a medium bowl, combine the bread cubes, shallot, tomatoes, rosemary, oil, and salt and toss to coat. Spread the bread evenly on the prepared baking sheet.

❸ Bake until the croutons are golden brown but not hard to the touch, about 15 minutes. Remove from the oven, toss once to redistribute, and continue to bake for 5 minutes more until the bread has dried out further and the croutons are firm. The fresher the bread, the longer the croutons will take to dry out. Let the croutons cool completely on the baking sheet, then transfer to an airtight container (see headnote, page 240).

DF   Vgt   V   SF   GF   use GF bread

Za'atar Pita Chip–Style Croutons

Za'atar, an herb mixture that includes toasted sesame seeds, dried sumac, thyme, and other spices, is one of the most popular carb companions in Middle Eastern cooking. It is often baked directly into fresh bread or pita, or used to garnish dipping sauces like hummus or labneh. If you eat gluten, you can make actual pita chip croutons with this recipe; otherwise use the bread of your choice. Cutting the bread into strips will allow you to serve it alongside **Muhammara Roasted Red Pepper Dip** (page 246) as a toast tip.

MAKES 4 CUPS

- 4 cups cubed gluten-free or regular bread (from 6 to 8 slices)
- ¼ cup extra-virgin olive oil
- 1 teaspoon dried oregano
- 1 teaspoon ground cumin
- 1 teaspoon ground coriander
- 1 teaspoon sesame seeds
- 1 teaspoon ground sumac
- 1 teaspoon dried thyme leaves
- ½ teaspoon sea salt
- Pinch Aleppo pepper (optional)

❶ Preheat the oven to 375°F. Line a baking sheet with parchment paper.

❷ In a medium bowl, toss together the bread cubes, oil, oregano, cumin, coriander, sesame seeds, sumac, thyme, salt, and pepper (if using) to coat. Spread the bread evenly on the prepared baking sheet.

❸ Bake until the croutons are golden brown but not hard to the touch, about 15 minutes. Remove from the oven, toss once to redistribute, and continue to bake for 5 minutes more until the bread has dried out further and the croutons are firm. The fresher the bread, the longer the croutons will take to dry out. Let the croutons cool completely on the baking sheet, then transfer to an airtight container (see headnote, page 240).

 LF **DF** **Vgt** **V** **SF** **GF** use GF bread

Sheet Pan Chicken BLT Panzanella with Vinegared Tomatoes

The best panzanella I ever ate involved bread that was baked together with chicken. The croutons were both crisp and soaked in drippings—kind of like a summer salad interpretation of stuffing. When I tried to recreate it, I thought, why not add some bacon grease to the pan for good measure? And that's how this BLT-style panzanella that can be, more or less, made start to finish on one sheet pan came to pass. I love entertaining at lunchtime with this salad since each element—the chicken, bacon, and bread—can be baked ahead, then tossed together with the marinated tomatoes when you're ready to serve. Although I usually can't say no to a good schmear of mayo on a BLT, the acid from the vinegared tomatoes works even better as a dressing in this dish.

*CARB SWAP: Use crispy diced polenta instead of the bread (see **Crispy Polenta Cakes**, page 272).*

MAKES 4 SERVINGS

4	boneless, skinless chicken thighs (about 1 ½ pounds)	6	slices gluten-free bread, crusts on, cut into 1-inch cubes (about 3 cups)	3	tablespoons balsamic or red wine vinegar
	Extra-virgin olive oil	1	pound heirloom or vine tomatoes (about 2 large), cut into rustic wedges	2	small Kirby or Persian cucumbers, sliced
	Sea salt			5	ounces baby arugula (about 4 cups, packed)
5	ounces pancetta, cubed (1 cup), or 4 nitrate-free uncured bacon slices	1	garlic clove, minced	½	cup torn fresh basil leaves

1. Preheat the oven to 400°F. Line a rimmed sheet pan with parchment paper.

2. Arrange the chicken, smooth-side down, on one side of the prepared sheet pan. Drizzle lightly with oil and season with salt. Scatter the pancetta on the other side of the pan, making sure each piece is touching the bottom.

3. Bake until the pancetta is crispy and nicely browned, 10 to 15 minutes. Remove from the oven and, using a slotted spatula, transfer the pancetta to paper towels, leaving behind as much grease as possible. If using bacon, once cool enough to touch, crumble or roughly chop it into bite-size pieces.

Loaves & Crusts

recipe continues →

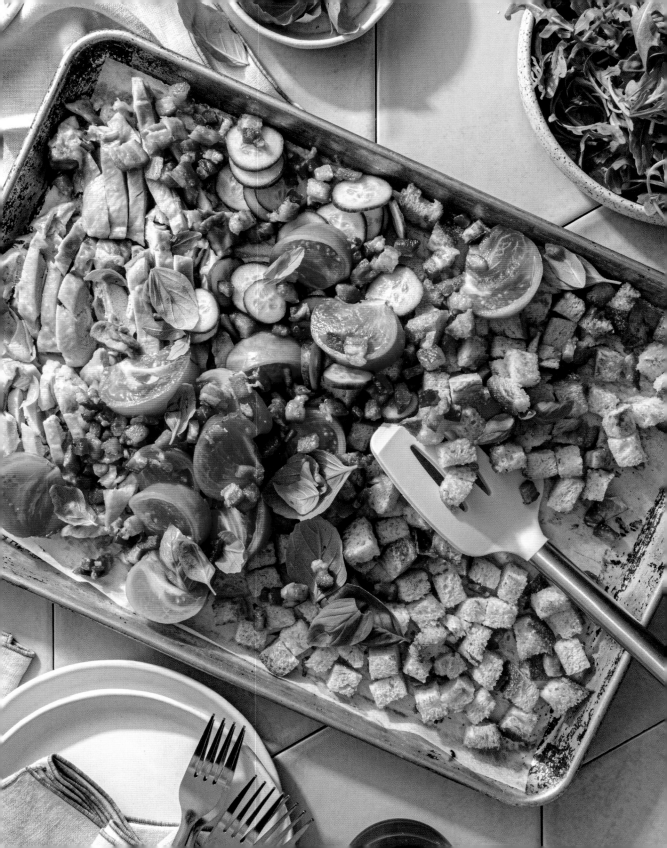

4 Flip the chicken with a spatula, smooth-side up. Season lightly with salt. Place the bread cubes on the pancetta side of the pan and toss to coat in the grease and chicken juices, then arrange in an even layer. Continue to bake until the bread is golden brown but not hard to the touch, 10 to 15 minutes. Transfer the chicken to a work surface and let rest for 10 minutes, then slice it.

5 Meanwhile, in a large salad bowl, toss together the tomatoes, garlic, vinegar, **3 tablespoons oil**, and **1 teaspoon salt**. Set aside to marinate for as long as you like.

6 When ready to serve, add the cucumbers, arugula, basil, bread, and chicken to the tomatoes and toss to combine. Taste for seasoning, and add more salt, as needed.

7 Scatter with the crispy pancetta bits and serve immediately.

GF   DF   SF   LF omit garlic

Muhammara Roasted Red Pepper Dip

If you want to add variety and color to a snack board, muhammara is the ticket. This spicy Syrian dip is made from a base of roasted red peppers, walnuts, and breadcrumbs. Pomegranate molasses is a common ingredient in Middle Eastern cooking and lends this dip a unique sweet tang (though more sour than sugary). If you can't find it, the dip will still taste great, just less like authentic muhammara. If you haven't already made the crumbs, begin this recipe by blitzing your bread in a small food processor. I usually take the shortcut of using store-bought jarred roasted red peppers, but you can also char and peel four large bell peppers from scratch. Any leftover dip will keep for at least a week in the fridge and can be repurposed as a sauce for morning eggs, chicken, fish, or **Millet & Zucchini Cakes** (page 145).

MAKES 1 ½ CUPS

⅔ cup fresh gluten-free breadcrumbs (see headnote)

4 whole roasted red peppers (from one 12- to 16-ounce jar, or fresh; see headnote)

½ cup raw walnuts, divided

1 small garlic clove, crushed

2 tablespoons extra-virgin olive oil

1 tablespoon fresh lemon juice

1 tablespoon pomegranate molasses (optional)

2 teaspoons Aleppo pepper, or ¼ teaspoon red pepper flakes

1 teaspoon ground cumin

½ teaspoon sea salt

Crudités, crusty bread, or pita

❶ In a small food processor, combine the breadcrumbs, roasted red peppers, **¼ cup walnuts**, garlic, oil, lemon juice, pomegranate molasses (if using), pepper, cumin, and salt and pulse until smooth, but still retaining some texture. Transfer to a serving bowl.

❷ Finely chop the remaining **¼ cup walnuts** and use them to garnish the dip, along with a drizzle of oil and a pinch of pepper, if desired. Serve alongside the dipper of your choosing.

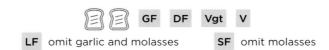

GF DF Vgt V

LF omit garlic and molasses   **SF** omit molasses

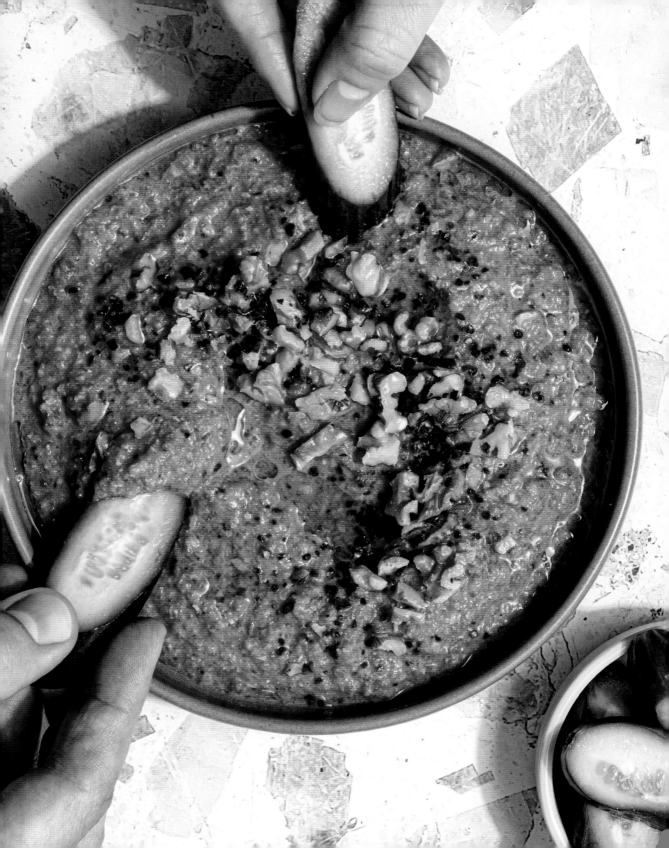

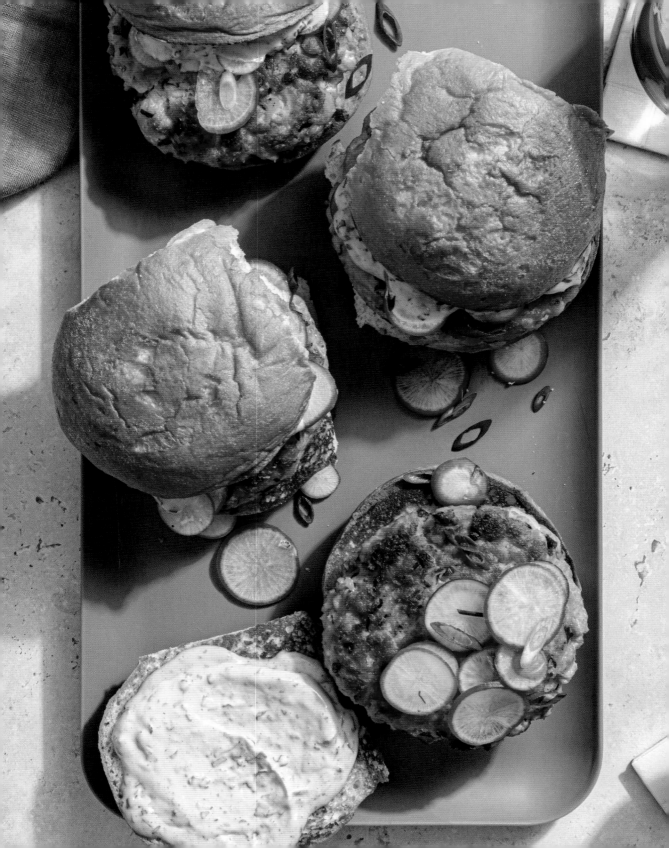

Ginger-Salmon Burgers

The first time I was ever paid as a private chef, I made a version of these salmon burgers. Like most of the choices I made during my early catering days, it was not the right one. When you're stressed out, I would not recommend pan-frying things that need to be served all at once. But despite arriving slightly broken on the table, the vibrant mix of ginger, Dijon, lime, and cilantro—won everyone over and remains a winner to this day.

MAKES 4 SERVINGS

- 1 pound salmon, skin removed, cut into 1-inch cubes
- ½ cup **Plain Jane Breadcrumbs** (page 237) or store-bought
- 6 scallions, thinly sliced, divided
- 2 tablespoons chopped fresh cilantro
- 2 tablespoons chopped fresh ginger
- 1 tablespoon fresh lime juice
- 1 tablespoon Dijon mustard
- 1 tablespoon mayonnaise
- 1 teaspoon hot sauce
  Sea salt
- 1 bunch pink radishes, thinly sliced
- 1 tablespoon rice vinegar
  Avocado oil
- 4 gluten-free burger buns, toasted, or Bibb lettuce leaves
- ½ cup **Cilantro-Sriracha Mayo** (page 70)

❶ In a small food processor, pulse the salmon until it's coarsely ground (you can also ask your fishmonger to do this for you), then transfer to a medium bowl. Add the breadcrumbs, half the scallions, cilantro, ginger, lime juice, mustard, mayonnaise, hot sauce, and **½ teaspoon salt**. Mix until completely incorporated. Form the salmon mixture into 4 equal balls and pat into 1-inch-thick patties about the size of your palm. Place the patties on a plate and refrigerate for at least 15 minutes to chill.

❷ Meanwhile, in a medium bowl, toss the radishes with the remaining scallions, vinegar, and **½ teaspoon salt** until coated. Set aside, stirring every 10 minutes or so to redistribute, until they are pink and pliable.

❸ When you're ready to cook, place a large nonstick or cast-iron skillet over medium-high heat and coat with a thin layer (about ⅛ inch) of oil. When the pan is hot, add the salmon patties and cook until nicely browned on the first side, about 3 minutes. Carefully flip, using two flat spatulas, and cook for 2 to 3 minutes more until opaque up the sides.

❹ Serve the burgers on the toasted buns and top with the mayo and radishes.

GF   DF   LF   green scallions only; LF hot sauce

Smoky Cauliflower Wedges with Zesty Old Bay Breadcrumbs

As far as "statement sides" go, a whole roasted cauliflower is a guaranteed stunner. But no matter how long I roast it, the stems always seem to be a touch on the tough side. A happy medium I've found is to cut the head into large wedges instead of florets. Simply drizzle your marinade over the wedges so the lemon-paprika mixture seeps into every nook and cranny. Halfway through the cooking process, I add a little water or stock to help steam those tough stems. Finally, the wedges get topped with a dusting of Old Bay breadcrumbs, which contrast nicely with the tangy capers. This is a fantastic side to pair with so many dinners in this book, but it also has enough star power on the plate to be rounded out with just a simple salad and grilled chicken breast.

*MAKE IT A MEAL: Serve alongside **Dijon Turkey Meat Loaf** (page 101), **Quinoa Paella** (page 151), **Mom's Millet Flour Fish Fry** (page 159)—the possibilities are endless!*

MAKES 4 SIDE SERVINGS

- 1 large head cauliflower (2 to 2 ½ pounds)
- 2 tablespoons avocado oil or extra-virgin olive oil
- 2 tablespoons fresh lemon juice
- 2 teaspoons smoked paprika
- ½ teaspoon sea salt
- 1 cup **Zesty Old Bay Breadcrumbs** (page 238)
- 1 cup vegetable stock or water
- 2 tablespoons capers
- 2 tablespoons unsalted butter, diced, or grass-fed ghee
- 1 tablespoon finely chopped fresh parsley (optional)

❶ Preheat the oven to 400°F.

❷ On a clean work surface, cut the cauliflower head into 8 wedges.

❸ In a 2-cup liquid measuring cup or small bowl, whisk together the oil, lemon juice, smoked paprika, and salt until combined.

❹ Lightly grease a large ovenproof cast-iron skillet (alternatively, use a baking dish, but I prefer a vehicle that is snugger around the cauliflower). Place the wedges in the skillet and slowly drizzle the sauce over them, allowing it to permeate every nook and cranny. Flip the wedges to ensure as much of the surface area is coated as possible. Arrange the wedges on one of their cut sides and transfer the skillet to the oven. Bake for 20 minutes until the bottoms of the wedges are nicely browned.

recipe continues →

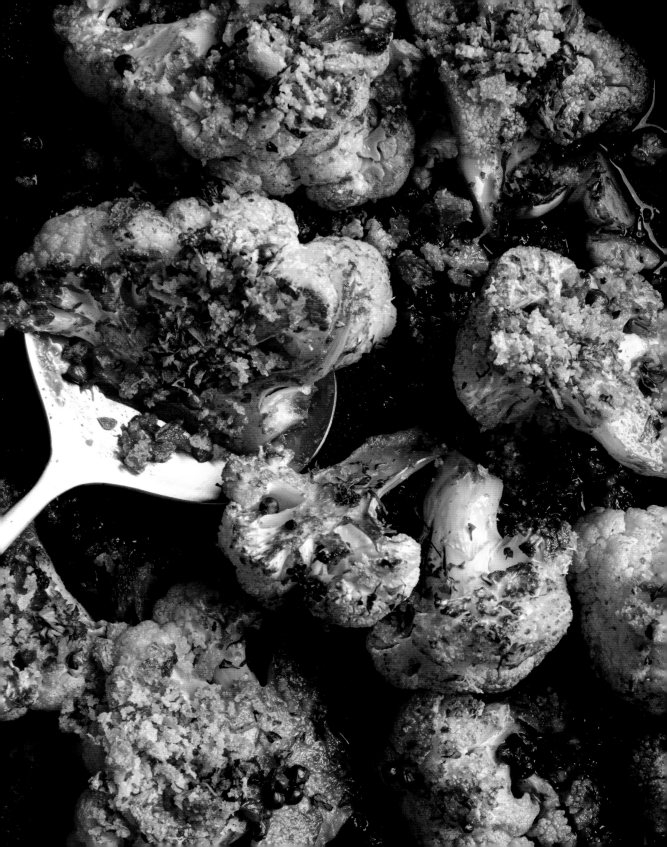

⑤ Meanwhile, make the **Zesty Old Bay Breadcrumbs**, if you haven't already.

⑥ Flip the cauliflower so each wedge is now sitting on its other cut side. Pour the stock over the cauliflower, sprinkle the capers around the skillet, and add the butter. Continue to bake for 20 minutes, or until the liquid is reduced to a pan sauce and the bottom of the cauliflower stems are tender enough to pierce easily with a knife. Using a spoon, baste the wedges with what remains of the caper butter.

⑦ Sprinkle the breadcrumbs over the wedges so they stick to the cauliflower as much as possible.

⑧ Serve directly from the skillet, garnished with parsley (if using), and enjoy warm or at room temperature.

GF Vgt SF   DF V   use plant-based butter

Grilled Balsamic Mushroom Melts

During my early twenties, fancy grilled cheese was my culinary medium of choice. I fell out of practice with my art once I became gluten-free but I'm picking up the reins again with these grilled mushroom melts. "Grilled" is the operative word here: The portobellos are grilled before being stuffed inside the bread, then the sandwiches themselves get grilled. I love the added effect of smoke on a meatless main course, but you can do this easily in a cast-iron pan if the grilling option isn't available. If you want to streamline things, simply grill the mushrooms with a splash of oil, salt, and balsamic, rather than the marinade.

MAKES 4 SERVINGS

- 4 large portobello mushrooms, stemmed
- ¼ cup **Charlie's Magic Grill Marinade** (page 71)
  Extra-virgin olive oil
- 8 slices gluten-free sourdough or whole-grain bread
- ½ cup **Arugula-Almond Pesto** (page 70) or store-bought pesto
- 8 slices white cheddar or mozzarella cheese (6 ounces)

① Arrange the mushroom caps on a large plate, or in a shallow baking dish, and drizzle with the marinade. Ensure every nook and cranny gets covered. The mushrooms can marinate all day, but aim for at least 10 minutes.

② Preheat an outdoor gas or charcoal grill to medium-high heat, or place a grill pan over medium-high heat on the stovetop.

③ Place the mushrooms on the grate, or in the pan, and grill for about 5 minutes per side, or until nicely charred. Transfer to the plate or baking dish with the marinade.

④ Arrange the bread on a work surface. Brush one side with oil and flip it over. Slather the naked side of the bread with pesto. Divide the cheese slices among the 8 bread slices. Top 4 of the slices with the mushrooms. Sandwich them together with the remaining bread, pesto-side down.

⑤ Place the sandwiches on the grill. Cook on the first side for 2 minutes, pressing down with a spatula. Rotate the sandwiches 90 degrees and cook for 1 minute more. Flip the sandwiches and repeat. Remove the sandwiches when the cheese is properly melted and you have a nice cross-hatch on the bread.

⑥ Cut the sandwiches in half and enjoy warm.

   GF Vgt SF DF V use plant-based cheese

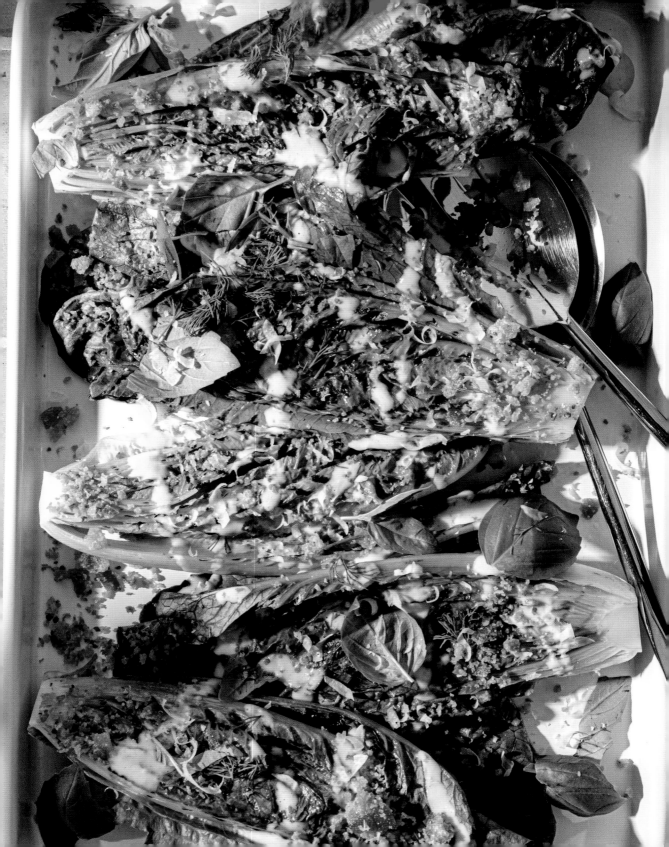

Grilled Romaine with Parmesan Pangritata & Caesar-ish Dressing

Pangritata is an Italian peasant garnish that is, essentially, poor man's parmesan. When money was tight in the old country, people would fry up coarsely chopped stale bread with garlic and herbs, and use that as a topping for pasta instead of grated cheese. In this recipe, I am combining poor man's parmesan with actual parmesan to create a dynamite topping for this salad. The charred romaine makes a sexy centerpiece, but it also tastes amazing raw if you don't want to bother with a flame.

MAKE IT A MEAL: This can easily be a main course salad with grilled shrimp or chicken added to it.

MAKES 6 SIDE SERVINGS

Breadcrumbs

¼	cup extra-virgin olive oil
1	garlic clove, minced
¾	cup fresh gluten-free breadcrumbs
⅓	cup grated parmesan cheese
¼	teaspoon sea salt

Salad

3	hearts of romaine lettuce, halved lengthwise
	Extra-virgin olive oil
½	cup **Caesar-ish Dressing** (page 63)
¼	cup torn fresh herbs (mint, dill, tarragon, or basil)

❶ **Make the breadcrumbs:** In a medium nonstick skillet, heat the oil over a medium flame. Add the garlic and breadcrumbs. Sauté until the crumbs are golden brown (if they brown too fast, turn the heat to low), about 5 minutes. Transfer to a bowl and immediately toss with the parmesan and salt. Set aside.

❷ **Make the salad:** Preheat an outdoor gas or charcoal grill to medium-high heat, or place a grill pan over medium-high heat on the stovetop. Dry the romaine with a clean kitchen towel and brush the cut sides lightly with oil. Place the lettuce, cut-side down, on the grate and grill until char marks form and the leaves begin to wilt slightly, 3 to 5 minutes. Transfer to a serving platter.

❸ Top the grilled romaine with a drizzle of dressing, followed by a pile of pangritata and herbs. Serve immediately.

GF SF Vgt LF omit garlic DF omit cheese

Greenhouse Gazpacho

Salmorejo is a Cordoban version of gazpacho using stale bread to override the slightly mealy texture of pureed raw vegetables. The result is the same orange-hued, velvety consistency as a cooked, pureed tomato soup. In this version, I use the stale bread trick to add volume and heft, but with all green vegetables. When we were living in Amsterdam, I had the best green gazpacho of my life at a restaurant called De Kas, which translates to The Greenhouse. Every day the soup is different, using any random herbs or greens grown on the premises that might otherwise go to waste. If you can't find green tomatoes, you can "recycle" other vegetables to bulk up the soup: avocado, celery, fennel, etc. You can also use parsley, basil, or chives for some of the spinach. This soup is truly a sippable salad—bright, tangy, and so good for you—and the bread creates a luscious, airy texture.

*CARB COMPANIONS: All you need for garnish is a drizzle of oil, but you can also add **Smoky Pumpkin-Hemp Sprinkles** (page 79), sliced avocado, a jammy egg, or flaked cooked fish.*

MAKES 4 SERVINGS

- 2 slices gluten-free sandwich bread, preferably stale or lightly toasted, cubed
- 2 medium green tomatoes (12 ounces), quartered
- 4 scallions, chopped
- 1 garlic clove
- 2 medium cucumbers (1 pound), unpeeled, quartered
- 2 cups packed baby spinach
- 2 tablespoons apple cider vinegar
- 2 tablespoons fresh lemon juice (from 1 lemon)
- 1 teaspoon sea salt
- ½ teaspoon ground cumin
- ½ cup extra-virgin olive oil, plus more for garnish

❶ In a blender or food processor, combine the bread, tomatoes, scallions, and garlic. Pulse until roughly combined.

❷ Add the cucumbers, spinach, vinegar, lemon juice, salt, cumin, and oil and puree until velvety green and frothy. Pour into bowls and garnish with a drizzle of oil and any carb companions you like.

GF DF Vgt V SF

LF omit garlic; green scallions only   **P** omit bread

Basque Tuna Salad Tartines

When I was traveling in the Basque region of Spain, I took a local cooking class, and among other dishes, I learned how to make a tuna salad that I've been riffing on ever since. The tweak is that instead of dried cranberries or raisins, the salad gets sweetness and acidity from tart green apples. If you dice them finely enough (which I recommend), you hardly notice them in the fish mixture until you take a bite, and there's a little something crunchy that you can't quite put your finger on. The benefit of a tartine is that you cut your carb consumption in half by using only one piece of bread. Because these are fancy sandwiches (they are open-face, after all), I recommend investing in a high quality tuna packed in olive oil.

MAKES 4 SERVINGS

8   ounces olive oil–packed tuna

1   small green apple, unpeeled, cored, and finely diced

1   small shallot, minced

¼   cup mayonnaise

2   tablespoons Dijon mustard

2   tablespoons fresh lemon juice (from 1 lemon)

2   tablespoons finely chopped fresh parsley or chives, divided

    Sea salt

4   slices gluten-free sourdough or whole-grain bread, toasted

❶ Place the tuna in a medium bowl (don't stress about draining all the liquid—some of that oil can carry over) and flake it into chunks with a fork. Stir in the apple, shallot, mayonnaise, mustard, lemon juice, and half the parsley until the tuna is fully incorporated. Taste for seasoning, and add salt, as needed.

❷ Scoop the tuna onto the toasted bread slices and smooth into an even layer. Sprinkle with the remaining parsley to serve.

  GF **DF** **SF** **P** serve in lettuce cups

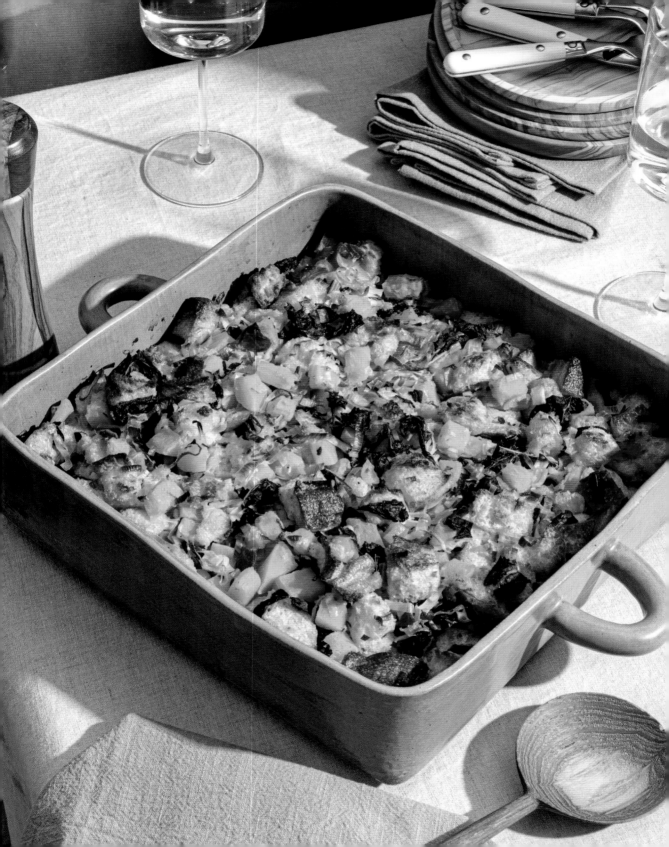

Butternut Squash & Leek Stuffing

Stuffing has been my contribution to our big fat Jewish Thanksgiving ever since I was a teenager. I've cycled through many variations over the years, but the equation has always been true to my Carbivore ethos: a crouton-packed veggie casserole. Two of the best years involved sweet, roasted butternut squash cubes and a silky, buttery leek confit, so for this immortalized Carbivore holiday side, you are getting BOTH. Each of the vegetable elements, along with the sautéed kale, can be made in advance and tossed together with the toasted bread on the day of. The stuffing itself can be baked (most of the way) a few hours ahead of the meal. Just wait until you're ready to eat to allow the top to crisp in the oven. I recommend using a good quality sourdough for this recipe, as bread is still the star of the show.

MAKES 10 SERVINGS

1	medium butternut squash (about 2 pounds), peeled and diced	3	large leeks, white and light green parts only, rinsed (see headnote, page 209), and thinly sliced		(preferably sourdough; from 1 large loaf)
	Extra-virgin olive oil	1	teaspoon chopped fresh rosemary or thyme leaves	2	large garlic cloves, minced
	Sea salt			4	cups chopped kale leaves (from 1 bunch)
4	tablespoons unsalted butter or plant-based alternative	1	cup dry white wine	3	large eggs, beaten
		8	cups cubed gluten-free bread	2	cups chicken or vegetable stock

❶ Preheat the oven to 425°F. Line a sheet pan with parchment paper.

❷ On the prepared sheet pan, toss together the butternut squash, **2 tablespoons oil**, and **½ teaspoon salt**. Arrange in an even layer and roast until nicely caramelized, about 30 minutes.

❸ Meanwhile, in a large Dutch oven or skillet over medium-low heat, melt the butter. Add the leeks and cook, stirring occasionally, until glassy and soft, about 10 minutes. Season with **½ teaspoon salt** and the rosemary. Continue cooking until the leeks melt into a sticky jam-like mixture, 15 minutes more. If they start to brown at any point, reduce the heat. Pour in the wine and simmer until the alcohol burns off, 3 minutes. Remove from the heat and taste for seasoning, adding more salt, as needed.

recipe continues →

④ When the butternut squash comes out of the oven, reduce the heat to 375°F. Transfer the squash to a large bowl and set aside. Reserve the sheet pan.

⑤ Add the cubed bread to the reserved sheet pan. Drizzle with 2 tablespoons oil and toss with the garlic. Arrange in an even layer and bake until the bread is lightly browned and dried out, 15 to 25 minutes, tossing once halfway through to redistribute. The fresher your bread, the longer it will take to toast.

⑥ Transfer the leeks to the bowl with the squash. Place the Dutch oven (no need to clean it) over medium heat. Add the kale and sauté until soft, about 5 minutes. Season lightly with salt and transfer to the bowl with the squash mixture. Everything up to this point can be made 2 days in advance, covered, and refrigerated.

⑦ When ready to bake the stuffing, preheat the oven to 375°F. Grease a 9 × 13-inch baking dish with oil.

⑧ In a 4-cup liquid measuring cup or medium bowl, whisk together the eggs and stock until smooth.

⑨ Toss the toasted bread with the veggie mixture, stock, and eggs. Let stand for 10 minutes, then toss again. When the liquid has been mostly absorbed by the bread, arrange the stuffing in an even layer in the prepared baking dish and cover with aluminum foil. Bake, covered, for 30 minutes. This can be done up to 4 hours in advance and set aside at room temperature.

⑩ When you're ready to eat, uncover the stuffing, and bake for 15 to 20 minutes until the top is crusty and brown.

GF   Vgt   DF   SF

Stuffed Artichokes with Italian Stallion Breadcrumbs

Instead of steaming artichokes whole, I hollow out the choke and stuff the cavity with seasoned breadcrumbs. The effort is worth it for the tender artichoke, crunchy bread morsels, and hit of acid (if you're dipping it) all in one bite. I like serving these with **Creamy Caper Dressing** (page 61) or **Basic Balsamic Vinaigrette** (page 60).

MAKES 2 TO 4 SERVINGS

2   large globe artichokes

½   lemon, cut into slices

1   bay leaf

1   garlic clove, crushed

1   cup **Italian Stallion Breadcrumbs** (page 239)

     Extra-virgin olive oil

     Sea salt

❶ Preheat the oven to 375°F.

❷ Trim the thick stem from the artichokes, leaving only a ½-inch stump. Using a serrated bread knife, cut the top 1 inch off the artichokes. With kitchen shears, snip off the thorny tips from all the remaining leaves. Pull open the center leaves of the artichokes. Using a small spoon (a serrated grapefruit spoon works well), uproot the tender yellow leaves and scrape out all of the fuzzy choke. Place the artichokes in a Dutch oven or lidded ovenproof pot that will hold them snugly, leaves facing up. Place the lemon slices, bay leaf, and garlic into the empty pockets around the artichokes. Spread the leaves apart and sprinkle the breadcrumbs over them so most get caught in the leaves or the center of the choke.

❸ Prepare a kettle of boiling water. Carefully pour the water between the artichokes (don't get the leaves wet!) until it comes ½ inch up the sides of the pot. Drizzle the tops of the artichokes with oil and season lightly with salt.

❹ Cover the pot and bake for 1 hour to 1 hour 10 minutes, or until the flesh of the outer petals is tender and easy to tear off with your teeth. If the crumbs have gone soggy (this doesn't usually happen), remove the lid and raise the oven to 450°F. Return the pot to the oven for a few minutes, until the crumbs are lightly browned. Enjoy alongside your favorite vinaigrette or aioli.

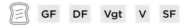 GF   DF   Vgt   V   SF

Pepperoni Pizza with Okra, Collards & Hot Honey

In spring 2020, we started a weekly tradition: TGIFPN (thank god it's Friday pizza night!). We became relative experts on the nuances of various toppings and gluten-free pizza crusts, both frozen and homemade. This pie straddles a salad and a pepperoni pizza, giving you the best of both worlds. Though there are collard greens and okra as carb companions, this is one of the few savory recipes in this book where I think adding a little sugar—in the form of spicy, sticky honey—is worth it. After all, you're eating pizza. Let's make that cheese count. If you start with dough instead of a frozen crust, simply roll it out and add your toppings. You may want to increase the oven temperature to 450° or 500°F. Otherwise, defer to the package directions. Lastly, if you have extra greens, well hallelujah, enjoy them as a starter while the pizza is in the oven!

CARB SWAP: Swap the hot honey for ½ cup fresh sweet corn kernels and 1 sliced jalapeño!

MAKES 2

- 1 bunch collard greens, thick stems removed, finely chopped
- 1 tablespoon fresh lime juice
- 1 tablespoon extra-virgin olive oil
- 1 garlic clove, minced
- ¼ teaspoon sea salt
- 2 gluten-free pizza crusts or dough (see headnote)
- ⅔ cup tomato sauce
- 1 cup shredded mozzarella cheese
- 8 okra pods, sliced
- 16 slices pepperoni or hard salami
- 1 teaspoon hot honey or honey with red pepper flakes

❶ Preheat the oven to 425°F. Line a baking sheet with parchment paper.

❷ In a medium bowl, combine the collards, lime juice, oil, garlic, and salt. Using clean hands, massage the collards until the leaves are coated well and wilted.

❸ Arrange the crusts on the prepared baking sheet. Spread ⅓ **cup tomato sauce** evenly over each crust. Sprinkle ¼ **cup mozzarella** over each, followed by a small handful of collard greens. Arrange the okra and pepperoni in an even layer. Top with the remaining cheese, divided evenly. Drizzle the pie with hot honey—the farther away you hold your spoon from the pie, the thinner the ribbons will be.

❹ Bake for about 15 minutes, or according to the package directions, if frozen, until the crust and cheese are lightly browned. Cut into slices and enjoy.

GF   **DF** use plant-based cheese   **Vgt** omit pepperoni   **SF** omit honey

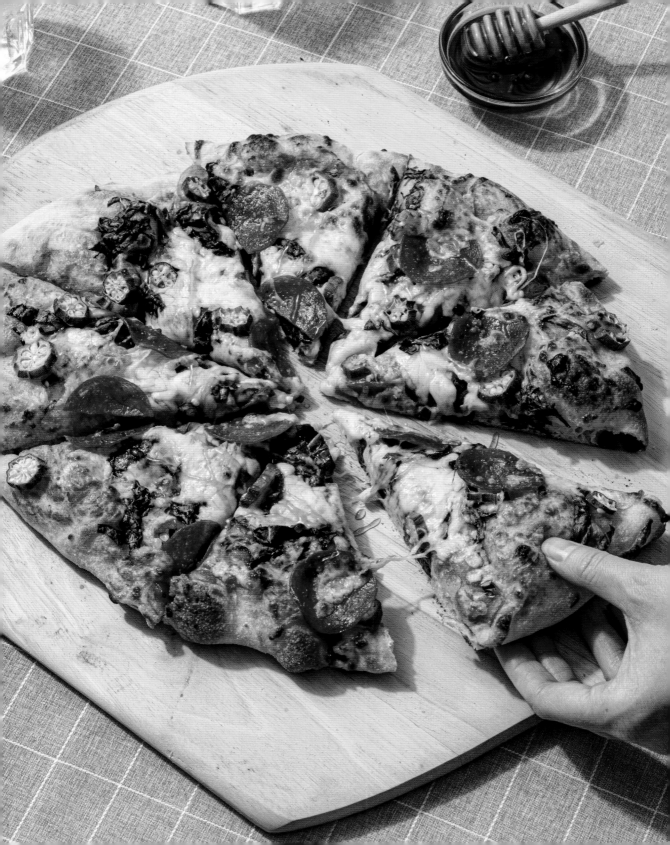

Apple-Cinnamon Baked French Toast

Baked French toast is more bread pudding than toast, but that's why I love it. The custard becomes one with the casserole and the top gives you that signature caramelization you expect. If you're serving this for dessert, it can be adjusted for sweetness by adding a drizzle of maple syrup on top. But I prefer, for obvious reasons, to keep things on the slightly savory side for breakfast. Though this recipe is easy enough for everyday meals, it is perfect for making ahead for a brunch spread and feeding a crowd. Enjoy it after one of the savory options like **Brussels Sprouts & Sweet Potato Hash with Eggs & Leftover Salsa** (page 212), **Chickpea Shakshuka with Summer Tomatoes** (page 306), or **Ham & Cheese Dutch Baby with Peas** (page 102) and you'll avoid any fructose frenzies.

CARB COMPANIONS: Serve topped with crème fraîche, full-fat plain Greek yogurt, coconut yogurt, or almond butter, and a sprinkle of chia seeds.

MAKES 8 SERVINGS

3 small Granny Smith apples (about 1 pound), unpeeled, cored, and finely diced into ⅛-inch pieces	½ cup unsweetened almond milk or oat milk	1 teaspoon ground ginger
1 tablespoon chia seeds	6 large eggs	½ teaspoon ground cardamom
1 ¾ teaspoons ground cinnamon, divided	¼ cup maple syrup	½ teaspoon sea salt
One 13.5-ounce can full-fat coconut milk	4 tablespoons coconut oil, unsalted butter, or grass-fed ghee, melted	1 loaf gluten-free sandwich bread (about 14 slices), preferably stale
	1 teaspoon vanilla extract	½ cup raw pecans, roughly chopped

❶ In a small saucepan over medium heat, combine the apples, chia seeds, **½ cup water**, and **¼ teaspoon cinnamon**. Bring the mixture to a boil, then reduce the heat to maintain a simmer. Cook until the apples are tender and most of the water has been absorbed, about 15 minutes, stirring every 3 to 5 minutes to prevent your compote from sticking or burning.

❷ Meanwhile, in a large bowl, whisk together the coconut milk, almond milk, eggs, maple syrup, coconut oil, vanilla, remaining **1 ½ teaspoons cinnamon**, ginger, cardamom, and salt until smooth. Don't worry if there are still some coconut cream chunks—they will dissolve in the oven.

③ Grease a 15-inch cast-iron skillet or 9 × 13-inch casserole dish with oil. Arrange half the bread slices in an even layer in the prepared dish, overlapping layers or tearing the bread into smaller pieces to fit. Top with the compote, then repeat the bread layer. Pour the custard evenly over the bread, using the back of a spoon to press down any rogue pieces so they are all, more or less, submerged. Let rest at room temperature for at least 30 minutes so the bread absorbs the custard, pressing down on the bread occasionally to flatten it. You can also cover the dish and refrigerate it overnight.

④ When ready to bake the apple French toast, preheat the oven to 400°F.

⑤ Bake for 20 minutes, then sprinkle with the pecans and continue to bake for 15 minutes, or until the bread is puffed like a soufflé and nicely browned on top. Let rest in the pan for at least 10 minutes before cutting into squares.

⑥ Dust the French toast with cinnamon and serve topped with any carb companions you like and additional maple syrup, as needed.

GF   DF   Vgt

LF   sub blueberries, strawberries, or raspberries for apple

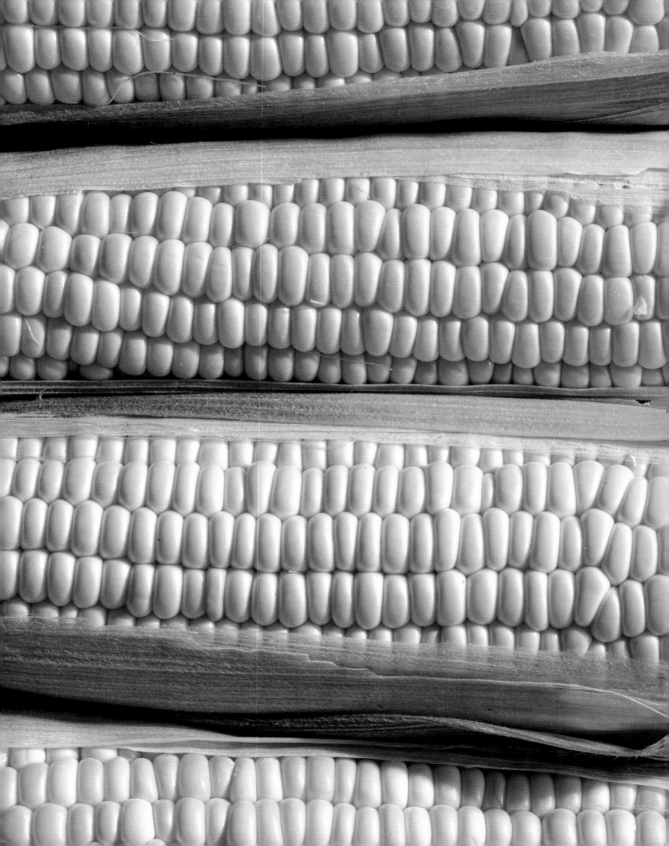

CORN

. . .

Mexican Street Corn & Collard Greens Salad

Crispy Polenta Cakes with Eggplant—Cherry Tomato Caponata

Zucchini Skillet Cornbread

Creamless Corn & Shrimp Chowder

Cajun Pork Tenderloin with Grits & Zucchini Hash

Jalapeño, Pumpkin & Corn Pudding

Seedy "Avocado Toast" Arepas

Summer Squash Succotash Enchiladas

Chicken Tinga Stew with Hominy & Kale

Baked Fish Tacos with Ginger-Mango Slaw

Upside-Down Strawberry-Rhubarb Polenta Cake

Sweet Corn

Sweet corn is at its peak midsummer and is best bought fresh and local, as close to harvesting time as you can get it. The kernels turn into nature's candy when slowly caramelized on the stove and are a wonderful accent to summer salads (see **Mexican Street Corn & Collard Greens Salad**, page 271). You can use the whole cobs to create a milky, flavorful vegetable stock, or blend some of the kernels into a soup to add creaminess and depth (see **Creamless Corn & Shrimp Chowder**, page 277). During winter months, frozen corn is easily accessible and perfect for casseroles. I've combined it with another seasonal favorite in my **Jalapeño, Pumpkin & Corn Pudding** (page 281).

Polenta or Grits

Popular preparation method: absorption

Ratio: 1 cup polenta or grits to 4 cups liquid

Cook time: 25 to 40 minutes

In Italy, polenta is derived from a specific type of corn, but you can equate it with any medium-ground cornmeal. Grits are traditionally more coarsely ground and take longer to cook as a result. These days, you can use the two interchangeably, using the absorption method in a large pot of water, milk, or stock to cook them. If you keep your cornmeal porridge on the soupy side, you'll have a perfect soft bed for shrimp or **Cajun Pork Tenderloin with Zucchini Hash** (page 279). If you allow the liquid to cook off a little longer, your creamy polenta will become easy to mold like a dough, which will allow you to cool and cut it into any shape you like (see **Crispy Polenta Cakes with Eggplant–Cherry Tomato Caponata**, page 272). You can often find store-bought polenta prepared up until this point in round tubes (like cookie dough), so feel free to use that shortcut if you are making polenta cakes. I find it much more useful and economical to store the dried grain in my pantry, which also comes in handy for making toothsome baked goods like **Upside-Down Strawberry-Rhubarb Polenta Cake** (page 293).

Cornmeal

More finely ground than grits or polenta, for baked goods (see **Zucchini Skillet Cornbread**, page 275 or **Jalapeño, Pumpkin & Corn Pudding**, page 281), you'll want to use cornmeal. This is perfect for giving cakes a sandy texture. White and yellow varieties are common, but like most grains, you'll get even more nutrient density if you opt for blue, red, or pink cornmeal.

Corn Flour & Masa Harina

Corn flour is the superfine ground version of cornmeal. It is light, fluffy, and similar in texture and volume to other gluten-free flours. You can use it in place of oat flour or rice flour to add sweetness to a recipe—I particularly like it in tart crusts. Masa harina is a type of corn flour made from nixtamalized hominy. The process allows the dough to bind better, which makes it the ideal base for making fresh tortillas for tacos, like my **Baked Fish Tacos with Ginger-Mango Slaw** (page 291). A special type of Colombian masa harina is sold specifically for arepas (see **Seedy "Avocado Toast" Arepas**, page 282).

Hominy

Hominy is dried whole corn kernels that have been nixtamalized (see preceding). When ground, they become the basis for masa harina, but you can also find them whole in the canned food aisle. The kernels taste very different from whole sweet corn—they are larger, slightly sour, and chewy. Hominy is used most commonly in soups and stews (like Mexican pozole) so the kernels can soften further and soak up the surrounding flavors. They add incredible texture to **Chicken Tinga Stew with Hominy & Kale** (page 288).

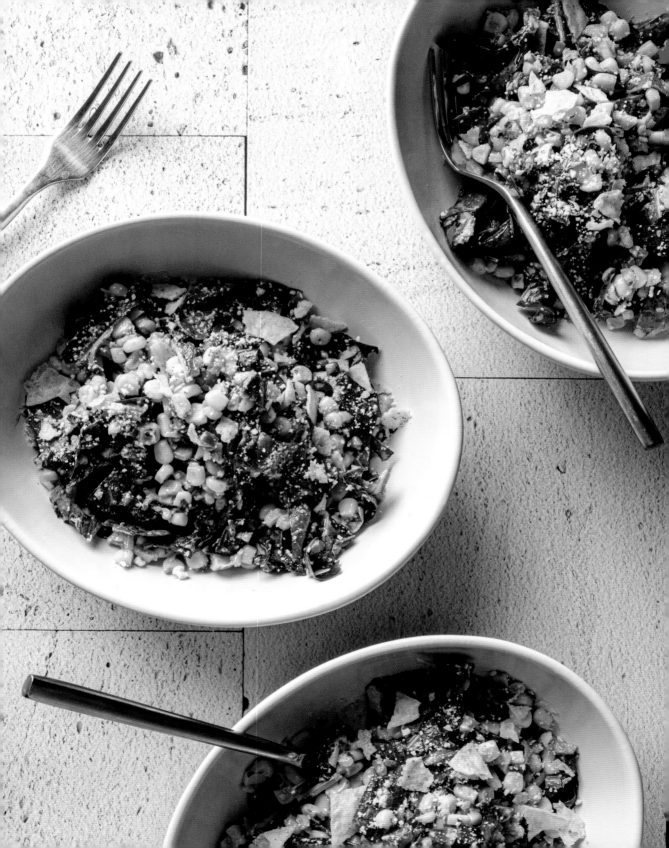

Mexican Street Corn & Collard Greens Salad

Elote, a staple of street vendors in Mexico, is, essentially, corn on the cob charred on a grill, then slathered with a spicy lime-y mayonnaise mixture and Cotija cheese. Because my face often looks like a feral, condiment-covered animal after eating elote, I prefer to enjoy it in salad form, with the kernels removed from the cobs and tossed with cilantro and scallions. If I'm being honest, it also ups the corn-to-mayo ratio in my favor. I've added collard greens massaged with a good dose of citrus, oil, and salt for a hearty base. Like kale, collards are one of the few salad options that can be dressed ahead and last a few days in the fridge, so feel free to make this in advance (omitting the tortilla topping).

CHANGE OF SEASON: In fall, sub roasted diced sweet potatoes or butternut squash for the corn.

MAKES 6 SIDE SERVINGS

1 bunch collard greens, thick stems removed, sliced into ribbons	4 scallions, thinly sliced, white and green parts separated	2 tablespoons mayonnaise
Extra-virgin olive oil		½ teaspoon chili powder
Sea salt	1 jalapeño, seeded and finely chopped	¼ cup finely crumbled Cotija cheese (optional)
3 tablespoons fresh lime juice, divided	1 garlic clove, minced	
3 cups fresh sweet corn kernels (from 4 ears)	½ cup roughly chopped fresh cilantro leaves	Handful corn tortilla chips (optional)

1 In a large bowl, combine the collard greens, **2 tablespoons oil, ½ teaspoon salt,** and **1 tablespoon lime juice.** Using clean hands, massage the oil into the leaves until they are fully coated and beginning to soften. Set aside.

2 Heat **2 tablespoons oil** in a large heavy-bottomed skillet over high heat. Add the corn and cook, allowing the corn to char undisturbed for a few minutes at a time, until nicely browned, about 10 minutes. Off the heat, add the white scallions, jalapeño, and garlic. Season lightly with salt and toss until combined, allowing the mixture to sizzle gently in the hot pan until fragrant, 1 minute.

3 Transfer the corn to another bowl and stir together with the remaining **2 tablespoons lime juice,** cilantro, green scallions, mayo, chili powder, and cheese (if using).

4 Add the corn mixture to the greens and toss to distribute. When you're ready to eat, crumble the tortilla chips (if using) on top to create small, crunchy shards.

GF Vgt SF DF omit cheese V use plant-based mayo; omit cheese

Crispy Polenta Cakes with Eggplant–Cherry Tomato Caponata

My days of catering large parties are long behind me, but when I was at my busiest, I was prepping for all my events out of a studio apartment with two feet of counter space. That meant that, often, my freezer was 80 percent polenta bites. Creamy polenta can become the ultimate blank canvas when turned out onto a sheet pan and chilled in the fridge. Having a party? Cut it into two-inch rounds for finger food or go with larger rectangles for a vegetarian main course. Whatever the shape, you can freeze the cakes, then bake them until crispy before the meal. This eggplant caponata is my go-to topping. What it lacks in beauty, it makes up for in flavor, especially with the addition of cherry tomatoes. Like the polenta, the caponata can be made a few days ahead and served on top of the reheated crispy cakes at room temperature.

MAKE IT A MEAL: **Back-Pocket Tricolore Salad** *(page 82) is all you need on the side. Leftovers make a great savory breakfast with a fried egg on top!*

MAKES 6 SERVINGS

Polenta

One 13.5-ounce can full-fat coconut milk, or 2 cups plant-based milk

4 cups vegetable stock or water

1 ½ cups polenta

1 tablespoon grass-fed ghee, unsalted butter, or coconut oil

Sea salt

Caponata

2 tablespoons extra-virgin olive oil

1 onion, finely diced

2 medium eggplants (2 pounds), cut into ½-inch cubes (about 8 cups)

2 garlic cloves, minced

1 ½ teaspoons sea salt

½ teaspoon red pepper flakes

1 pint cherry tomatoes, halved

¼ cup golden raisins

2 tablespoons balsamic vinegar

⅓ cup coarsely chopped fresh basil

❶ Line a 9 × 13-inch baking dish with parchment paper using two sheets, one for the length and one for the width, so there's at least a 2-inch flap up the sides of the pan. Clear a shelf in the refrigerator and line it with a towel.

❷ **Make the polenta:** In a large Dutch oven or stockpot over high heat, combine the coconut milk and stock and bring to a boil. Be careful once it starts steaming that it doesn't foam over. Pour in the polenta. Reduce the heat to low and cook, whisking frequently, until the polenta has thickened to the point of clumping inside the whisk when you lift it, about 15 minutes, depending on the coarseness of the polenta.

recipe continues →

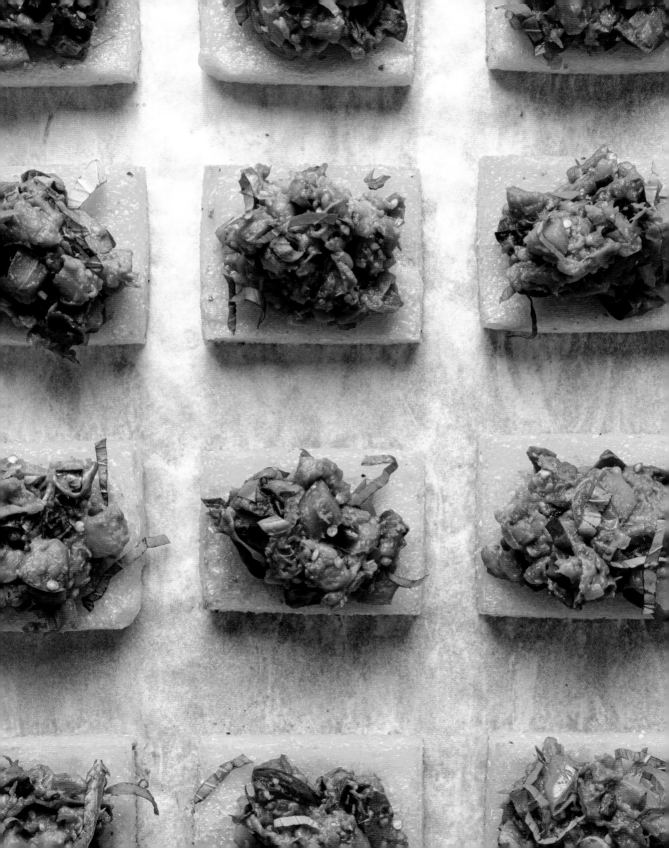

Stir in the ghee until melted and taste for seasoning, adding salt, as needed (if you used water, you will need about 1 teaspoon).

3 Pour the polenta into the prepared pan and smooth it into an even layer with a rubber spatula. Refrigerate the polenta, uncovered, until cool and very firm, at least 30 minutes, or overnight.

4 Preheat the oven to 425°F. Line a baking sheet with parchment paper.

5 Cut the polenta into 12 even rectangles, triangles, or circles. Arrange the polenta cakes, leaving a little room between each, on the prepared baking sheet.

6 Bake until the edges are crispy but the cakes are still pillowy to the touch, 30 to 40 minutes. If you begin with frozen cakes, or prefer them crunchy and lightly browned, aim for 40 minutes to 1 hour.

7 **Make the caponata:** Meanwhile, in a large Dutch oven or saucepan, heat the oil over medium heat. Add the onion and eggplant and sauté, stirring occasionally, until the eggplant is al dente, about 10 minutes. Add more oil to the pan, as needed, but don't worry about the browned bits on the bottom—those will come up later. Add the garlic, salt, and red pepper flakes and cook for 2 minutes. Add the cherry tomatoes and cook for about 8 minutes until the acidity of the tomatoes has cooked off and the eggplant is beginning to fall apart. Off the heat, stir in the raisins, vinegar, and half the basil. The eggplant mixture can be made 2 days ahead and kept refrigerated.

8 Transfer the polenta cakes to a serving platter and top with the caponata. Garnish with the remaining basil and enjoy warm or at room temperature.

  GF **DF** **Vgt** **V** **LF** omit onion and garlic **SF** omit raisins

Zucchini Skillet Cornbread

If the zucchini in the title didn't already warn you, this is your savory cornbread PSA! The vegetables melt away (similar to zucchini bread) but help keep the cornbread moist. It also makes this ordinarily sweet, simple carb confection a little friendlier for your blood sugar. If in season, fresh corn kernels add more sweetness and heft to the bread. Another addition in the savory department would be ½ cup shredded cheddar cheese sprinkled on top before baking.

*MAKE IT A MEAL: Serve with **Chicken Tinga Stew** (page 288) or **BBQ Chicken Thighs** (page 303).*

MAKES 8 SERVINGS

5   tablespoons grass-fed ghee or unsalted butter, divided

1   cup brown rice flour

¾   cup stone-ground cornmeal

2 ½ teaspoons baking powder

1 ¼ teaspoons sea salt

2   large eggs, beaten

1   cup unsweetened oat or almond milk

2   tablespoons honey or maple syrup

1   large (12-ounce) zucchini, coarsely grated

1   cup fresh sweet corn kernels (optional)

¼   cup fresh cilantro, finely chopped

1   jalapeño, thinly sliced (optional)

① Preheat the oven to 400°F. Place a large (12- to 15-inch) cast-iron skillet on the center rack.

② In a large microwave-safe bowl, melt **4 tablespoons ghee** in the microwave. Let cool.

③ Meanwhile, in a medium bowl, stir together the rice flour, cornmeal, baking powder, and salt.

④ Add the eggs, milk, and honey to the cooled melted ghee and stir until blended. Stir in the zucchini, corn (if using), and cilantro. Stir the flour mixture into the wet ingredients until just combined.

⑤ Remove the skillet from the oven, add the remaining **1 tablespoon ghee** to melt, and swirl until it coats the pan. Pour the batter into the hot skillet. Arrange the jalapeño slices (if using) on top.

⑥ Bake for 30 to 40 minutes, or until the sides are golden brown, the top is crackly, and a wooden toothpick inserted into the center comes out clean. Let the cornbread rest in the skillet for 10 minutes, or until cool enough to touch. Cut into slices and serve directly in the pan. It's best warm or at room temperature.

GF   DF   Vgt   LF omit corn kernels   SF omit sweetener

Corn

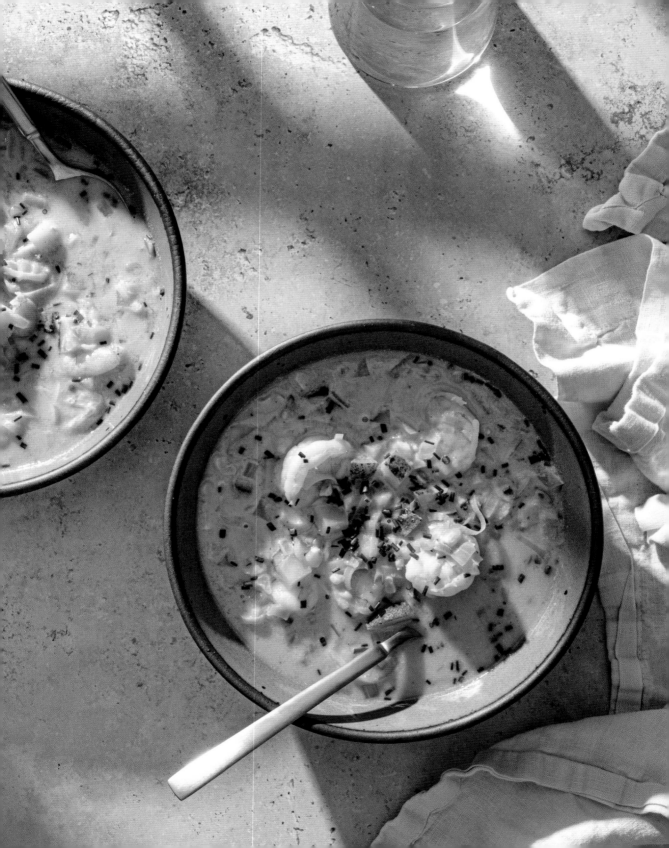

Creamless Corn & Shrimp Chowder

Although I eat dairy-free most of the time, I can never turn down a good chowder. At home, I use coconut milk and diced potato to add creaminess. The trick is to puree a few cups of soup and whisk it back into the pot. Corn and shrimp is a classic pairing because their sweetness complements each other. If you want to level up this chowder even more, save the corn cobs and shrimp tails and turn them into stock! For more fiber, top the soup with diced avocado or add 2 cups of chopped kale (in step 5).

MAKES 4 SERVINGS

2	tablespoons extra-virgin olive oil or unsalted butter
1	Vidalia onion, finely diced
1	leek, white and light green parts only, thinly sliced
1	garlic clove, minced
1	medium Yukon Gold potato, finely diced
½	cup dry white wine
1	cup clam juice
One 13.5-ounce can full-fat coconut milk	
2	cups fish, chicken, or vegetable stock
1	teaspoon sea salt
3	cups fresh sweet corn kernels
12	ounces large shrimp, peeled, deveined, and tails removed
2	tablespoons fresh lemon juice
1	teaspoon hot sauce
2	tablespoons finely chopped fresh chives

❶ In a large Dutch oven or saucepan, heat the oil over medium heat. Add the onion and leek; sauté until translucent and just beginning to caramelize, 8 minutes. Add the garlic and cook for 1 minute.

❷ Stir in the potato, then pour in the wine, clam juice, coconut milk, and stock. Add the salt. Increase the heat to medium-high and bring to a simmer. Simmer for about 15 minutes, or until the potatoes are fork-tender.

❸ Stir in the corn and cook for 3 minutes until just vibrant in color.

❹ With a stand or immersion blender, puree 2 cups of soup (or roughly one-fourth of the pot) until smooth. Reincorporate the pureed soup into the pot—the broth will thicken immediately.

❺ Stir in the shrimp and return the soup to a gentle simmer over medium-low heat. Cook until the shrimp are pink and curled, about 3 minutes. Off the heat, stir in the lemon juice, hot sauce, and half the chives.

❻ Ladle the chowder into bowls and garnish with the remaining chives.

GF DF SF   P omit corn

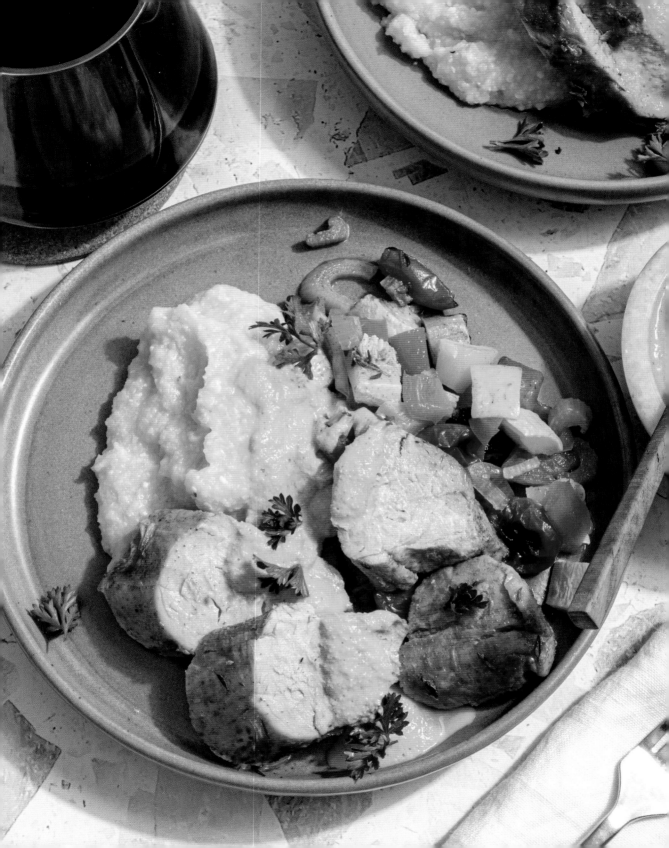

Cajun Pork Tenderloin with Grits & Zucchini Hash

When I'm making a sheet pan meal, I try to avoid dirtying other cookware. But, occasionally, the additional elements are so good they are impossible to resist. In this case, an assortment of summer vegetables are roasted beneath a Cajun-inspired pork tenderloin and served over a simple pot of well-seasoned grits. The creamy tomato vinaigrette is optional, since the grits in some ways are a sauce in and of themselves (and . . . dirty pans), but the bright acidity offsets the spicy pork and rich corn porridge. If you're the type of person who plans in advance, the pork can be marinated all day or overnight—it will just get better as it sits. The vinaigrette, similarly, can be done ahead. And the grits cook up in roughly the same amount of time as the pork hangs out in the oven.

*CARB SWAP: Serve the pork over brown rice, quinoa, or **Braised Lemony Colcannon** (page 213).*

MAKES 4 SERVINGS

2 tablespoons apple cider vinegar	2 medium celery stalks, thinly sliced	4 cups chicken stock or water
1 garlic clove, minced	1 shallot, thinly sliced	1 cup uncooked grits or polenta (not instant or quick cooking)
1 teaspoon paprika	1 red bell pepper, diced	
1 teaspoon fresh thyme leaves, or ½ teaspoon dried	1 medium zucchini (8 ounces), diced	2 tablespoons unsalted butter, grass-fed ghee, or extra-virgin olive oil
¼ teaspoon cayenne pepper	1 medium summer squash (8 ounces), diced	½ cup **Summer Tomato-Cashew Dressing** (page 59; optional)
Extra-virgin olive oil	1 pint cherry tomatoes, halved, or 10 ounces vine tomatoes (2 medium), diced	2 tablespoons fresh flat-leaf parsley leaves
Sea salt		
1 pound pork tenderloin		

❶ Preheat the oven to 450°F. Line a rimmed sheet pan with parchment paper.

❷ In a medium bowl, whisk together the vinegar, garlic, paprika, thyme, cayenne, **2 tablespoons oil**, and **½ teaspoon salt**. Add the pork and swish around until coated in the marinade. Set aside to marinate at room temperature. This can also be done overnight in the fridge, covered.

❸ On the prepared sheet pan, toss together the celery, shallot, bell pepper, zucchini, summer squash, cherry tomatoes, **2 tablespoons oil**, and **½ teaspoon salt** until coated. Arrange in an even layer.

recipe continues →

Corn

④ Remove the pork from the marinade and nestle it on the vegetables. Drizzle the remaining marinade over the veggies.

⑤ Roast for 25 to 30 minutes until the pork is nicely browned on top and firm to the touch, or the internal temperature reads 145°F. Transfer the pork to a work surface and let rest for at least 10 minutes, then thinly slice on a diagonal. If the veggies aren't caramelized enough, return them to the oven for 5 minutes.

⑥ While the pork roasts, make the grits. In a medium saucepan or Dutch oven over high heat, bring the stock to a boil. Add **½ teaspoon salt,** then slowly stream in the grits, stirring constantly. Reduce the heat to low and simmer, stirring occasionally, until the grits are creamy and tender, 15 to 20 minutes. Off the heat, stir in the butter. If the polenta finishes before the pork, add some stock or water in ¼-cup increments and whisk over low heat until hot and loose again when you're ready to eat.

⑦ Divide the grits, vegetables, and sliced pork among four bowls or plates. Drizzle with the tomato vinaigrette (if using), and garnish with parsley.

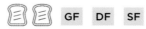 GF DF SF

LF omit garlic, shallot, and celery   P omit grits

Jalapeño, Pumpkin & Corn Pudding

It's always surprising to me that corn pudding is a winter holiday staple when corn is so far from its peak season. That said, frozen corn is available year-round, so there should be no stopping you! You know what else is available year-round? Pumpkin puree. This vegetable pairing is wonderfully delicious, whether you enjoy it in summer with fresh corn or during winter months with frozen. The pumpkin turns the pudding a luscious golden color and adds another layer of natural sweetness and creamy body. But other than that and the nutrients it provides, you'd hardly know it's there. Naturally sweet with plenty of fat and protein from the eggs and coconut oil to round out the carbs, this pudding is a model year-round Carbivore side.

*MAKE IT A MEAL: Serve with **BBQ Chicken Thighs** (page 303), **Roasted Sweet Potatoes with Beans & Greens** (page 311), or **Dijon Turkey Meat Loaf** (page 101).*

MAKES 6 TO 8 SERVINGS

One 15-ounce can (or 1 ½ cups) unsweetened pumpkin puree

4   large eggs

1   tablespoon honey or maple syrup

¼   cup melted coconut oil, unsalted butter, or grass-fed ghee, at room temperature

1   cup unsweetened almond or oat milk

¼   cup stone-ground cornmeal

1   teaspoon sea salt

4   cups (1 pound) fresh or frozen sweet corn kernels

4   scallions, thinly sliced

1   jalapeño, seeded and thinly sliced

① Preheat the oven to 375°F. Lightly grease a 9 × 13-inch baking dish or a large (15-inch) ovenproof cast-iron skillet with oil.

② In a large bowl, beat the pumpkin puree and eggs until smooth. Stir in the honey and melted coconut oil until incorporated. Fold in the milk, followed by the cornmeal, salt, corn kernels (no need to thaw if frozen), scallions, and jalapeño until just combined. Pour the corn mixture into the prepared pan.

③ Bake until the pudding is set and the sides are browned, about 30 minutes. If you want the top to have more color, place the dish under the broiler for 1 minute. Let the pudding rest in the pan for 5 minutes to firm up, then serve warm.

  GF **DF** **Vgt**   **SF** omit sweetener

Seedy "Avocado Toast" Arepas

Avocado toast is a staple workweek savory breakfast for me, and it's fun to have another vehicle on hand that's packed with fiber. Arepas are thin, crispy corn cakes that are common in northern South America, often sliced in half and stuffed like a sandwich. In this version, I've taken a hard left turn from tradition by adding some carb companions to the dough: flaxseed meal and hemp seeds. The arepas can be pan-fried in advance and reheated (or thawed—they freeze well) in a 400°F oven until their shells become hard again.

MAKES 4 SERVINGS

1 cup masa harina, areparina, or masarepa (not cornmeal or corn flour)

¼ cup flaxseed meal

¼ cup hemp seeds

Sea salt

Avocado oil

2 avocados

2 tablespoons fresh lemon or lime juice

4 red radishes, thinly sliced

Hot sauce

1¼ cups **Smoky Pumpkin-Hemp Sprinkles** (page 79)

❶ Preheat the oven to 400°F. Line a baking sheet with parchment paper.

❷ In a medium bowl, combine the masa harina, flaxseed meal, hemp seeds, and **½ teaspoon salt**. Stir in **1¼ cups water** (at room temperature), then let sit for 5 minutes. Form the dough into a ball and pat it smooth. Divide the ball in half, and each half into quarters so you have 8 balls, about ¼ cup dough per ball. Flatten balls between your palms to form ¼-inch patties. Pat out any cracks and place the patties on the prepared baking sheet.

❸ In a large cast-iron skillet, heat a thin layer of oil over medium-high heat. Working in batches, add the arepas to the skillet and cook for 3 to 5 minutes per side until a golden crust forms, adjusting the heat if they start to burn. Transfer to the prepared baking sheet. Repeat with the remaining arepas, adding more oil, as needed.

❹ Bake the arepas for about 10 minutes, or until fully cooked through and hard on the outside. Set aside to cool.

❺ Meanwhile, in a medium bowl, mash together the avocados, lemon juice, and **1 teaspoon salt**.

❻ Top each arepa with some mashed avocado and sliced radishes. Season lightly with salt and a dash of hot sauce. Garnish with the pumpkin-hemp sprinkles.

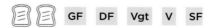 GF DF Vgt V SF

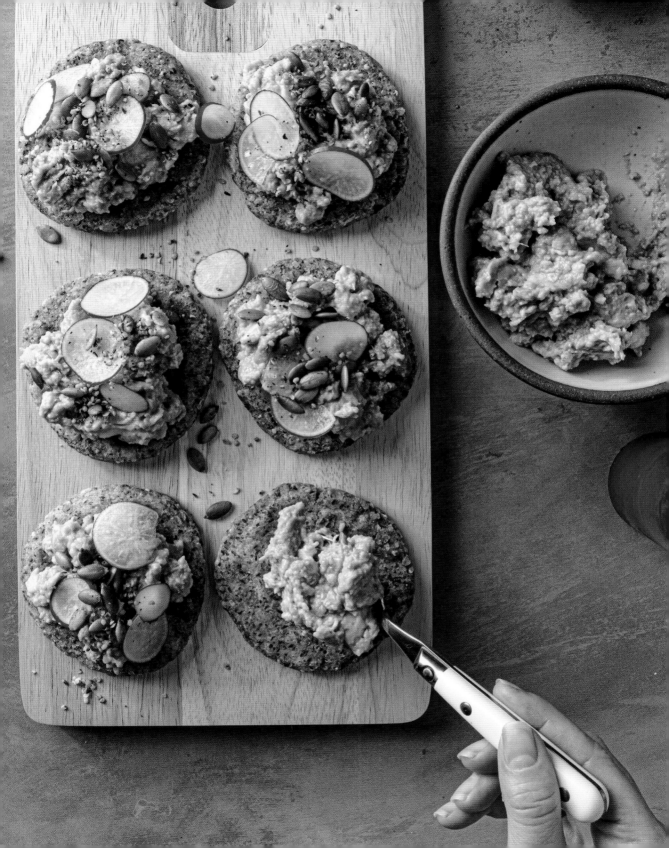

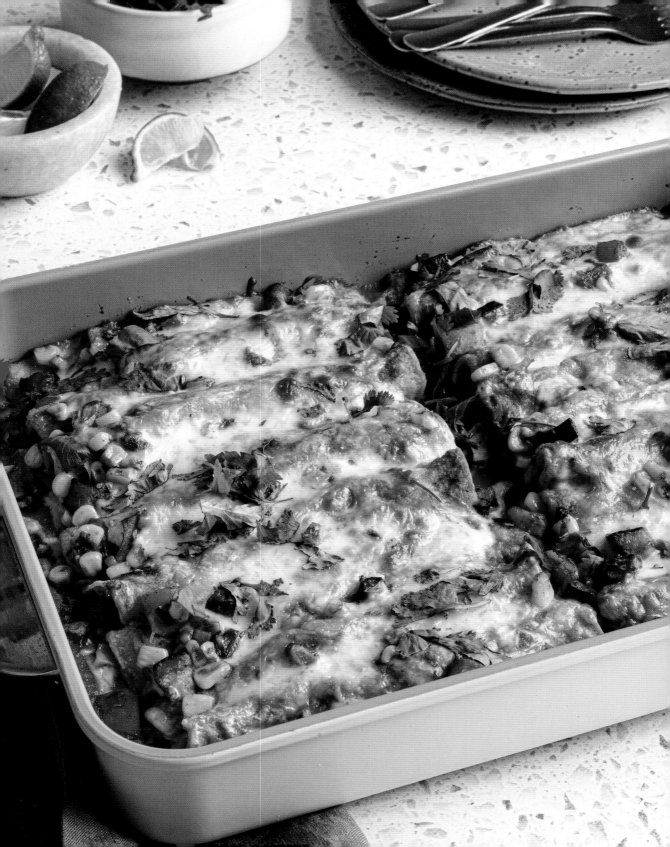

Summer Squash Succotash Enchiladas

I tend to think of most casseroles as fall or winter comfort foods, but these enchiladas are ideal for summer's end, when nights are getting a little cooler, yet tomatoes, corn, and summer squash are still popping off at the farmers' market. Since enchiladas often cook down into a deliciously soft, gooey mess, the fresh corn gives the casserole much-needed texture in addition to sweetness. Though I've designed this recipe to suit more ubiquitous six-inch corn tortillas, my favorite gluten-free option for enchiladas is Siete Foods' cassava or almond flour varieties. Their pliability is closer to a flour tortilla and they are a little larger (about eight inches). If using traditional corn tortillas, warm them, per the instructions, to avoid any splitting. If this happens, though, any imperfections can be covered with sauce and cheese!

*CARB COMPANIONS: Top with **Smoky Pumpkin-Hemp Sprinkles** (page 79) or diced avocado.*

MAKES 6 SERVINGS

Sauce

⅓ cup raw unsalted cashews

24 ounces marinara or tomato sauce (about 3 cups)

2 scallions, roughly chopped

1 jalapeño, seeded

1 teaspoon ground cumin

1 teaspoon chili powder

¾ teaspoon sea salt

Filling

2 tablespoons extra-virgin olive or avocado oil

1 medium zucchini (8 ounces), finely diced

1 medium summer squash (8 ounces), finely diced

4 scallions, sliced

2 garlic cloves, minced

2 cups fresh corn kernels

1 teaspoon sea salt

½ teaspoon ground turmeric

½ teaspoon ground cumin

½ teaspoon chili powder

2 medium vine or Roma tomatoes (8 ounces), diced

2 tablespoons fresh lime juice

Enchiladas

Twelve 6-inch corn tortillas (see headnote)

1 ½ cups shredded sharp white cheddar or Monterey Jack cheese

½ cup roughly chopped fresh cilantro

1 lime, cut into 8 wedges

1 Preheat the oven to 425°F.

2 **Begin the sauce:** Bring a kettle of water to a boil. Place the cashews in a blender or food processor and cover with **⅔ cup boiling water**. Set aside for at least 10 minutes.

recipe continues →

Corn

③ **Make the filling:** In a large skillet or Dutch oven, heat the oil over medium heat. Add the zucchini and summer squash and sauté until tender and beginning to brown, about 10 minutes. Stir in the scallions, garlic, corn, salt, turmeric, cumin, and chili powder. Cook for about 3 minutes until fragrant. Add the tomatoes and cook for about 5 minutes until they just begin to release their juices. Off the heat, stir in the lime juice.

④ **Finish the sauce:** Pour the tomato sauce into the blender with the cashews and add the scallions, jalapeño, cumin, chili powder, and salt. Puree until smooth, creamy, and orange in hue. Taste for seasoning, and add more salt, as needed. Pour 1 ½ cups of the sauce into a 9 × 13-inch baking dish and spread it evenly to cover the bottom.

⑤ **Make the enchiladas:** Wrap the tortillas in a clean kitchen towel and warm them in the microwave for 30 seconds until pliable. Alternatively, warm them in the oven for 10 minutes, or individually on the stovetop.

⑥ Divide the succotash among the tortillas, along with 1 tablespoon cheese. Roll the tortillas tightly around the filling and line them up snugly, seam-side down, in the baking dish. If they crack, don't worry. Slather the remaining sauce over the enchiladas and sprinkle with the remaining cheese and any leftover filling.

⑦ Bake until the cheese is melted and golden brown and the sauce is bubbling, about 15 minutes. Let the enchiladas rest for a few minutes, then garnish with the cilantro and serve alongside the lime wedges.

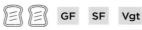

GF   **SF**   **Vgt**

LF omit cashews and garlic; green scallions only   **DF**   **V** use plant-based cheese

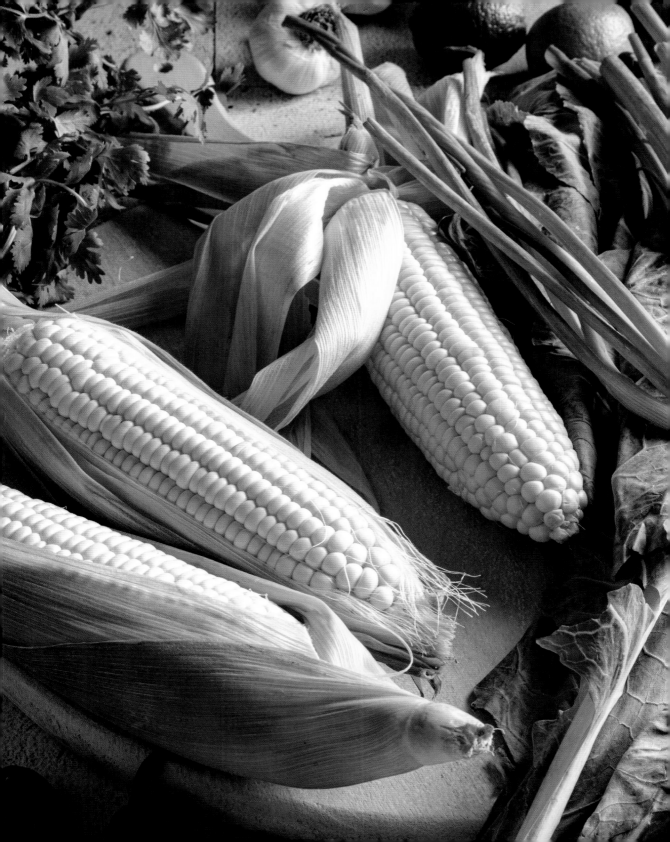

Chicken Tinga Stew with Hominy & Kale

You'll usually find chicken tinga, a concoction of tomatoes and chipotles in adobo, on restaurant menus as a taco filling. But since it's shredded and saucy, the base lends itself well to a low and slow stew with lots of greens and a few carbs thrown in for bulk. Hominy is a whole, dried corn kernel that can be found in the canned section of the supermarket. It's often used in soups (like pozole) as it stands up well to long cooking times, becoming even more tender and soaking up all the intense spices. This stew is ideal on a sick day (I love it when I need to open my sinuses with a little heat), and it freezes well for later.

CARB SWAP: If you can't find hominy, use black beans or chickpeas. Or, omit the hominy and serve the stew as a taco filling with warm tortillas.

MAKES 4 SERVINGS

2	tablespoons avocado oil	1	teaspoon ground cumin	1	bunch kale, roughly chopped
2	pounds boneless, skinless chicken thighs	2	cups crushed tomatoes (about 18 ounces)		One 15-ounce can hominy, rinsed and drained
	Sea salt	2	chipotle chiles in adobo, coarsely chopped	1	lime, cut into wedges
1	small red onion, thinly sliced			1	cup roughly chopped fresh cilantro
2	garlic cloves, minced	4	cups chicken stock	1	avocado, sliced

❶ In a large Dutch oven or heavy-bottomed pot, heat the oil over a medium-high flame. Season the chicken all over with salt and sear, in batches if needed, until nicely browned on both sides, about 10 minutes total. Transfer to a plate.

❷ Reduce the heat to medium and add the onion, garlic, cumin, and more oil, as needed. Sauté until the onion softens and the garlic is golden brown, about 3 minutes. Stir in the tomatoes, scraping up any browned bits from the bottom of the pan. Add the chipotles, stock, and **1 teaspoon salt**.

❸ Fold in the kale and hominy, then nestle the chicken back in the pot so it's submerged in the liquid. Bring to a boil, then reduce the heat to medium-low and simmer, uncovered, for 45 minutes, or until the sauce thickens and the chicken falls apart easily when nudged with a spoon.

④ Off the heat, using two forks, shred the chicken roughly in the pot.

⑤ Serve the stew in bowls with a lime wedge, a generous handful of cilantro, and a few avocado slices.

Slow-Cooker Instructions: At the end of step 2, transfer everything to a slow cooker. Add the chicken and hominy. Cook for 2 hours on high, or 4 hours on low. Add the kale during the last 30 minutes of cooking.

Electric Pressure Cooker Instructions: After step 2, add the chicken and hominy. Cook on high pressure for 15 minutes. Let the pressure release naturally. Add the kale and simmer for 5 minutes.

GF   DF   SF   P   omit hominy

Corn

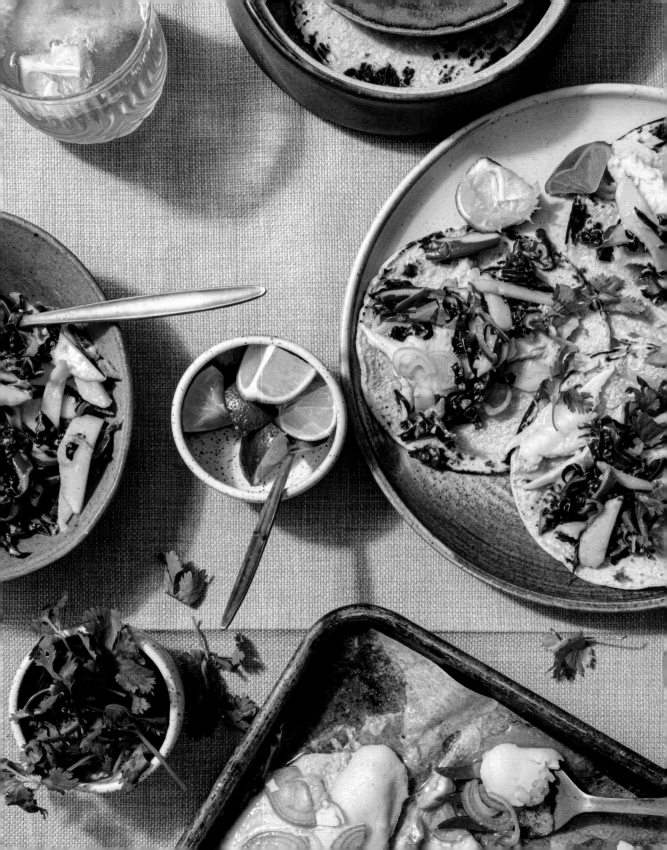

Baked Fish Tacos with Ginger-Mango Slaw

When I'm cooking just for my immediate family, I prefer my fish tacos on the crispy side—usually, some variation of **Mom's Millet Flour Fish Fry** (page 159). But when it's for a larger crowd, my economical (and easy) go-to is a baked fish buffet using thin white fillets (which tend to be cheaper—you can even use tilapia!), lime juice, shallots, and hot sauce. I like Cholula as a basic option, or Queen Majesty for something smaller batch and high end. The kale-mango slaw adds sweetness and crunch to the flaky fish and can hang out on the buffet table until you're ready to eat. When it's go time, the fish needs only five minutes in the oven and you can warm the tortillas alongside it.

---

*MAKE IT A MEAL: You can round out the buffet with sliced avocado, **Zucchini Skillet Cornbread** (page 275), or **Gazpacho Rice & Bean Pilaf** (page 317).*

MAKES 4 SERVINGS

Slaw

- 2 cups thinly sliced purple cabbage (from ½ small head)
- 2 cups tightly packed thinly sliced Lacinato or Tuscan kale, thick stems removed
- 1 large jalapeño, seeded and minced
- 1 tablespoon grated or minced fresh ginger
- ¼ cup fresh lime juice (from 2 or 3 limes)
- 2 tablespoons extra-virgin olive oil
- ½ teaspoon sea salt
- 1 slightly underripe mango, julienned
- 2 tablespoons mayonnaise

Tacos

- 2 pounds thin white fish fillets (flounder, fluke, sole, or similar)

  Sea salt
- 1 tablespoon hot sauce (see headnote)
- ⅓ cup fresh lime juice (from 3 limes)
- 2 small shallots, sliced
- 4 tablespoons unsalted butter, diced, or extra-virgin olive oil

  Twelve 6-inch corn tortillas
- ½ cup fresh cilantro leaves

① Preheat the oven to 425°F. Line a rimmed sheet pan or baking dish with parchment paper.

② **Make the slaw:** In a large bowl, combine the cabbage, kale, jalapeño, ginger, lime juice, oil, and salt. Using clean hands, toss until the kale and cabbage are coated well and starting to wilt. Set aside while you prepare the remaining ingredients. The slaw can be made a day ahead until this point, covered, and refrigerated.

Corn

recipe continues →

3 **Make the tacos:** Arrange the fish in an even layer on the prepared sheet pan, overlapping slightly to fit, as needed. Season generously with salt.

4 In a small bowl, whisk together the hot sauce and lime juice. Pour the sauce over the fish. Scatter the shallots over the fillets, followed by the butter pieces.

5 Bake for about 5 minutes, or until the fish is completely white and cooked through.

6 Simultaneously, wrap the tortillas in aluminum foil and place on a baking sheet. Bake until heated through, about 5 minutes. Alternatively, wrap them in a clean kitchen towel and microwave for 30 seconds.

7 When ready to serve, add the mango and mayonnaise to the slaw and toss to combine.

8 Arrange the fish, slaw, warm tortillas, and cilantro on a table and serve family-style.

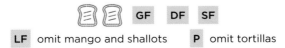

GF   DF   SF

LF omit mango and shallots   **P** omit tortillas

Upside-Down Strawberry-Rhubarb Polenta Cake

This strawberry-rhubarb cake is proof that gluten-free baking is much more forgiving than people give it credit for. Between my recipe testers and me, we've tried this cake a dozen different ways, including using (accidentally) a precooked roll of polenta instead of the dried sack. Somehow that cake still turned out delicious (though presumably involved a LOT of whisking . . .). To clarify, you are looking for medium-ground cornmeal, which is most frequently called polenta (avoid the "instant" kind). I love the combination of the gritty cornmeal with rich, nutty almond flour, but you can use a finer cornmeal, or substitute buckwheat, white rice, or oat flour for the almond flour. The cake is not too sweet, and the combination of strawberry and rhubarb adds a tart finish. Though I discourage eating cake on an empty stomach, my friend aptly called it an "everyday snacking cake."

CHANGE OF SEASON: Sub fresh blueberries, raspberries, thinly sliced peaches (2 small), thinly sliced Meyer lemons, or blood oranges for the strawberry-rhubarb combination.

MAKES ONE 9-INCH CAKE

1	pint fresh strawberries, quartered (about 2 cups)	1	cup polenta (see headnote)	1	teaspoon vanilla extract
½	rhubarb stalk (about 1 ounce), thinly sliced (about ½ cup)	1	cup almond flour	½	cup extra-virgin olive oil
⅓	cup shelled pistachios, finely chopped, divided	1	teaspoon baking powder		Full-fat plain yogurt, sour cream, or crème fraîche (optional)
		½	teaspoon sea salt		
		3	large eggs		
		⅓	cup honey or maple syrup		

❶ Preheat the oven to 350°F. Line a 9-inch round or square cake pan with parchment paper and lightly grease it with oil.

❷ Layer the strawberries, rhubarb, and half the pistachios (in that order) evenly in the prepared pan.

❸ In a medium bowl, whisk together the polenta, almond flour, baking powder, and salt until there are no lumps.

❹ In a second medium bowl, whisk together the eggs, honey, vanilla, and oil until smooth and all the sweetener is incorporated.

Corn

5 Fold the dry ingredients into the wet ingredients and stir until just combined—the batter will be thick. Pour the batter into the prepared pan over the fruit and spread it evenly into the corners with a spatula.

6 Bake for 25 to 35 minutes until golden brown around the edges and a toothpick inserted into the center comes out clean. Let the cake cool in the pan for at least 15 minutes, then invert it onto a serving platter. Discard the parchment.

7 Cut the cake into slices or squares, garnish with the remaining pistachios, and serve as is or with a dollop of yogurt.

GF **Vgt** **DF** use coconut yogurt

LF use coconut yogurt and maple syrup; omit pistachios

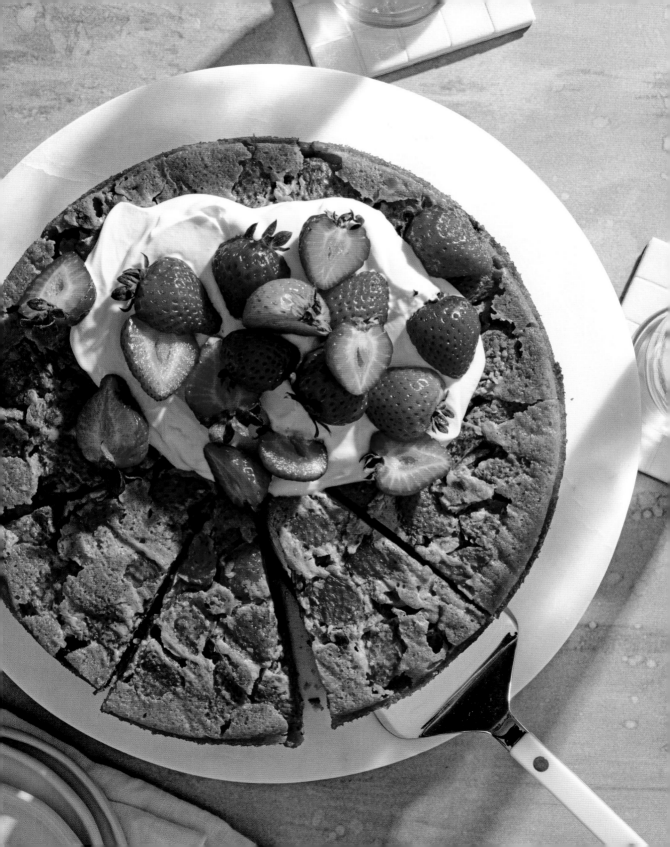

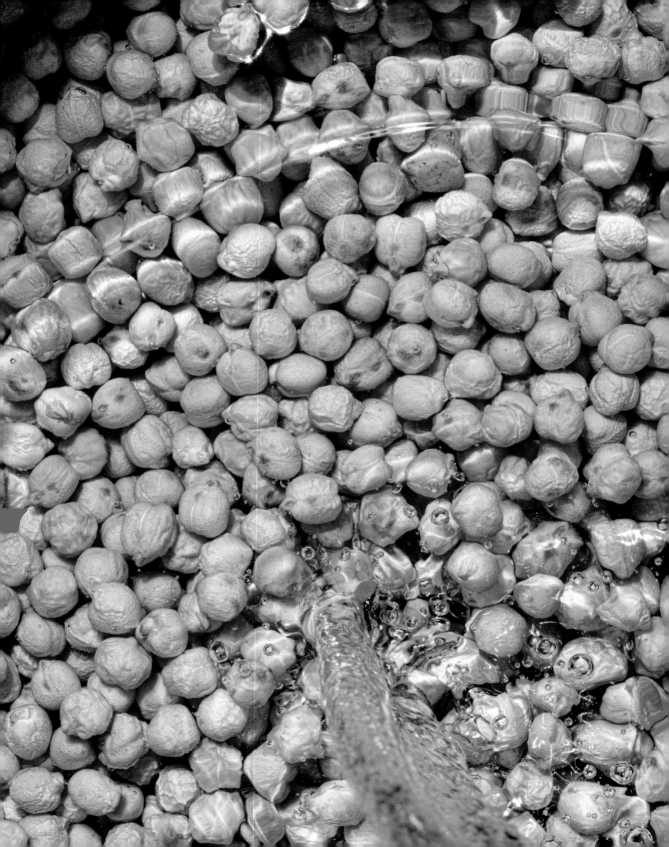

LEGUMES

. . .

All-Day Brothy Beans, 3 Ways

BBQ Chicken Thighs with Black-Eyed Peas & Collards

French Onion White Bean Dip with Rosemary

Smashed Chickpea Shakshuka with Summer Tomatoes

Lazy-Day Dal with Butternut Squash & Kale

Roasted Sweet Potatoes with Beans & Greens

Sausage & Greens Minestrone Soup

French Lentil & Beet Salad with Garlicky Walnuts

Gazpacho Rice & Bean Pilaf

Pesto Socca with Antipasti Salad

Seared Scallops with White Beans, Watercress &
Kefir Green Goddess Dressing

Braised Chickpeas & Broccolini with Golden Raisins

TYPES & PREPARATION TIPS

Beans

Varieties: black, great northern, cannellini, gigante, kidney, pinto, adzuki

There are so many culinary uses for beans, it would be hard to put them down on paper. Pureed, they become a thick, creamy dip (see **French Onion White Bean Dip with Rosemary**, page 305). Boiled with other ingredients in soups or stews, they lend their starch as a natural gluten-free thickener (see **Sausage & Greens Minestrone Soup**, page 312). And mixed with vegetables and proteins alike, they are a cheap way to bulk up a meal, add textural variety, and give you another way to soak up a delicious sauce like in **Roasted Sweet Potatoes with Beans & Greens** (page 311) and **Seared Scallops with White Beans, Watercress & Kefir Green Goddess Dressing** (page 321).

Peas

Varieties: black-eyes peas, crowder peas, split field peas

Most cowpeas in the world are grown in Africa, but they were brought to the Americas by enslaved people and now are a staple of Southern cooking. Despite their name, cowpeas resemble many common beans in both shape and lineage. Feel free to use any of the recipes for **All-Day Brothy Beans** (page 301) to cook black-eyed peas from scratch, or just use a canned variety to make **BBQ Chicken Thighs with Black-Eyed Peas & Collards** (page 303). Split field peas, on the other hand, are yellow or green and are known for their ability to be boiled with a ham hock into soupy oblivion. Not that there's anything wrong with that.

Lentils

Varieties: brown lentils, French green lentils, black or beluga lentils, red lentils, yellow lentils

Like beans, lentils come in all colors and sizes. I'm partial to cooking them al dente and tossing them in green salads, or using them as the main event in sides like my **French Lentil & Beet Salad with Garlicky Walnuts** (page 315). When fall hits, I start craving lentils, simmered into porridge like the Indian-inspired **Lazy-Day Dal with Butternut Squash & Kale** (page 309). If you start with split lentils, your soup will be ready in 15 minutes. But even whole lentils are true weeknight pulses, cooking up from their dried form in under 40 minutes, rather than the hours it takes beans and peas.

Chickpeas (Garbanzo Beans)

Chickpeas are found all over, but are, perhaps, most ubiquitous in Middle Eastern and Indian cuisine. In addition to adding them to braises and stews (see **Braised Chickpeas & Broccolini with Golden Raisins**, page 323, or **Smashed Chickpea Shakshuka with Summer Tomatoes**, page 306), when dried chickpeas are ground into flour, they become one of the most versatile gluten-free ingredients. I love using chickpea flour for fritters or battered vegetables. But it also becomes an easy one-ingredient pizza crust. Socca or farinata is a chickpea pancake eaten all over the Mediterranean in various thicknesses and crepe-like consistencies (see **Pesto Socca with Antipasti Salad**, page 318).

All-Day Brothy Beans, 3 Ways

Though canned beans are incredibly practical and affordable, once you've begun boiling your own dried beans from scratch, it's hard to go back. Today, I keep my freezer stocked with various varieties in the same way I used to stack cans on my pantry shelves.

These all-day legume recipes are completely hands-off—set, forget, and simmer. They are flavorful enough to enjoy on their own, but they aren't too ostentatiously seasoned that they can't be used in any recipe that calls for regular canned beans. There's no need to presoak, which opens up a world of impulsivity. The larger the bean, the longer it needs to cook. The resulting broth is almost as big a treasure as the cooked beans themselves, so store them in their liquid or strain it and use as a starchy stock for future soups and stews.

All-Day Brothy Black Beans

Though there are many ways to use these black beans, I must mention that the whole pot can be the basis for a black bean soup if you throw in some diced vegetables. Otherwise, I love using the cooked beans in **Gazpacho Rice & Bean Pilaf** (page 317), **Roasted Sweet Potatoes with Beans & Greens** (page 311), or as a substitute for black-eyed peas in **BBQ Chicken Thighs** (page 303).

MAKES 8 CUPS

1	pound (about 2 ½ cups) dried black beans, rinsed and sorted
1	medium shallot, unpeeled, halved
1	jalapeño, halved (optional)
2	teaspoons sea salt
1	teaspoon smoked paprika
1	teaspoon ground cumin
¼	cup extra-virgin olive oil

❶ In a slow cooker, combine the dried beans, shallot, jalapeño (if using), salt, smoked paprika, cumin, and oil. Pour **8 cups filtered water** over the beans and cover the pot. Cook on high heat for 5 to 7 hours, or until the beans are tender but not mushy or falling apart. To be safe, begin checking at hour 4. The older the beans, the longer they'll take.

❷ Taste the beans and "pot liquor" and add more salt, as needed. Discard the shallot and jalapeño.

❸ Refrigerate the beans in their liquid in an airtight container for up to 2 weeks, or freeze for later.

All-Day Brothy Chickpeas

Have these turmeric-sunned chickpeas at the ready for **Smashed Chickpea Shakshuka with Summer Tomatoes** (page 306), **Braised Chickpeas & Broccolini with Golden Raisins** (page 323), and **Sweet & Sour Moroccan Chicken-Rice Casserole** (page 119).

VARIATION: Sub dried chickpeas for black beans and add **4 garlic cloves**, *unpeeled,* **one 2-inch piece fresh ginger**, *unpeeled and sliced,* **1 teaspoon ground turmeric, 1 teaspoon ground coriander,** *and* **¼ teaspoon cayenne pepper**. *Omit shallot, jalapeño, paprika, and cumin.*

All-Day Brothy White Beans

Tinged with anise and heat from the red pepper flakes, these brothy beans work wonderfully in **French Onion White Bean Dip with Rosemary** (page 305), **Sausage & Greens Minestrone Soup** (page 312), and **Seared Scallops with White Beans, Watercress & Kefir Green Goddess Dressing** (page 321). The cook time may vary but the spice mix works with any variety of white bean: navy, great northern, or cannellini.

VARIATION: Sub dried white beans for black beans and add **4 garlic cloves**, *unpeeled,* **2 teaspoons fennel seeds, 4 rosemary or thyme sprigs**, *and* **½ teaspoon red pepper flakes** *(optional). Omit jalapeño, paprika, and cumin.*

Stovetop Method: In a large Dutch oven or heavy-bottomed stockpot over high heat, bring all the ingredients to a boil. Reduce the heat to low and simmer, uncovered, until the beans are tender, 1 to 3 hours. Add more water, if needed, along the way if the beans start to dry out.

Oven Method: Preheat the oven to 325°F. In a large Dutch oven or lidded heavy-bottomed stockpot, combine all the ingredients. Bake, covered, until the beans are tender, 1 to 3 hours. Add more water, if needed, along the way if the beans start to dry out.

GF   DF   Vgt   V   SF

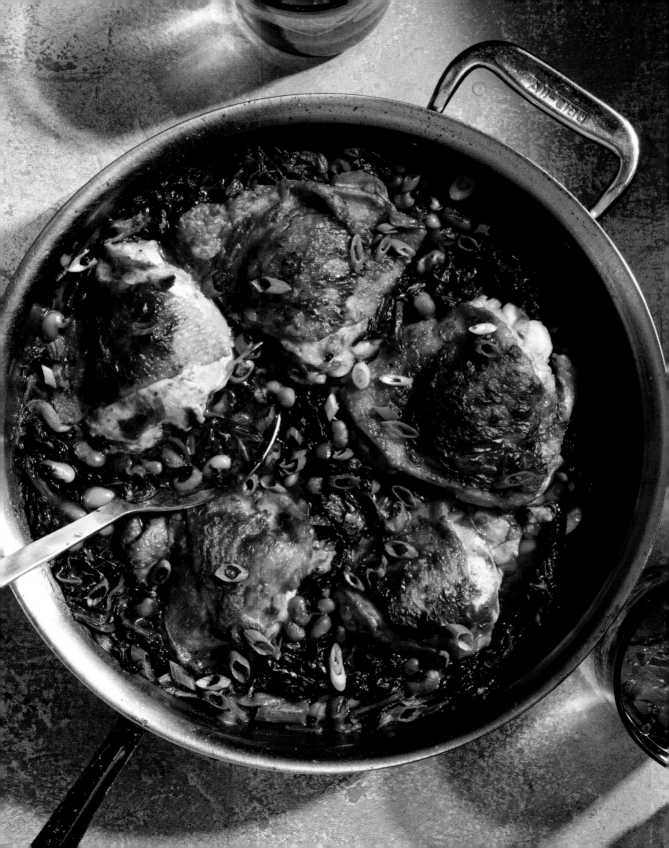

BBQ Chicken Thighs with Black-Eyed Peas & Collards

My husband's family congregates for the holidays in South Carolina, and when I'm down there, I have a few one-pan meals on rotation that feed a crowd. This smoky skillet chicken is always the most requested. Collard greens offset the sugar-laden shortcut of store-bought barbecue sauce. Unless you're making homemade **Low-Fructose BBQ Sauce** (page 67) from scratch, you'll benefit from taking extra care here to use the greens leaf to stem because the woody parts of your vegetables always have the most fiber! If you're not a fan of black-eyed peas (at least, of the non-Fergie variety), substitute black, white, or pinto beans, or even cooked green lentils. But these little two-tone peas, apparently, look like coins (at least, if you've consumed enough bourbon), and, therefore, the Southern lore is that they guarantee a prosperous year ahead. So, there's that to consider.

---

*MAKE IT A MEAL: This dish is already a one-pan meal, but you can stretch it by serving alongside **Big Leaf Lettuces** (page 81) and **Zucchini Skillet Cornbread** (page 275).*

MAKES 4 SERVINGS

1	bunch collard greens	1	teaspoon paprika	2	tablespoons apple cider vinegar
1	bunch red chard	¼	teaspoon cayenne pepper		
	Avocado oil			1	cup chicken or vegetable stock
2	pounds bone-in, skin-on chicken thighs	2	cups cooked black-eyed peas (from one 14-ounce can, rinsed and drained)	1	cup store-bought BBQ sauce or **Low-Fructose BBQ Sauce** (page 67), divided
	Sea salt				
1	large shallot, thinly sliced	4	scallions, thinly sliced		

❶ Preheat the oven to 425°F.

❷ On a clean work surface, separate the collard greens from their stalks by grabbing hold of the stem and pulling upward to sever the leaf. Thinly slice the stalks and set aside. Stack the collard leaves, with the largest at the bottom and smallest at the top. Roll the leaves widthwise into a cigar shape and thinly slice—the result will be beautiful ribbons of greens.

❸ Cut off the bottom inch from the chard stalks and discard (no need to remove the vein from the leaves). Thinly slice the remainder of the stalks and set aside with the collard stems. Repeat the cigar method from step 2 and thinly slice the chard leaves.

recipe continues →

④ In a large ovenproof skillet, heat a thin layer (about ⅛ inch) of oil over a medium-high flame. Season the chicken with salt and place it in the skillet, skin-side down. Sear the chicken until some of the fat has rendered and the skin is golden brown, about 5 minutes. Transfer the chicken to a plate, skin-side up, and set aside. Don't worry, we will fully cook the chicken later.

⑤ Turn the heat down to medium and add the shallot, along with the chopped collard and chard stems, to the skillet. Sauté until soft, about 3 minutes. Add the collard and chard leaves, in batches, if needed, to the skillet. Season with the paprika, **½ teaspoon salt,** and the cayenne. Continue to cook, redistributing occasionally, until vibrant and wilted, 5 minutes.

⑥ Fold in the black-eyed peas, half the scallions, the vinegar, stock, and **¾ cup BBQ sauce.**

⑦ Arrange the chicken, skin-side up, in the bean mixture, nestling them into the pan. Slather the top with the remaining **¼ cup BBQ sauce.**

⑧ Bake for 20 minutes, or until the chicken is cooked through. Garnish with the remaining scallions and serve immediately.

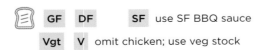

GF **DF**   **SF** use SF BBQ sauce

Vgt **V** omit chicken; use veg stock

French Onion White Bean Dip with Rosemary

One of the iconic recipes from my first cookbook is a three-onion dip. For those who don't like mayo, I've experimented with making it with other fillers, like full-fat yogurt, but pureed white beans are perhaps the most versatile. Simply grab a can from the pantry and any dairy-free or vegan folks coming to your party are covered. Regardless of dietary restriction, this dip is always the first thing to disappear.

The key to this recipe is the three types of alliums: onion, shallot, and leek. Using sweet Vidalia or Spanish onion helps with the caramelization, but a regular yellow onion will work too. The most time-consuming part is getting the onions to melt into a darkened, sweet state, but a dash of tamari shaves off 15 minutes at the stove.

MAKES 2 CUPS

Extra-virgin olive oil

1 medium sweet Vidalia or Spanish onion, thinly sliced

1 large leek, white and light green parts only, halved lengthwise, rinsed (see headnote, page 209), and thinly sliced

1 medium shallot, thinly sliced

1 tablespoon gluten-free tamari

Sea salt

2 cups cooked cannellini or white beans (from one 15-ounce can, rinsed and drained) or **All-Day Brothy White Beans** (page 301)

2 tablespoons fresh lemon juice

2 teaspoons chopped fresh rosemary leaves

¼ teaspoon red pepper flakes (optional)

Potato chips, taro chips, crackers, or crudités

❶ In a large skillet, heat **2 tablespoons oil** over medium-high heat. Sauté the onion, leek, and shallot until translucent and beginning to brown, 7 minutes. Turn the heat to low and cook, stirring occasionally, until the onion mixture is dark and caramelized, 20 to 30 minutes. Add the tamari and continue to cook until the liquid has evaporated, 1 minute. Season with salt to taste and set aside.

❷ Meanwhile, in a small food processor, puree the beans, lemon juice, rosemary, red pepper flakes (if using), **½ teaspoon salt**, and **2 tablespoons oil** until smooth.

❸ Transfer all but 1 tablespoon of the onion mixture to a medium bowl and stir in the bean puree. Taste for seasoning, and add more salt, as needed. Spoon the dip into a serving bowl and garnish with the reserved caramelized onions and a drizzle of oil.

❹ Serve alongside your dippers of choice. Leftover dip, refrigerated in an airtight container, can be repurposed as a spread on a roasted veggie sandwich the next day!

GF DF Vgt V SF

Smashed Chickpea Shakshuka with Summer Tomatoes

North African shakshuka has long been a favorite when making a slightly elevated brunch. There's no cooking eggs to order, you simply add them to a simmering spiced tomato sauce and your meal can be served directly from the skillet. I've bulked up this version by adding chickpeas to the sauce. It's a nod to another favorite dish from across the Mediterranean, *espinacas con garbanzos*, the smoky, tomatoey Andalusian chickpea tapa. Although shakshuka is a great dish year-round, it's especially delicious in summer months when bell peppers and tomatoes are at their peak. If you're making this recipe out of season, sub one 28-ounce can or jar of diced tomatoes for the fresh. The most time-consuming part of this recipe is the chopping, so if it's too much labor for you in the morning, make the sauce in advance. It tastes even better the next day. Simply heat it up and crack your eggs in the wells when you're ready to serve.

CARB COMPANIONS: For more fiber, add 5 ounces baby spinach to the chickpea tomato mixture at the end of step 2. Serve with crumbled feta cheese or a dollop of yogurt on top.

MAKES 4 SERVINGS

- 2 tablespoons extra-virgin olive oil
- 1 small red onion, finely diced
- 1 red bell pepper, seeded and finely diced
- 2 garlic cloves, minced
- 1 ½ teaspoons smoked paprika

- 1 teaspoon ground cumin
- 1 tablespoon harissa paste, or 1 teaspoon Aleppo pepper (optional)
- 1 teaspoon sea salt
- 4 medium plum or vine tomatoes (1 pound), diced

- 2 cups cooked chickpeas (from one 15-ounce can, rinsed and drained) or **All-Day Brothy Chickpeas** (page 301)
- ½ cup vegetable stock or water
- 4 large eggs
- ¼ cup roughly chopped fresh cilantro

❶ In a large (at least 12-inch), lidded heavy-bottomed skillet, heat the oil over a medium-high flame. Add the onion and bell pepper and sauté until soft, about 8 minutes. Stir in the garlic, smoked paprika, cumin, harissa (if using), and salt. Cook for 2 minutes until very fragrant.

❷ Add the tomatoes and chickpeas to the skillet and cook, stirring occasionally, until the tomatoes release their juices and begin to caramelize, about 5 minutes.

Carbivore

recipe continues →

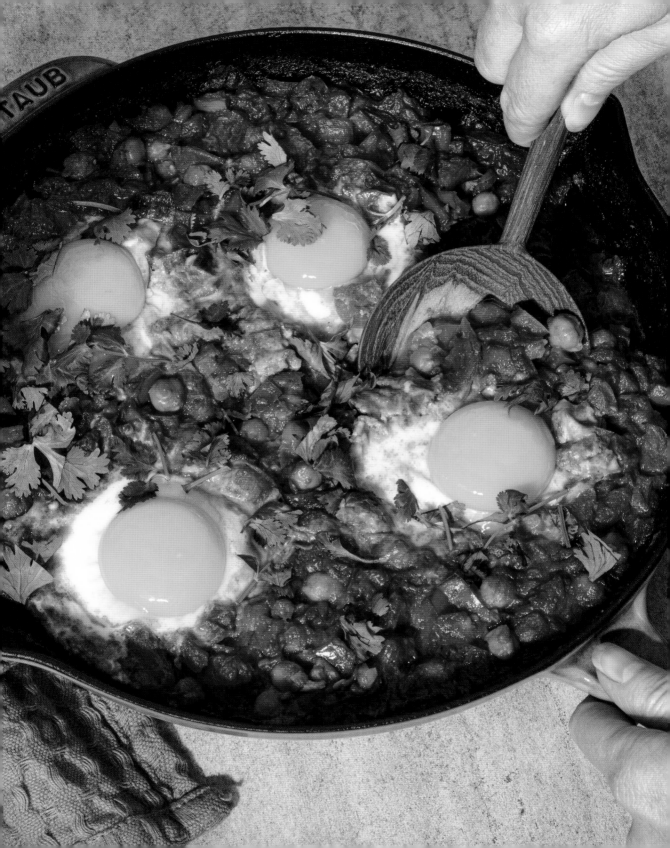

3 Pour the stock into the skillet, scraping up any browned bits from the bottom. Using a fork or potato masher, crush half the tomatoes and chickpeas to release even more liquid and create a saucy consistency. Continue to cook over medium-high heat until the sauce has thickened and the tomatoes have lost their acidity, about 5 minutes more.

4 With the back of a spoon or spatula, create 4 wells in the tomato mixture. Crack 1 egg into each well and season lightly with salt. Cover the pan to trap the steam and simmer over low heat until the egg whites have set but the yolks are still runny, about 5 minutes.

5 Garnish with the cilantro and serve directly from the skillet.

GF   **DF**   **Vgt**   **SF**   **LF** omit onion, garlic, and chickpeas

P omit chickpeas   **V** omit eggs

Lazy-Day Dal with Butternut Squash & Kale

I call this lazy-day dal because, although there's a bit of chopping involved, the recipe flows in a way that you can casually dice everything as you cook and the resulting bowl is as easy to spoon down as it was to prepare. Dal is a blanket term in Indian cuisine for split pulses—red or yellow lentils, in this case—that cook quickly and do not require any presoaking. Though these ingredients are prepared differently depending on the region, most often, the lentils or peas melt away into something between a soup and a stew. The squash and kale add texture and make this dish into a full, warming meal.

MARKE IT A MEAL: Serve with brown rice and top with diced avocado or **Smoky Pumpkin-Hemp Sprinkles** *(page 79).*

MAKES 4 TO 6 SERVINGS

- 2 tablespoons avocado oil or coconut oil
- 1 red onion, diced
- 1 garlic clove, minced
- 1 tablespoon minced fresh ginger
- 1 serrano chile, seeded and minced
- 1 teaspoon ground cumin
- 1 teaspoon garam masala
- ½ teaspoon ground coriander
- 3 cups finely diced butternut squash (from one 1 ½-pound squash)
- 1 ½ cups crushed tomatoes (from one 15-ounce can or jar)
- One 13.5-ounce can full-fat coconut milk
- 1 teaspoon sea salt
- 1 cup split red or yellow lentils
- 1 bunch kale, finely chopped
- ⅓ cup fresh cilantro leaves

  Full-fat plain Greek or coconut yogurt

1 In a large stockpot or Dutch oven over a medium-high flame, heat the oil. Add the onion and sauté until soft, about 5 minutes. Stir in the garlic, ginger, serrano, cumin, garam masala, and coriander. Cook until very fragrant, 2 minutes.

2 Add the butternut squash and tomatoes, scraping up any browned bits from the bottom of the pan. Pour in the coconut milk, salt, and **2 cups water**. Bring to a boil over high heat. Stir in the lentils and reduce the heat to medium-low. Cook, uncovered, for 20 minutes, stirring occasionally to prevent the lentils from sticking to the bottom of the pan, or until the lentils are al dente and the squash is soft. Add the kale (and more water, as needed) and continue to cook until wilted, 5 minutes.

3 Divide into bowls and garnish with the cilantro and yogurt.

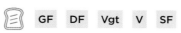 GF DF Vgt V SF

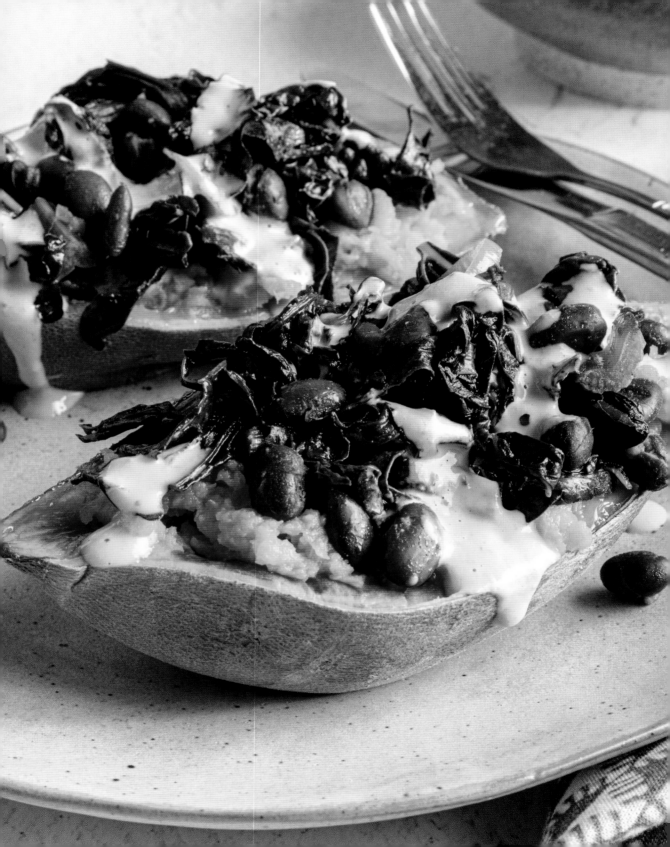

Roasted Sweet Potatoes with Beans & Greens

If you're looking for a quicker, healthier spin on a classic baked potato, these halved sweet potatoes with wilted kale and a creamy Southwestern drizzle are beloved by carnivores and plant-heads alike. The fiery tahini sauce helps jazz up the blank canvas of black beans, which, unless you're using **All-Day Brothy Black Beans** (page 300), don't have a ton of built-in flavor. For an even more decadent dish, melt a small handful of shredded sharp cheddar cheese on each potato half, then pile on the toppings.

CARB SWAP: Nix the sweet potatoes and serve over toasted gluten-free sourdough bread with mashed avocado as the base for a Carbivore-approved beans on toast.

MAKES 4 SERVINGS

4	medium sweet potatoes (2 pounds), halved lengthwise
	Extra-virgin olive oil
1	shallot, sliced
2	bunches chard or kale (or a mix), leaves and stems separated, finely sliced
1	teaspoon smoked paprika
½	teaspoon ground cumin
½	teaspoon sea salt
2	cups cooked black beans (from one 15-ounce can, rinsed and drained) or **All-Day Brothy Black Beans** (page 300)
2	tablespoons fresh lime juice
1	cup **Chipotle-Tahini Sauce** (page 68)
	Fresh cilantro leaves

❶ Preheat the oven to 400°F. Line a baking sheet with parchment paper.

❷ Brush the flesh of the sweet potatoes with oil and place them, cut-side down, on the prepared baking sheet. Bake until fork-tender, 25 to 30 minutes. Flip the sweet potatoes so they are flesh-side up and set aside to cool. (Transfer to the refrigerator for 20 minutes to help develop the resistant starch, if you like.)

❸ Meanwhile, heat **2 tablespoons oil** in a large cast-iron skillet over medium heat. Sauté the shallot and chard stems until soft, 3 minutes. Add the smoked paprika, cumin, and salt and cook for 2 minutes until vibrant. Fold in the chard leaves, in batches, and cook until quite wilted, about 3 minutes. Stir in the beans and cook for 2 minutes more. Off the heat, stir in the lime juice.

❹ When the sweet potatoes are cool enough to handle, use a fork to fluff the flesh and mash it toward the sides to create a well for the filling. Divide the beans and greens among the potato halves, patting the filling gently into the center.

❺ Drizzle the sweet potatoes with **chipotle-tahini sauce** and garnish with cilantro to serve.

GF   DF   Vgt   V   SF   P   omit beans

Sausage & Greens Minestrone Soup

Minestrone is a fantastic "meal in a bowl" strategy—a way to use up whatever odds and ends you have in the fridge or balance a handful of this or that carb with this or that vegetable. I find that super tomatoey soups can irritate my gut, so I opt for tomato paste to impart richness without a whole mess of tomatoes to contend with. The sleeper star of this recipe is the hot Italian sausage, which allows you to imbue lots of spice into the broth. Use whichever sturdy greens you have, and if there are no fresh herbs, a tablespoon or two of pesto is perfect in a pinch.

CARB SWAP: Sub 1 small russet potato, diced, or 1 cup short pasta for the beans.

MAKES 4 SERVINGS

Extra-virgin olive oil

1 small onion, diced

2 medium carrots, finely diced

8 ounces uncooked hot Italian sausage (chicken, pork, or turkey), casings removed

2 tablespoons tomato paste

2 garlic cloves, minced

1 teaspoon sea salt

1 teaspoon paprika

8 cups vegetable or chicken stock

4 cups cooked cannellini beans (from two 15-ounce cans, drained and rinsed) or **All-Day Brothy White Beans** (page 301)

1 bunch leafy greens (kale, chard, collards, spinach, or even broccoli rabe), stems and leaves, chopped

½ cup fresh herbs (basil, chives, parsley, dill, or a mix), roughly chopped or torn

2 tablespoons fresh lemon juice

❶ In a large Dutch oven or stockpot, heat a thin layer (⅛ inch) of oil over medium-high heat. Sauté the onion and carrots until soft, about 5 minutes. Push the veggies to the sides of the pan and add the sausage. Cook, breaking apart the meat with a spatula, until crumbled and browned, about 5 minutes. Stir in the tomato paste, garlic, salt, and paprika and cook until quite fragrant and coating the meat like a paste, 2 minutes.

❷ Stir in the stock and beans. Bring to a boil, then reduce the heat to medium-low. Simmer for 15 minutes, or until the broth thickens slightly and the soup is flavorful. Mash some of the beans with the back of a spoon to thicken it further.

❸ Add the greens to the pot and cook for 5 to 10 minutes until tender and wilted. Off the heat, stir in the herbs and lemon juice. Ladle into bowls and garnish with a drizzle of oil.

GF DF SF   P omit beans   Vgt   V omit sausage

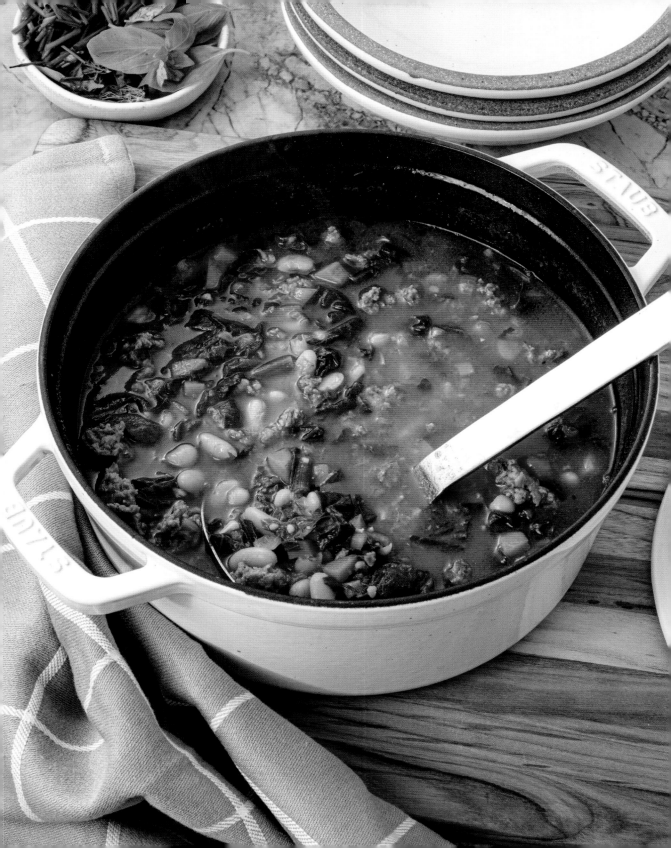

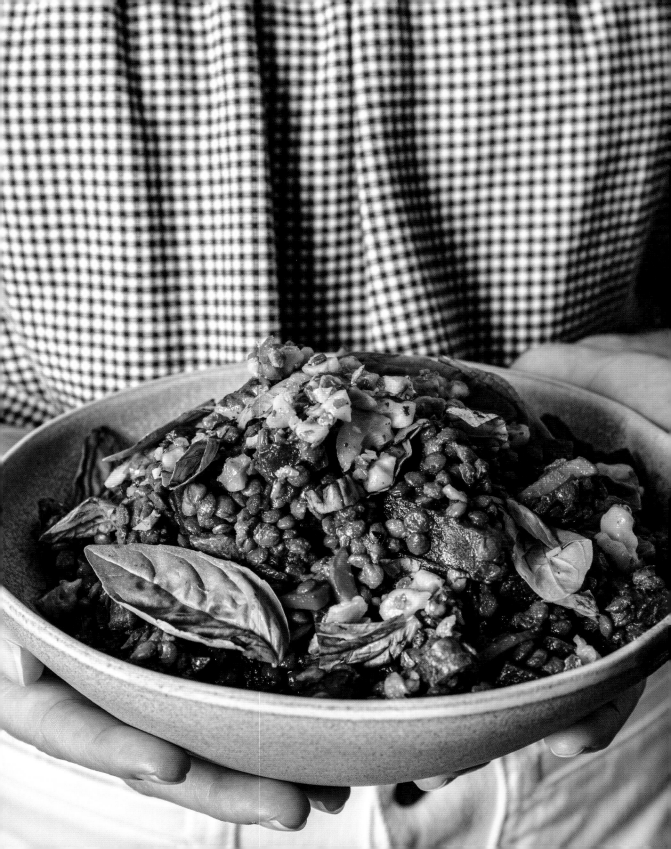

French Lentil & Beet Salad with Garlicky Walnuts

Boiled green lentils tossed with crunchy carrots and a biting Dijon dressing is an iconic French side dish to eat alongside a piece of poached salmon or chicken. But it often looks like a stodgy brown mess. This recipe dresses up those drab legumes with all the colors of the spring rainbow: pink radishes, green sugar snaps, and garnet (or golden) roasted beets. The latter can be roasted a few days in advance to save time, and you can do the rest of the chopping and whisking while the lentils cook. The salad is finished with a little Italian flair—balsamic vinaigrette and torn basil. Garlicky walnuts add crunch, and if you're angling for another carb companion, add shaved parmesan or ricotta salata.

*MAKE IT A MEAL: Bulk up this salad by tossing it with marinated kale or baby arugula, or serve it alongside chicken, fish, or grilled portobellos (see **Grilled Balsamic Mushroom Melts**, page 253).*

MAKES 6 SIDE SERVINGS

- 4 medium beets (1 pound), scrubbed
- Sea salt
- 1 cup dried small French green lentils (Puy lentils), rinsed
- 1 bay leaf
- 1 shallot, unpeeled, halved
- ½ cup thinly sliced red radishes (8 ounces)
- ½ cup thinly sliced sugar snap peas (4 ounces)
- ¾ cup **Basic Balsamic Vinaigrette** (page 60)
- 2 tablespoons extra-virgin olive oil
- 2 garlic cloves, minced
- 1 cup chopped raw unsalted walnuts
- ½ cup loosely packed torn basil leaves

1 Preheat the oven to 375°F.

2 Divide the beets between two 10-inch squares of aluminum foil, season generously with salt, and wrap so the beets are sealed—taking care not to puncture the foil. You want all the steam kept inside. Place the packets on a baking sheet and roast the beets until fork-tender, about 1 hour. Let the beets cool to room temperature, then slip off their skins. This can be done a few days in advance.

3 Meanwhile, bring a large pot of salted water to a boil over high heat. Add the lentils, bay leaf, and shallot. Turn the heat to medium and simmer until al dente, about 15 minutes. Drain the lentils and shake out as much moisture as possible. Discard the bay leaf and shallot. Transfer to a large bowl.

recipe continues →

④ Finely dice the beets and add to the bowl with the lentils, along with the radishes, snap peas, and **½ cup vinaigrette.** Toss to combine. The salad can be made a day ahead up to this point, covered, and refrigerated.

⑤ In a small skillet, heat a thin layer (⅛ inch) of oil over medium-low heat. Add the garlic and walnuts and sauté until the nuts are toasted and the garlic is golden brown, about 3 minutes. Season lightly with salt.

⑥ Taste the lentils for seasoning, and add more salt or dressing, as needed (especially if it's cooled). Top with the torn basil and garlicky toasted nuts. Enjoy warm or at room temperature.

Gazpacho Rice & Bean Pilaf

Pilaf is a fantastic technique for adding more flavor and plants to your grains. Of course, the more veggies involved, the more chopping. One day, I thought how wonderful it would be to just puree lots of water-laden vegetables and use their moisture to cook the rice itself. And thus gazpacho rice was born. Cooking the rice in the tomato mixture takes the edge off the alliums, but still retains an air of brightness. The dish is finished with chopped, lemony cucumbers. Serve it as a summertime accompaniment to grilled meats or a more low-key alternative to paella with seafood on the side.

CARB SWAP: To use brown rice, add an extra tomato and increase the cook time to 45 minutes.

MAKES 6 TO 8 SERVINGS

3   medium vine tomatoes (1 ⅓ pounds), quartered

1   red bell pepper, roughly chopped

1   jalapeño, seeded and roughly chopped

1   small red onion, roughly chopped

Extra-virgin olive oil

2   garlic cloves, minced

1 ½ cups long-grain white rice

1   teaspoon smoked paprika

1 ¾ cups cooked black beans (from one 15-ounce can, rinsed and drained) or **All-Day Brothy Black Beans** (page 300)

Sea salt

1   English cucumber, finely diced

1   tablespoon fresh lemon juice

¼   cup chopped fresh cilantro or parsley

① In a blender or food processor, combine the tomatoes, bell pepper, jalapeño, and onion and pulse until you have a coarse puree. You should have 4 cups puree. If not, add water until you reach that measurement. Set aside.

② In a medium Dutch oven or lidded saucepan, heat **2 tablespoons oil** over medium heat. Add the garlic, rice, and smoked paprika and sauté until fragrant and slightly toasted, 2 minutes. Add the gazpacho puree, beans, and **1 ½ teaspoons salt**. Bring to a simmer over medium-high heat, then cover the pot, turn the heat to low, and cook until the rice is tender and all the liquid is absorbed, about 25 minutes. You can remove the lid to check on it—pilafs are not fussy. Be warned that this is a sticky rice dish not a dry, fluffy one. When the rice is cooked, remove the pot from the heat and let stand for 10 minutes, covered.

③ Meanwhile, in a small bowl, combine the cucumber, lemon juice, and cilantro. Season generously with salt.

④ To serve, fluff the rice with a fork and transfer to a serving platter. Garnish with the cucumbers and a drizzle of oil. Enjoy warm or at room temperature.

GF   DF   Vgt   V   SF

Pesto Socca with Antipasti Salad

Since it involves only two ingredients—chickpea flour and water—socca has been a weeknight savior for me over the years, especially as a last-minute gluten-free pizza crust that can be cooked directly in a hot skillet. This version adds pesto to the batter (turning it green), then tops the crusty, buttery pancake with more pesto, creamy ricotta, and a briny salad of radicchio and crushed green olives. It's best eaten with a knife and fork, which is okay, since a salad pizza might be the only type of slice that a self-respecting New Yorker would dare eat with a knife and fork anyway.

MAKES 2 TO 4 SERVINGS

- 1 cup chickpea flour
  Sea salt
- 1 cup **Arugula-Almond Pesto** (page 70) or store-bought, divided
  Extra-virgin olive oil
- 1 shallot, thinly sliced
- 4 oil-packed sun-dried tomatoes, thinly sliced
- 2 cups baby arugula
- 1 cup thinly sliced radicchio
- ¼ cup (about 8) Castelvetrano olives, pitted and roughly torn
- 1 tablespoon fresh lemon juice
- ¼ cup ricotta or plant-based alternative (optional)

❶ Adjust an oven rack to the upper position and preheat the oven to 450°F. Place a large (15-inch) ovenproof cast-iron skillet on the upper rack.

❷ In a medium bowl, whisk together the chickpea flour and **1 teaspoon salt** until incorporated. While whisking, slowly pour in **1 cup lukewarm water** (test it on your forearm—it should feel slightly warm on your skin), whisking until the liquid is absorbed and the batter is smooth. Let sit until the oven is hot, then stir **3 tablespoons pesto** into the batter until smooth.

❸ Remove the hot skillet from the oven and pour in 2 tablespoons oil. Swirl around to coat the skillet well. Pour in the batter and shake the pan so it forms an even layer. Scatter the shallot and sun-dried tomatoes over the surface.

❹ Bake the chickpea pancake for 15 to 20 minutes until firmly set and crispy around the edges.

❺ Meanwhile, in a medium bowl, toss together the arugula, radicchio, olives, **1 tablespoon oil**, and lemon juice until well combined. Season generously with salt.

❻ Remove the socca from the oven and dot with the remaining pesto and ricotta (if using), then top with the salad. Enjoy immediately with extra pesto on the side.

 GF DF Vgt V SF

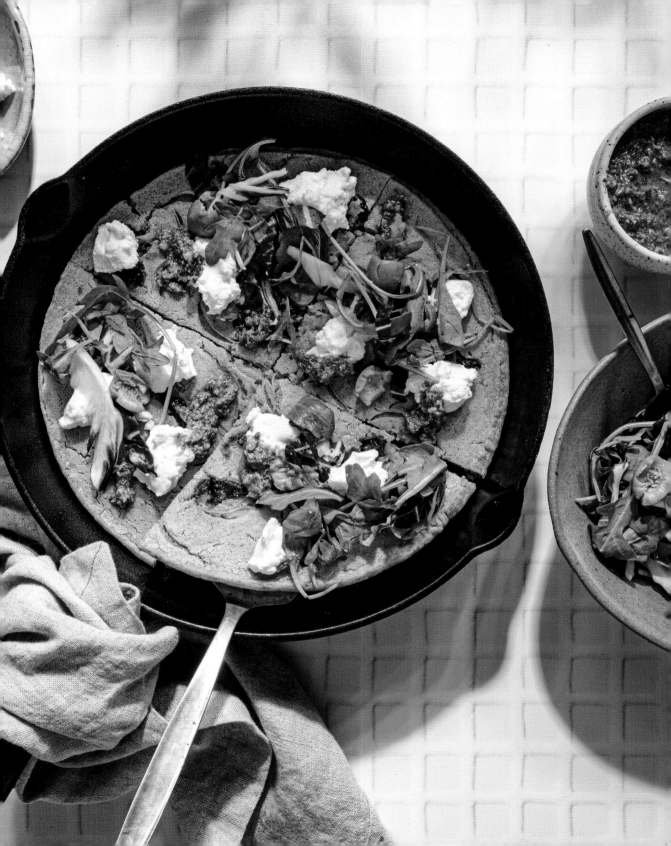

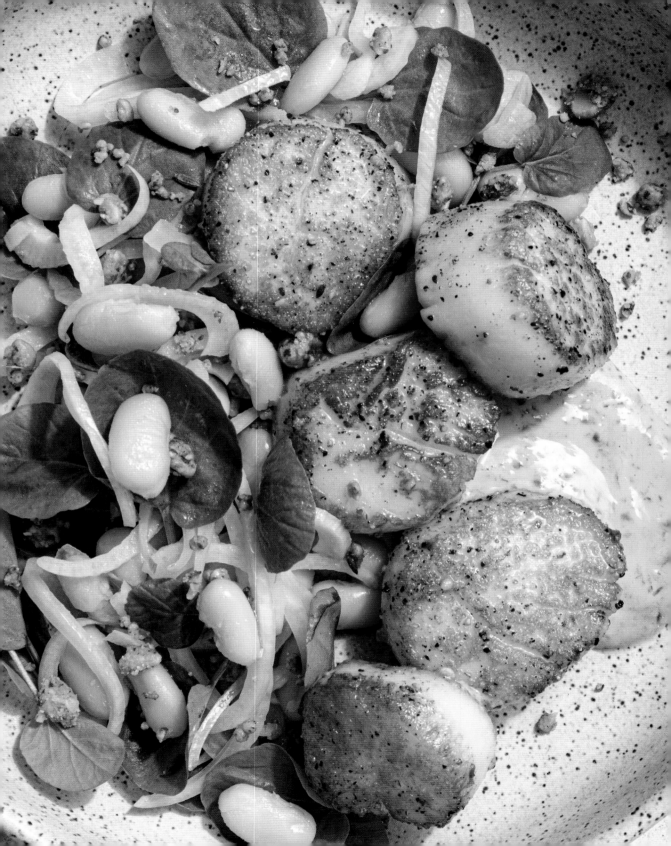

Seared Scallops with White Beans, Watercress & Kefir Green Goddess Dressing

I may have been hopeless at fluffy omelets and cutting carrots into perfect squares, but searing scallops was one of the first "chef-y" techniques I mastered. And I did so when I was a teenager—long before I was ever paid for my labor—by the simple act of love and repetition. If you are intimidated by the prospect of searing scallops, hopefully this fun fact, along with the slightly painstaking instructions below, can put you at ease. If not, sautéed shrimp also work well with the herby probiotic-rich dressing and marinated, crunchy fennel. Briny and bright, this plate of scallops is an ideal "clean" meal when you're craving something on the lighter side or want to make a beautiful presentation for company. Cannellini is my white bean of choice here, but you could also get creative with gigante beans for an even creamier bite.

CARB SWAP: Sub 1 pound roasted halved fingerling potatoes for the beans.

MAKES 4 SERVINGS

- 1 medium fennel bulb, shaved with a mandoline or very thinly sliced
- 3 tablespoons fresh lemon juice (from 1 or 2 lemons)
- 3 tablespoons extra-virgin olive oil
- Sea salt

- 1 ½ cups cooked white beans (from one 15-ounce can, rinsed and drained) or **All-Day Brothy White Beans** (page 301)
- 1 pound sea scallops
- Avocado oil
- 5 ounces watercress or arugula (about 4 cups, packed)

- 1 cup **Kefir Green Goddess Dressing** (page 65)
- ¼ cup **Anise-y Pine Nut–Almond Crunch** (page 77; optional)

❶ In a large bowl, combine the fennel, lemon juice, olive oil, and **½ teaspoon salt** and toss to combine. Stir in the beans. Set aside.

❷ Rinse the scallops under cold water. If there is a skinny tendon on the sides of the scallops, remove and discard it. Set aside on a clean kitchen towel.

❸ In a large nonstick or cast-iron skillet, heat a thin layer (about ⅛ inch) of avocado oil over a medium-high flame. Pat the scallops gently with a paper towel so they are nice and dry and season them with salt. When the oil is quite hot, add the scallops (you will likely need to do this in two batches), making sure not to crowd the pan.

recipe continues →

DO NOT move the scallops until they have properly browned, 2 to 3 minutes, depending on their size. When they have a dark brown crust on the bottom, flip them and cook for another minute. The scallops should still be slightly translucent in the center—if they are opaque throughout, they will likely be overcooked by the time you serve them. Transfer the scallops to a plate, beautiful seared-side up. Repeat with the remaining scallops, adding more oil, as needed.

4 Just before you're ready to eat, add the watercress to the bean and fennel mixture and toss to combine.

5 On a serving platter or individual plates, slather half the green goddess dressing. Arrange the salad on top, followed by the scallops. Drizzle with the remaining dressing and sprinkle with the crunch (if using).

SF **GF** **DF** use plant-based kefir

Braised Chickpeas & Broccolini with Golden Raisins

This is one of those deceptively simple, but stunning, vegetarian dishes that can do double duty as a main course served over grains or as a side dish for a dinner party. The combination of broccolini and chickpeas in a Moroccan-inspired broth is light enough for summer, but really shines in cooler temperatures. Like a lot of braises, this dish tastes better after a few days of hanging around the fridge, and both the broccolini and the chickpeas can stand up to the make-ahead treatment. If you can't find long-stemmed broccolini or broccoli rabe, use regular broccoli cut into florets. Choose a dry white wine— something you would drink—that's not too fruity. The sweetness in this recipe comes from a scant amount of golden raisins, which we get away with because this dish is completely made up of fibrous plants.

MAKE IT A MEAL: Serve as a side dish alongside **Spicy Beef Tagine** *(page 220),* **Sweet & Sour Moroccan Chicken-Rice Casserole** *(page 119),* **Quinoa Paella with Sausage & Shrimp** *(page 151), or* **Spaghetti with Harissa Bolognese** *(page 185).*

MAKES 4 SIDE SERVINGS

1	medium shallot, thinly sliced	½ teaspoon ground coriander
2	garlic cloves, minced	½ teaspoon ground ginger
½	cup extra-virgin olive oil	½ teaspoon sea salt
½	cup dry white wine	¼ teaspoon cayenne pepper
2	tablespoons fresh lemon juice	1 pound broccolini or broccoli rabe
½	teaspoon ground turmeric	

1 ½ cups cooked chickpeas (from one 15-ounce can, rinsed and drained) or **All-Day Brothy Chickpeas** (page 301)

2 tablespoons golden raisins

2 tablespoons fresh mint leaves, torn

① Preheat the oven to 375°F.

② In a 9 × 13-inch casserole dish or large lidded ovenproof saucepan, combine the shallot, garlic, oil, wine, lemon juice, turmeric, coriander, ginger, salt, and cayenne. Whisk with a fork until well mixed.

③ On a clean work surface, trim the bottom inch from the broccolini and discard. If your stalks are thick, halve the broccolini lengthwise into two skinnier trees. You can also thinly slice the base of the stalks to make the trees shorter and easier to fit in your dish.

recipe continues →

Legumes

Add the broccolini, chickpeas, and golden raisins to the dish and toss until the veggies are coated well in the oil and spices. Arrange in an even layer, cover the pan with aluminum foil or a lid, and transfer to the oven.

④ Bake for 15 to 20 minutes until the broccolini stems are tender. Give the vegetables a toss and continue to bake, uncovered, for 5 to 10 minutes more until the sauce has reduced slightly (it will be on the brothy side) and the broccoli is completely wilted.

⑤ Garnish with the mint to serve.

GF　DF　Vgt　V　　SF　omit raisins

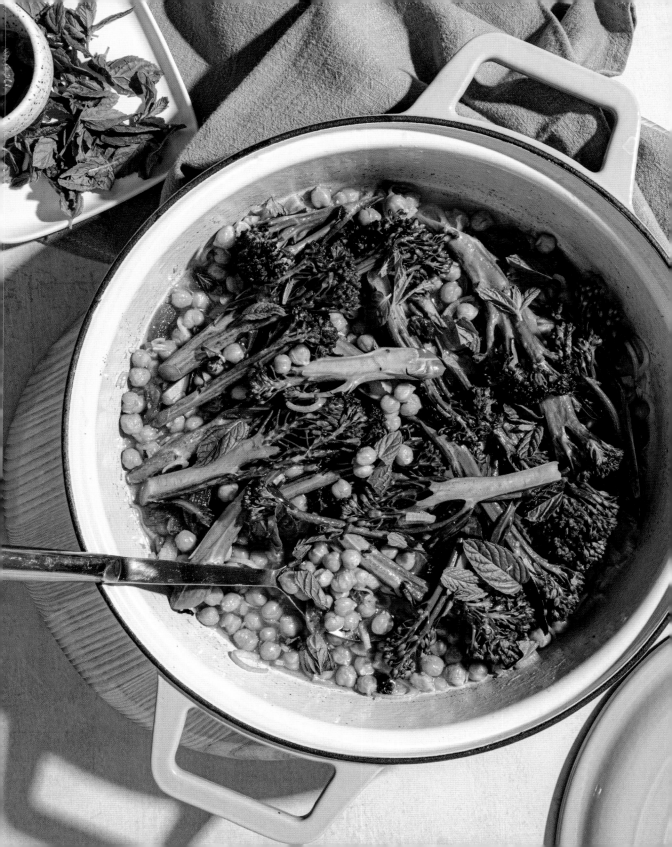

Recipe Index by Type

Appetizers & Finger Food

Basque Tuna Salad Tartines, 257

Crispy Rice with Spicy Beet Tartare, 125

French Onion White Bean Dip with
Rosemary, 305

Hemp-Crusted Chicken Tenders with Dill
Aioli, 136

Maple Walnut–Pecan Spice Brittle, 78

Millet & Zucchini Cakes, 145

Muhammara Roasted Red Pepper Dip, 246

Parsnip-Potato Latkes, 225

Prelude-to-Summer Rolls with Ginger-
Walnut Sauce, 131

Seedy "Avocado Toast" Arepas, 282

Tangy Peanut-Cashew Crunch, 76

Breakfast

Apple-Cinnamon Baked French Toast, 264

Banana–Nut Crunch Granola, 91

Black Sesame–Buckwheat Banana Bread, 164

Brussels Sprouts & Sweet Potato Hash with
Eggs & Leftover Salsa, 212

Buckwheat Crepes with Leek Confit,
Salmon & Eggs, 149

Carrot Cake Baked Steel Cut Oats, 96

Everything Bagel Granola, 92

Ham & Cheese Dutch Baby with Peas, 102

Kasha Pilaf with Mushrooms, Bacon &
Greens, 162

Lemon Poppy Overnight Oats, 95

Savory Yogurt & Granola Bowls with
Avocado & Eggs, 94

Seed Cracker Granola, 92

Seedy "Avocado Toast" Arepas, 282

Smashed Chickpea Shakshuka with
Summer Tomatoes, 306

Steel Cut Oat Congee with Bok Choy, 99

Sweet Potato & Cabbage Rosti with
Kimchi Aioli, 231

Violet's Big Blueberry-Oat Muffins, 103

Salads

Back-Pocket Tricolore Salad with Lemon
Poppy Vinaigrette, 82

Basic Bitch Kale Salad with Liquid Gold
Turmeric-Tahini Dressing, 85

Big Leaf Lettuces with Summer
Tomato-Cashew Dressing, 81

Brussels Sprouts & Wild Rice Salad with
Maple Walnut–Pecan Spice Brittle, 139

Creamy Sesame Noodle Salad with
Smashed Cucumbers, 183

Eggs Mimosa Pasta Salad with Crispy
Prosciutto, Asparagus & Piles of Herbs, 191

French Lentil & Beet Salad with Garlicky
Walnuts, 315

Grilled Romaine with Parmesan Pangritata
& Caesar-ish Dressing, 255

Mexican Street Corn & Collard Greens
Salad, 271

Peanut & Lime Slaw, 83

Roasted Cauliflower Salad with Quinoa,
Arugula & Creamy Romesco Dressing, 146

Seared Tuna Niçoise-ish Salad with Creamy
Caper Dressing, 215

Sheet Pan Chicken BLT Panzanella with
Vinegared Tomatoes, 243

Soups & Stews

Spring Potato-Leek Soup with Asparagus,
209

Chicken Tinga Stew with Hominy & Kale, 288

Creamless Corn & Shrimp Chowder, 277

Ginger-Scallion Chicken Soba Noodle Soup,
196

Greenhouse Gazpacho, 256

Lazy-Day Dal with Butternut Squash & Kale,
309

Sausage & Greens Minestrone Soup, 312

Spicy Beef Tagine with Apricots &
Rosemary, 220

Turmeric-Pumpkin Fall Reset Soup, 160

Warming Mushroom & Wild Rice Soup, 127

Poultry

BBQ Chicken Thighs with Black-Eyed Peas & Collards, 303

Chicken Satay Meatballs, 155

Chicken Tinga Stew with Hominy & Kale, 288

Dijon Turkey Meat Loaf with Spinach, 101

Ginger-Scallion Chicken Soba Noodle Soup, 196

Hemp-Crusted Chicken Tenders with Dill Aioli, 136

One-Pan Provençal Chicken Thighs & Slivered Potatoes, 207

Sheet Pan Chicken BLT Panzanella with Vinegared Tomatoes, 243

Sweet & Sour Moroccan Chicken-Rice Casserole, 119

Beef & Pork

Cajun Pork Tenderloin with Grits & Zucchini Hash, 279

Chili con Carne Shepherd's Pie with Sweet Potato Mash, 217

Eggs Mimosa Pasta Salad with Crispy Prosciutto, Asparagus & Piles of Herbs, 191

Grilled Skirt Steak & Vermicelli Bowls with Nuoc Cham, 198

Inside-Out Egg Roll Noodles, 175

Linguine with Chorizo, Clams & Kale, 193

Pepperoni Pizza with Okra, Collards & Hot Honey, 262

Quinoa Paella with Sausage & Shrimp, 151

Spaghetti with Harissa Bolognese & Mint-Almond Gremolata, 185

Spicy Beef Tagine with Apricots & Rosemary, 220

Fish & Seafood

Baked Fish Tacos with Ginger-Mango Slaw, 291

Basque Tuna Salad Tartines, 257

Buckwheat Crepes with Leek Confit, Salmon & Eggs, 149

Cod & Orzo Arrabbiata, 178

Crab Cake Twice-Baked Potatoes, 223

Ginger-Salmon Burgers with Quick-Pickled Radishes, 249

Mom's Millet Flour Fish Fry with Tarragon-Chive Tartar Sauce, 159

Oven Risotto with Shrimp, Asparagus & Peas, 128

Quinoa Paella with Sausage & Shrimp, 151

Salmon & Broccoli Noodle Casserole, 188

Seared Scallops with White Beans, Watercress & Kefir Green Goddess Dressing, 321

Seared Tuna Niçoise-ish Salad with Creamy Caper Dressing, 215

The Simplest Poke Bowls, 123

Vegetarian Main Courses

Brussels Sprouts & Sweet Potato Hash with Eggs & Leftover Salsa, 212

Creamy Sesame Noodle Salad with Smashed Cucumbers, 183

Crispy Polenta Cakes with Eggplant–Cherry Tomato Caponata, 272

Gnocchi Primavera with Peas & Lemon "Cream" Sauce, 229

Green Curry Ramen with Eggplant & Green Beans, 181

Grilled Balsamic Mushroom Melts, 253

Kimchi & Cashew Fried Brown Rice, 133

Lazy-Day Dal with Butternut Squash & Kale, 309

Pesto Socca with Antipasti Salad, 318

Ratatouille Quinoa Bake, 163

Roasted Sweet Potatoes with Beans & Greens, 311

Smashed Chickpea Shakshuka with Summer Tomatoes, 306

Spanakopita Lasagna, 201

Spinach-Artichoke Dip Mac & Cheese, 173

Summer Squash Succotash Enchiladas, 285

Sides

All-Day Brothy Black Beans, 300

All-Day Brothy Chickpeas, 301

All-Day Brothy White Beans, 301

Braised Chickpeas & Broccolini with Golden Raisins, 323

Braised Coconut-Lime Sweet Potatoes & Bok Choy, 226

Braised Lemony Colcannon, 213

Brussels Sprouts & Wild Rice Salad with Maple Walnut-Pecan Spice Brittle, 139

Butternut Squash & Leek Stuffing, 259

Crab Cake Twice-Baked Potatoes, 223

French Lentil & Beet Salad with Garlicky Walnuts, 315

Gazpacho Rice & Bean Pilaf, 317

Grilled Romaine with Parmesan Pangritata & Caesar-ish Dressing, 255

Jalapeño, Pumpkin & Corn Pudding, 281

Kasha Pilaf with Mushrooms, Bacon & Greens, 162

Low-Sugar Sushi Rice, 121

Mexican Street Corn & Collard Greens Salad, 271

Millet & Zucchini Cakes, 145

Minty Green Rice Pilaf with Chiles & Peanuts, 134

Miso–Red Curry Black Rice with Kale & Delicata Squash, 120

Parsnip-Potato Latkes, 225

Roasted Cauliflower Salad with Quinoa, Arugula & Creamy Romesco Dressing, 146

Roasted Sweet Potatoes with Beans & Greens, 311

Smoky Cauliflower Wedges with Zesty Old Bay Breadcrumbs, 250

Stuffed Artichokes with Italian Stallion Breadcrumbs, 239

Sweet Potato & Cabbage Rosti with Kimchi Aioli, 231

Zucchini Skillet Cornbread, 275

Dessert

Apple-Cinnamon Baked French Toast, 264

Black Sesame–Buckwheat Banana Bread, 164

Ginger-Pear Cake with Oat Crumble, 109

PB & J Cups with Crunchy Quinoa, 167

Raspberry Lime Rickey Curd Tart, 111

Upside-Down Strawberry-Rhubarb Polenta Cake, 293

Violet's Big Blueberry-Oat Muffins, 103

Year-Round Fruit & Almond Crisp, 106

Sauces and Condiments

Arugula-Almond Pesto, 70

Basic Balsamic Vinaigrette, 60

Caesar-ish Dressing, 63

Charlie's Magic Grill Marinade, 71

Chipotle-Tahini Sauce, 68

Cilantro-Sriracha Mayo, 70

Creamy Caper Dressing, 61

Dill Aioli, 69

Ginger-Walnut Sauce, 66

Harissa Yogurt, 68

Kefir Green Goddess Dressing, 65

Lemon Poppy Vinaigrette, 64

Liquid Gold Turmeric-Tahini Dressing, 62

Low-Fructose BBQ Sauce, 67

Raspberry-Chia Jam, 73

Spicy Sesame Dressing, 60

Sugar-Free Ginger Applesauce, 72

Summer Tomato-Cashew Dressing, 59

Tarragon-Chive Tartar Sauce, 69

Toppings and Garnishes

Anise-y Pine Nut–Almond Crunch, 77

Italian Stallion Breadcrumbs, 239

Plain Jane Breadcrumbs, 237

Rosemary-Shallot Focaccia-Style Croutons, 241

Salty Sesame–Sunflower Gomasio, 75

Simple Sourdough Croutons, 240

Smoky Pumpkin-Hemp Sprinkles, 79

Za'atar Pita Chip–Style Croutons, 242

Zesty Old Bay Breadcrumbs, 238

Acknowledgments

The gestation period for this book overlapped with that of our first child, which meant that the editing process was very much caught in the crosshairs of new motherhood. I will always look back fondly on this chaotic juggling period, and am even more grateful to the patient and tenacious team that helped make this book a beautiful, well-punctuated masterpiece when my brain was nothing more than a well-scrambled egg.

A huge thank you to Sally Ekus for being the most hands-on agent, best gifter of gluten-free bagels, and a calm fielder of way too many panic texts.

To Renée Sedliar for joining me for the sequel, insisting that every recipe stay in, and advocating for a higher page count. My books are always better because of you. I am also so appreciative of the hard work of Melanie Gold, Nzinga Temu, and the rest of the Hachette Go team who helped make my vision for this book come to life and usher it into the world.

To Haley Hunt Davis and Ryan Norton for being a creative dream team, letting me take over your home for a full week, and agreeing to a jam-packed shoot schedule. I couldn't have asked for more gorgeous pictures or better people to spend time with in the kitchen.

To Erica Adler for always ironing out the kinks when a recipe isn't going my way, and the literal hundreds of members of the Carbivore recipe testing cohort that made these dishes during their nascency and sent invaluable feedback. I made so many changes thanks to your advice, and still can't believe the overwhelming outpouring of support when it came time to roll up your sleeves and cook these carbs.

Finally, to my family, for helping me carve out time to write, feed myself, and shower—sometimes all in one day! And especially to my husband, Charlie, and number one Carbivore, piglet. You both changed my life forever and nothing brings me more joy than watching you inhale a piece of sourdough.

Resources

Carbivore Symptom & Activity Tracker
CarbivoreCookbook.com

Blood Sugar Testing
Levels | LevelsHealth.com

Zoe | JoinZoe.com

Legumes
Heirloom Beans | Rancho Gordo | RanchoGordo.com

Oats
Gluten-Free Steel Cut Oats, Rolled Oats & Oat Flour | Bob's Red Mill | BobsRedMill.com

Ancient Grains
Buckwheat Groats & Roasted Kasha | Skvira | Amazon.com

Organic Whole Millet | Arrowhead Mills | ArrowheadMills.com

Quinoa | Ancient Harvest | AncientHarvest.com

Bread
Gluten-Free Sourdough | Bread Srsly | Breadsrsly.com

| Knead Love | Kneadlovebakerynyc.com

| Superbloom Bakery | SuperbloomBakery.com

Corn
Gluten-Free Yellow Corn Polenta | Bob's Red Mill | BobsRedMill.com

Heirloom Masa Harina | Masienda | Masienda.com

Organic Gluten-Free Yellow Cornmeal | Arrowhead Mills | ArrowheadMills.com

Pasta
Almond Flour Gnocchi & Lasagna Sheets | Cappello's | Cappellos.com

Brown Rice Penne, Fusilli & Spaghetti | Jovial Foods | JovialFoods.com

Buckwheat Soba Noodles | King Soba | KingSoba.com

Gluten-Free Lasagna Sheets & Linguine | Taste Republic | TasteRepublicGlutenFree.com

Gluten-Free Orzo Pasta | DeLallo | DeLallo.com

Millet & Brown Rice Ramen | Lotus Foods | LotusFoods.com

Organic Brown Pad Thai Rice Noodles | Lotus Foods | LotusFoods.com

Rice Vermicelli Noodles | Star Anise Foods | StarAniseFoods.com

Rice
Black Rice & Jade Rice | Lotus Foods | LotusFoods.com

Sprouted Brown GABA Rice | Koshihikari | Amazon.com

Sushi Rice | Nishiki | Ricenco.com

Wild Rice | Red Lake Nation Foods | RedLakeNationFoods.com

DIY CARBIVORE BLOOD SUGAR EXPERIMENTS

To get a clear read on how a meal affects your blood sugar, you must do the following:

1. Test the first meal of the day. You want your experiments to be done after fasting overnight. If using a continuous glucose monitor or other testing system, take your fasting glucose reading before beginning so you can see the change. Don't eat or drink anything before your meal.

2. Avoid exercise or activity for 2 hours before and after eating. As you learned, moving your muscles can affect blood sugar levels. Unless explicitly part of your experiment, stay sedentary.

3. Log your levels (or symptoms) 1 to 2 hours after a meal. This is when your highest blood sugar spike is likely to occur, since it takes insulin about an hour to enter the bloodstream in response to a meal.

4. Note any volatility throughout the day. Pay attention to how your blood sugar and symptoms change throughout the day. The tracker makes this easier to monitor and log.

Sample Experiments

Day 1: Simple Carbs
Choose a food item from the simple carbs and eat it for your first meal of the day.

Day 2: Carb Companions
Eat that same simple carb with the carb companion.

Day 3: Fiber First
Eat your carb companion first. Wait 10 minutes, then eat the simple carb.

Day 4: Moving After Your Meal
Eat your simple carb solo again, then go for a brisk 15-minute walk afterward.

Day 5: Caffeine on Empty Stomach
Enjoy your morning coffee or caffeinated tea on an empty stomach, followed by your simple carb.

Day 6: Water with Your Meal
Enjoy your simple carb and drink 8 ounces of water during your meal.

SIMPLE CARBS | CARB COMPANIONS

1 cup white rice + 1 medium avocado

1 cup pasta + 1 cup steamed broccoli, roasted carrots, or sautéed spinach

1 slice white toast + 2 tablespoons nut butter

1 cup oatmeal + 2 tablespoons nuts + ¼ cup full-fat plain yogurt

Notes

1. Lenoir, Magalie, et al. "Intense Sweetness Surpasses Cocaine Reward." PLOS One 8, no. 2 (August 2007): e698. doi:10.1371/journal.pone.0000698. www.ncbi.nlm.nih.gov/pmc/articles/PMC1931610/.

2. Lennerz, B. S., et al. "Effects of Dietary Glycemic Index on Brain Regions Related to Reward and Craving in Men." American Journal of Clinical Nutrition 98, no. 3 (September 2013): 641–647. doi:10.3945/ajcn.113.064113. https://pubmed.ncbi.nlm.nih.gov/23803881/.

3. Ebbeling, C. B., et al. "Effects of Dietary Composition on Energy Expenditure During Weight-Loss Maintenance." JAMA 307, no. 24 (June 2012): 2627–2634. doi:10.1001/jama.2012.6607. https://jamanetwork.com/journals/jama/fullarticle/1199154.

4. National Institute of Diabetes and Digestive and Kidney Diseases. "A Tale of Two Sugars—Fructose and Glucose Cause Differing Metabolic Effects." News Release, October 3, 2017. www.niddk.nih.gov/news/archive/2017/tale-two-sugars-fructose-glucose-cause-differing-metabolic-effects.

5. Chang, C. R., et al. "Restricting Carbohydrates at Breakfast Is Sufficient to Reduce 24-Hour Exposure to Postprandial Hyperglycemia and Improve Glycemic Variability." *American Journal of Clinical Nutrition* 109, no. 5 (May 2019): 1302–1309. doi:10.1093/ajcn/nqy261. www.ncbi.nlm.nih.gov/pmc/articles/PMC6499564/.

6. Suez, J., et al. "Artificial Sweeteners Induce Glucose Intolerance by Altering the Gut Microbiota." *Nature* 514, no. 7521 (October 2014): 181–186. doi:10.1038/nature13793. https://pubmed.ncbi.nlm.nih.gov/25231862/.

7. Pang, M. D., et al. "The Impact of Artificial Sweeteners on Body Weight Control and Glucose Homeostasis." *Frontiers in Nutrition* (January 2021): 598340. doi:10.3389/fnut.2020.598340. www.ncbi.nlm.nih.gov/pmc/articles/PMC7817779/.

8. Kim, Y., et al. "Combination of Erythritol and Fructose Increases Gastrointestinal Symptoms in Healthy Adults." *Nutrition Research* 31, no. 11 (November 2011): 836–841. doi:10.1016/j.nutres.2011.09.025. www.ncbi.nlm.nih.gov/pubmed/22118754.

9. Shukla, A. P., et al. "Food Order Has a Significant Impact on Postprandial Glucose and Insulin Levels." *Diabetes Care* 38, no. 7 (July 2015): e98–e99. doi:10.2337/dc15-0429. www.ncbi.nlm.nih.gov/pmc/articles/PMC4876745/.

10. Torsdottir, I., et al. "Effect on the Postprandial Glycaemic Level of the Addition of Water to a Meal Ingested by Healthy Subjects and Type 2 (Non-Insulin-Dependent) Diabetic Patients." *Diabetologia* 32, no. 4 (April 1989): 231–235. doi:10.1007/BF00285289. https://pubmed.ncbi.nlm.nih.gov/2759361/.

11. Smith, H. A., et al. "Glucose Control upon Waking Is Unaffected by Hourly Sleep Fragmentation during the Night, but Is Impaired by Morning Caffeinated Coffee." *British Journal of Nutrition* 124, no. 10 (November 2020): 1114–1120. doi:10.1017/S0007114520001865. https://pubmed.ncbi.nlm.nih.gov/32475359/.

12. Church, T. S., et al. "Effects of Aerobic and Resistance Training on Hemoglobin A1c Levels in Patients with Type 2 Diabetes: A Randomized Controlled Trial." *JAMA* 304, no. 20 (November 2010): 2253–2262. doi:10.1001/jama.2010.1710. https://pubmed.ncbi.nlm.nih.gov/21098771/.

13. Spiegel, K., et al. "Sleep Loss: A Novel Risk Factor for Insulin Resistance and Type 2 Diabetes." *Journal of Applied Physiology* 99, no. 5 (November 2005): 2008–2019. doi:10.1152/japplphysiol.00660.2005. https://pubmed.ncbi.nlm.nih.gov/16227462/.

14. Kuo, B., et al. "Genomic and Clinical Effects Associated with a Relaxation Response Mind-Body Intervention in Patients with Irritable Bowel Syndrome and Inflammatory Bowel Disease." *PLOS One* 10, no. 4 (2015): e0123861. https://doi.org/10.1371/journal.pone.0123861. https://journals.plos.org/plosone/article?id=10.1371/journal.pone.0123861. See also National Center for Complementary and Integrative Health, Selected Research Results. https://nccih.nih.gov/research/results/spotlight/031912.

15. World Health Organization. "IARC Monographs Evaluate Consumption of Red Meat and Processed Meat." News Release, October 26, 2016. www.iarc.fr/wp-content/uploads/2018/07/pr240_E.pdf.

16. Godman, Heidi. "Are Sprouted Grains More Nutritious Than Regular Whole Grains?" *Harvard Health*. www.health.harvard.edu/blog/sprouted-grains-nutritious-regular-whole-grains-2017110612692.

Index

Added Sugar Cheat Sheet, 20, 22
adrenaline, 34
agave, 25
alcohol, 21, 36
almond flour, 44
    Strawberry-Rhubarb Polenta Cake, 293
    Blueberry-Oat Muffins, 103
almond milk, 24, 29
    Carrot Cake Baked Oats, 96
    Ginger-Pear Cake, 109
    Lemon Poppy Overnight Oats, 95
almonds
    Anise-y Pine Nut–Almond Crunch, 77
    Arugula-Almond Pesto, 70
    Banana–Nut Crunch Granola, 91
    Basic Bitch Kale Salad, 85
    Spaghetti with Harissa Bolognese, 185
    Moroccan Chicken-Rice Casserole, 119
    Fruit & Almond Crisp, 106
anchovies, Caesar-ish Dressing, 63
antibiotics, 36
antimicrobials, 36
apples
    Apple-Cinnamon Baked French Toast, 264
    Basque Tuna Salad Tartines, 257
    Ginger Applesauce, 72
arborio rice, 117
    Oven Risotto, 128
    Moroccan Chicken-Rice Casserole, 119
artichokes
    Spinach-Artichoke Dip Mac & Cheese, 173
    Stuffed Artichokes, 261
artificial sweeteners, 25
arugula
    Arugula-Almond Pesto, 70
    Tricolore Salad, 82
    Gnocchi Primavera, 229
    Ham & Cheese Dutch Baby, 102
    Pesto Socca with Antipasti Salad, 318
    Prelude-to-Summer Rolls, 131
    Roasted Cauliflower Salad, 146
    Seared Tuna Niçoise-ish Salad, 215
    Chicken BLT Panzanella, 243
asparagus
    Eggs Mimosa Pasta Salad, 191
    Oven Risotto, 128
    Prelude-to-Summer Rolls, 131
    Spring Potato-Leek Soup, 209
autoimmune diseases, ix, x, 7, 14

avocados
    Basic Bitch Kale Salad, 85
    Crispy Rice with Spicy Beet Tartare, 125
    Kefir Green Goddess Dressing, 65
    Prelude-to-Summer Rolls, 131
    Savory Yogurt & Granola Bowls, 94
    Seedy "Avocado Toast" Arepas, 282
    Simplest Poke Bowls, 123

bacon
    Kasha Pilaf, 162
    Chicken BLT Panzanella, 243
balsamic vinegar
    Basic Balsamic Vinaigrette, 60
    Charlie's Magic Grill Marinade, 71
    Grilled Balsamic Mushroom Melts, 253
bananas
    Banana–Nut Crunch Granola, 91
    Black Sesame–Buckwheat Banana Bread, 164
basil
    Chicken BLT Panzanella, 243
    Cod & Orzo Arrabbiata, 178
    Crispy Polenta Cakes, 272
    Eggs Mimosa Pasta Salad, 191
    French Lentil & Beet Salad, 315
    Gnocchi Primavera, 229
    Grilled Romaine with Parmesan Pangritata, 255
    Grilled Steak & Vermicelli Bowls, 198
    Italian Stallion Breadcrumbs, 239
    Kefir Green Goddess Dressing, 65
    Prelude-to-Summer Rolls, 131
    Ratatouille Quinoa Bake, 163
    Sausage & Greens Minestrone, 312
beans, about, 51, 298–99
bedtime and eating schedule, 33
beef
    Chili con Carne Shepherd's Pie, 217
    Grilled Skirt Steak & Vermicelli Bowls, 198
    Spaghetti with Harissa Bolognese, 185
    Spicy Beef Tagine, 220
beets
    Crispy Rice with Spicy Beet Tartare, 125
    French Lentil & Beet Salad, 315
bell peppers
    Cajun Pork Tenderloin with Grits, 279
    Gazpacho Rice & Bean Pilaf, 317
    Green Curry Ramen, 181
    Egg Roll Noodles, 175

    Minty Green Rice Pilaf, 134
    Muhammara Roasted Red Pepper Dip, 246
    Quinoa Paella with Sausage & Shrimp, 151
    Ratatouille Quinoa Bake, 163
    Roasted Cauliflower Salad, 146
    Smashed Chickpea Shakshuka, 306
    Spaghetti with Harissa Bolognese, 185
beverages
    skipping sweetened, 24
    sugar-free homemade ideas, 24
black or forbidden rice, 47, 116
    Miso–Red Curry Black Rice, 120
black beans, 298
    All-Day Brothy Black Beans, 300
    Chili con Carne Shepherd's Pie, 217
    Gazpacho Rice & Bean Pilaf, 317
    Roasted Sweet Potatoes with Beans & Greens, 311
black-eyed peas, 298
    BBQ Chicken Thighs, 303
blood sugar, x, 2, 10–14, 15–16, 37
    DIY carbivore blood sugar experiments, 331
    eating speed and, 27–28
    sleep and, 32–33
blueberries
    Blueberry-Oat Muffins, 103
    Fruit & Almond Crisp, 106
bok choy
    Braised Coconut-Lime Sweet Potatoes & Bok Choy, 226
    Ginger-Scallion Chicken Soba Noodle Soup, 196
    Oat Congee with Bok Choy, 99
brain and sugar, 9–10
bread
    about, 49–50
    Apple-Cinnamon Baked French Toast, 264
    Basque Tuna Salad Tartines, 257
    Butternut Squash & Leek Stuffing, 259
    Ginger-Salmon Burgers, 249
    Greenhouse Gazpacho, 256
    Grilled Balsamic Mushroom Melts, 253
    Grilled Romaine with Parmesan Pangritata, 255
    Italian Stallion Breadcrumbs, 239
    Muhammara Roasted Red Pepper Dip, 246
    Pepperoni Pizza, 262

Plain Jane Breadcrumbs, 237
Rosemary-Shallot Focaccia-Style
  Croutons, 241
Chicken BLT Panzanella, 243
Smoky Cauliflower Wedges, 250
sourdough, 43, 49
Stuffed Artichokes, 261
Za'atar Pita Chip–Style Croutons, 242
Zesty Old Bay Breadcrumbs, 238
breakfasts
  empty stomach and sugar, 23
  fiber in, 27
  savory, slow carb, 23
broccoli, **broccolini**, or **broccoli rabe**
  Braised Chickpeas & Broccolini, 323
  Salmon & Broccoli Noodle Casserole,
    188
  Sausage & Greens Minestrone, 312
  Fall Reset Soup, 160
brown rice, 46–47, 116
  Kimchi & Cashew Fried Brown Rice,
    133
Brussels sprouts
  Brussels Sprouts & Sweet Potato
    Hash, 212
  Brussels Sprouts & Wild Rice Salad,
    139
buckwheat, 46, 48, 142
  Black Sesame–Buckwheat Banana
    Bread, 164
  Buckwheat Crepes, 149
  Kasha Pilaf, 162
butternut squash
  Butternut Squash & Leek Stuffing,
    259
  Lazy-Day Dal, 309

cabbage
  Fish Tacos with Ginger-Mango Slaw,
    291
  Braised Lemony Colcannon, 213
  Egg Roll Noodles, 175
  Kimchi & Cashew Fried Brown Rice,
    133
  Peanut & Lime Slaw, 83
  Simplest Poke Bowls, 123
  Sweet Potato & Cabbage Rosti, 231
  Mushroom & Wild Rice Soup, 127
caffeine, 21, 25
  on empty stomach, 31, 36, 331
capers
  Creamy Caper Dressing, 61
  Provençal Chicken Thighs & Slivered
    Potatoes, 207
  Smoky Cauliflower Wedges, 250
  Tarragon-Chive Tartar Sauce, 69
carb (carbohydrates), 2
  anatomy of, 4–5
  healthy relationship with, ix–x

measuring tolerance, 15–16
problem with cutting all, 16–17
carb companions, 2, 331
  adding to meal, 28
  dessert with, 44
  go-to, 29
  nuts and seeds, 42
Carbivore Symptom & Activity Tracker,
  19, 34, 330
carrots, 31
  Carrot Cake Baked Oats, 96
  Grilled Skirt Steak & Vermicelli Bowls,
    198
  Egg Roll Noodles, 175
  Peanut & Lime Slaw, 83
  Moroccan Chicken-Rice Casserole, 119
  Fall Reset Soup, 160
cashews
  Egg Roll Noodles, 175
  Kimchi & Cashew Fried Brown Rice,
    133
  Summer Squash Succotash
    Enchiladas, 285
  Summer Tomato-Cashew Dressing, 59
  Tangy Peanut-Cashew Crunch, 76
cauliflower
  Roasted Cauliflower Salad, 146
  Smoky Cauliflower Wedges, 250
celiac disease, 37, 43, 45, 88
chard
  BBQ Chicken Thighs, 303
  Cod & Orzo Arrabbiata, 178
  Kasha Pilaf, 162
  Quinoa Paella with Sausage & Shrimp,
    151
  Roasted Sweet Potatoes with Beans
    & Greens, 311
  Sausage & Greens Minestrone, 312
cheddar
  Chili con Carne Shepherd's Pie, 217
  Grilled Balsamic Mushroom Melts, 253
  Spinach-Artichoke Dip Mac & Cheese,
    173
  Summer Squash Succotash
    Enchiladas, 285
cheese. *See specific cheeses*
chia seeds
  Lemon Poppy Overnight Oats, 95
  Raspberry-Chia Jam, 73
  Seed Cracker Granola, 92
chicken
  BBQ Chicken Thighs, 303
  Chicken Satay Meatballs, 155
  Chicken Tinga Stew, 288
  Ginger-Scallion Chicken Soba Noodle
    Soup, 196
  Hemp-Crusted Chicken Tenders with
    Dill Aioli, 136
  Egg Roll Noodles, 175

Provençal Chicken Thighs & Slivered
  Potatoes, 207
Chicken BLT Panzanella, 243
Moroccan Chicken-Rice Casserole, 119
chickpea flour, 299
  Pesto Socca with Antipasti Salad, 318
chickpeas (garbanzo beans), 299
  All-Day Brothy Chickpeas, 301
  Braised Chickpeas & Broccolini, 323
  Smashed Chickpea Shakshuka, 306
  Moroccan Chicken-Rice Casserole, 119
chipotle chiles
  Chicken Tinga Stew, 288
  Chipotle-Tahini Sauce, 68
chives
  Basque Tuna Salad Tartines, 257
  Creamless Corn & Shrimp Chowder,
    277
  Eggs Mimosa Pasta Salad, 191
  Ham & Cheese Dutch Baby, 102
  Kefir Green Goddess Dressing, 65
  Mushroom & Wild Rice Soup, 127
  Oven Risotto, 128
  Sausage & Greens Minestrone, 312
  Tarragon-Chive Tartar Sauce, 69
chocolate
  PB & J Cups, 167
  using higher percentage of cacao, 44
cilantro
  Chicken Satay Meatballs, 155
  Chicken Tinga Stew, 288
  Chili con Carne Shepherd's Pie, 217
  Cilantro-Sriracha Mayo, 70
  Fall Reset Soup, 160
  Fish Tacos with Ginger-Mango Slaw,
    291
  Gazpacho Rice & Bean Pilaf, 317
  Green Curry Ramen, 181
  Grilled Skirt Steak & Vermicelli Bowls,
    198
  Lazy-Day Dal, 309
  Mexican Street Corn & Collard Greens
    Salad, 271
  Minty Green Rice Pilaf, 134
  Miso–Red Curry Black Rice, 120
  Simplest Poke Bowls, 123
  Smashed Chickpea Shakshuka, 306
  Summer Squash Succotash
    Enchiladas, 285
  Zucchini Skillet Cornbread, 275
clams or **clam juice**
  Creamless Corn & Shrimp Chowder,
    277
  Linguine with Chorizo, Clams & Kale,
    193
coconut, shredded
  Banana–Nut Crunch Granola, 91
  Tangy Peanut-Cashew Crunch, 76
  Fruit & Almond Crisp, 106

Index

coconut milk
Apple-Cinnamon Baked French Toast, 264
Braised Coconut-Lime Sweet Potatoes & Bok Choy, 226
Chicken Satay Meatballs, 155
Creamless Corn & Shrimp Chowder, 277
Crispy Polenta Cakes, 272
Green Curry Ramen, 181
Lazy-Day Dal, 309
Salmon & Broccoli Noodle Casserole, 188
Fall Reset Soup, 160

collard greens
BBQ Chicken Thighs, 303
Mexican Street Corn & Collard Greens Salad, 271
Pepperoni Pizza, 262
Quinoa Paella with Sausage & Shrimp, 151
Sausage & Greens Minestrone, 312
continuous glucose monitors (CGMs), 2, 16, 19, 32

corn
about, 49–50, 268–69
Creamless Corn & Shrimp Chowder, 277
Jalapeño, Pumpkin & Corn Pudding, 281
Mexican Street Corn & Collard Greens Salad, 271
Summer Squash Succotash Enchiladas, 285
Zucchini Skillet Cornbread, 275
cornmeal, 269
Jalapeño, Pumpkin & Corn Pudding, 281
Zucchini Skillet Cornbread, 275
cortisol, 17, 34

cucumbers
Creamy Sesame Noodle Salad, 183
Gazpacho Rice & Bean Pilaf, 317
Greenhouse Gazpacho, 256
Chicken BLT Panzanella, 243
Simplest Poke Bowls, 123

curry paste
Green Curry Ramen, 181
Miso–Red Curry Black Rice, 120

dairy, full-fat, 43
deep belly breathing, 35
diabetes, x, 7, 10, 12, 14, 16, 37
digestive system, 11, 14, 15, 31
dill
Braised Lemony Colcannon, 213
Buckwheat Crepes, 149
Dill Aioli, 69
Eggs Mimosa Pasta Salad, 191

Grilled Romaine with Parmesan Pangritata, 255
Kasha Pilaf, 162
Kefir Green Goddess Dressing, 65
Sausage & Greens Minestrone, 312
Spanakopita Lasagna, 201
distractions, 28, 33, 35
drinking water, 31, 36, 331

eggplant
Crispy Polenta Cakes, 272
Green Curry Ramen, 181
Ratatouille Quinoa Bake, 163
eggs
Apple-Cinnamon Baked French Toast, 264
Brussels Sprouts & Sweet Potato Hash, 212
Buckwheat Crepes, 149
Eggs Mimosa Pasta Salad, 191
Ham & Cheese Dutch Baby, 102
hard boiled, for snacking, 31
Kimchi & Cashew Fried Brown Rice, 133
Savory Yogurt & Granola Bowls, 94
Smashed Chickpea Shakshuka, 306
Oat Congee with Bok Choy, 99
empty stomach
caffeine on, 31, 36, 331
consuming sugar on, 22–23
estrogen, 14, 34
exercise, 10, 32, 331

fasting glucose, 2, 10–11
fennel
Seared Scallops with White Beans, 321
Spring Potato-Leek Soup, 209
fennel seeds
Anise-y Pine Nut–Almond Crunch, 77
Italian Stallion Breadcrumbs, 239
feta, Spanakopita Lasagna, 201
fiber, 5, 8, 15, 331
eating first, 26–27
peeling vegetables and, 41
fish
Fish Tacos with Ginger-Mango Slaw, 291
Basque Tuna Salad Tartines, 257
Buckwheat Crepes, 149
Cod & Orzo Arrabbiata, 178
Ginger-Salmon Burgers, 249
Mom's Millet Flour Fish Fry, 159
Salmon & Broccoli Noodle Casserole, 188
Seared Tuna Niçoise-ish Salad, 215
Simplest Poke Bowls, 123
five-day sugar break, 21
FODMAP, 2, 25, 52–53

fructose, 4, 12, 25
fruit juices, 8, 20, 24

ginger
Fish Tacos with Ginger-Mango Slaw, 291
Ginger-Pear Cake, 109
Ginger-Salmon Burgers, 249
Ginger-Scallion Chicken Soba Noodle Soup, 196
Ginger-Walnut Sauce, 66
Ginger Applesauce, 72
glucose, 4, 10–11
glucose intolerance, 25, 33
glucose spikes, 3, 15–16, 26, 37
gluten-free, ix, xiii, 39, 43, 45, 48, 49, 52
glycemic index, 3, 25
Gouda, Ham & Cheese Dutch Baby, 102
grains, soaking and sprouting, 42
green beans (or haricots verts)
Green Curry Ramen, 181
Minty Green Rice Pilaf, 134
Prelude-to-Summer Rolls, 131
Seared Tuna Niçoise-ish Salad, 215
gut microbiome. *See* microbiome

harissa
Harissa Yogurt, 68
Smashed Chickpea Shakshuka, 306
Spaghetti with Harissa Bolognese, 185
Spicy Beef Tagine, 220
headaches, 14, 21
hemp seeds
Hemp-Crusted Chicken Tenders with Dill Aioli, 136
Seed Cracker Granola, 92
Seedy "Avocado Toast" Arepas, 282
Smoky Pumpkin-Hemp Sprinkles, 79
high fructose corn syrup, 3, 25
hominy, 269
Chicken Tinga Stew, 288
hydration, 31, 36, 331
hypoglycemia, 3

IBS (irritable bowel syndrome), 2, 14, 25, 35, 37, 49, 52–53
inflammation, 12–14, 37
ingredient labels
how to read, 22
sugar on, 8, 20, 22
insulin, 3, 11–12, 14, 34
insulin resistance, 7, 49
intermittent fasting, 30

kale
Fish Tacos with Ginger-Mango Slaw, 291
Basic Bitch Kale Salad, 85

Butternut Squash & Leek Stuffing, 259
Chicken Tinga Stew, 288
Lazy-Day Dal, 309
Linguine with Chorizo, Clams & Kale, 193
Miso–Red Curry Black Rice, 120
Sausage & Greens Minestrone, 312
kasha, Kasha Pilaf, 162
kefir, Kefir Green Goddess Dressing, 65
keto diet, x, 16–17
keto insomnia, 33
kimchi
Kimchi & Cashew Fried Brown Rice, 133
Sweet Potato & Cabbage Rosti, 231
kombucha, 24

leaky gut syndrome, 14, 25, 51
leeks
Buckwheat Crepes, 149
Butternut Squash & Leek Stuffing, 259
Creamless Corn & Shrimp Chowder, 277
Parsnip-Potato Latkes, 225
Salmon & Broccoli Noodle Casserole, 188
Spring Potato-Leek Soup, 209
legumes. *See also specific legumes*
about, 51, 298–99
lemons
Braised Lemony Colcannon, 213
Creamy Caper Dressing, 61
Gnocchi Primavera, 229
Lemon Poppy Overnight Oats, 95
Lemon Poppy Vinaigrette, 64
Turmeric-Tahini Dressing, 62
lentils, 51, 298
French Lentil & Beet Salad, 315
Lazy-Day Dal, 309
lettuces
Big Leaf Lettuces with Summer Tomato-Cashew Dressing, 81
Grilled Skirt Steak & Vermicelli Bowls, 198
limes
Braised Coconut-Lime Sweet Potatoes & Bok Choy, 226
Chipotle-Tahini Sauce, 68
Grilled Skirt Steak & Vermicelli Bowls, 198
Peanut & Lime Slaw, 83
Raspberry Lime Rickey Curd Tart, 111
Tangy Peanut-Cashew Crunch, 76
liver, 11, 12–13, 14

magnesium, 33
mangoes, Fish Tacos with Ginger-Mango Slaw, 291

masa harina, 269
Seedy "Avocado Toast" Arepas, 282
mayonnaise
Cilantro-Sriracha Mayo, 70
Dill Aioli, 69
Tarragon-Chive Tartar Sauce, 69
meditation, 35
menstrual cycle and diet, 34
metabolism, 3, 12
microbiome, 3
fiber and, 5
sugars and, 25, 35
supporting, 35–36
migrating motor complex (MMC), 30
millet, 46, 142
Millet & Zucchini Cakes, 145
Mom's Millet Flour Fish Fry, 159
Seed Cracker Granola, 92
mindful eating, 27–28
mint
Grilled Skirt Steak & Vermicelli Bowls, 198
Harissa Yogurt, 68
Kefir Green Goddess Dressing, 65
Millet & Zucchini Cakes, 145
Minty Green Rice Pilaf, 134
Peanut & Lime Slaw, 83
Prelude-to-Summer Rolls, 131
Spaghetti with Harissa Bolognese, 185
Spanakopita Lasagna, 201
miso paste, Miso–Red Curry Black Rice, 120
mozzarella
Grilled Balsamic Mushroom Melts, 253
Pepperoni Pizza, 262
Ratatouille Quinoa Bake, 163
Spanakopita Lasagna, 201
mushrooms
Grilled Balsamic Mushroom Melts, 253
Kasha Pilaf, 162
Salmon & Broccoli Noodle Casserole, 188
Oat Congee with Bok Choy, 99
Mushroom & Wild Rice Soup, 127

natural sweeteners, 25
noodles
Cod & Orzo Arrabbiata, 178
Creamy Sesame Noodle Salad, 183
Eggs Mimosa Pasta Salad, 191
Ginger-Scallion Chicken Soba Noodle Soup, 196
Green Curry Ramen, 181
Grilled Skirt Steak & Vermicelli Bowls, 198
Egg Roll Noodles, 175
Linguine with Chorizo, Clams & Kale, 193

Salmon & Broccoli Noodle Casserole, 188
Spaghetti with Harissa Bolognese, 185
Spanakopita Lasagna, 201
Spinach-Artichoke Dip Mac & Cheese, 173
nut crunches, 42, 75–76
nutritional ketosis, 17

oat flour, 89
Black Sesame–Buckwheat Banana Bread, 164
Ginger-Pear Cake, 109
Ham & Cheese Dutch Baby, 102
Raspberry Lime Rickey Curd Tart, 111
Blueberry-Oat Muffins, 103
oat milk, 43, 89
Ginger-Pear Cake, 109
oats, 45, 88–89
Banana–Nut Crunch Granola, 91
Carrot Cake Baked Oats, 96
Dijon Turkey Meat Loaf with Spinach, 101
Ginger-Pear Cake, 109
Lemon Poppy Overnight Oats, 95
Savory Yogurt & Granola Bowls, 94
Seed Cracker Granola, 92
Oat Congee with Bok Choy, 99
Blueberry-Oat Muffins, 103
Fruit & Almond Crisp, 106
olives
Provençal Chicken Thighs & Slivered Potatoes, 207
Pesto Socca with Antipasti Salad, 318
Seared Tuna Niçoise-ish Salad, 215

paleo diet, ix, 52
parmesan
Grilled Romaine with Parmesan Pangritata, 255
Spinach-Artichoke Dip Mac & Cheese, 173
parsley
Creamy Caper Dressing, 61
Eggs Mimosa Pasta Salad, 191
Gazpacho Rice & Bean Pilaf, 317
Kefir Green Goddess Dressing, 65
Linguine with Chorizo, Clams & Kale, 193
Sausage & Greens Minestrone, 312
Spanakopita Lasagna, 201
parsnips
Parsnip-Potato Latkes, 225
Fall Reset Soup, 160
pasta, 48
Eggs Mimosa Pasta Salad, 191
Linguine with Chorizo, Clams & Kale, 193
resources, 330

Salmon & Broccoli Noodle Casserole, 188

Spaghetti with Harissa Bolognese, 185

Spinach-Artichoke Dip Mac & Cheese, 173

substitutions for paleo diet, 52

PCOS (polycystic ovary syndrome), x, 12, 14

peanut butter
Chicken Satay Meatballs, 155
PB & J Cups, 167

peanuts
Minty Green Rice Pilaf, 134
Peanut & Lime Slaw, 83
Tangy Peanut-Cashew Crunch, 76

pecans
Apple-Cinnamon Baked French Toast, 264
Banana–Nut Crunch Granola, 91
Maple Walnut–Pecan Spice Brittle, 78

perfectionism myth, 37

perioral dermatitis, 12–13

pesticides, 36, 50

pine nuts, Anise-y Pine Nut–Almond Crunch, 77

pistachios
Spicy Beef Tagine, 220
Strawberry-Rhubarb Polenta Cake, 293

polenta or **grits**, 51, 268
Cajun Pork Tenderloin with Grits, 279
Crispy Polenta Cakes, 272
Strawberry-Rhubarb Polenta Cake, 293

pomegranate
Brussels Sprouts & Wild Rice Salad, 139
Muhammara Roasted Red Pepper Dip, 246

poppy seeds
Everything Bagel Granola, 92
Lemon Poppy Overnight Oats, 95
Lemon Poppy Vinaigrette, 64

pork
Cajun Pork Tenderloin with Grits, 279
Eggs Mimosa Pasta Salad, 191
Ham & Cheese Dutch Baby, 102
Egg Roll Noodles, 175
Kasha Pilaf, 162
Chicken BLT Panzanella, 243

potatoes
about, 48–49, 204–5
Braised Lemony Colcannon, 213
Crab Cake Twice-Baked Potatoes, 223
Creamless Corn & Shrimp Chowder, 277
Provençal Chicken Thighs & Slivered Potatoes, 207
Parsnip-Potato Latkes, 225

Seared Tuna Niçoise-ish Salad, 215

Spring Potato-Leek Soup, 209

potato starch, 49

processed deli meats, 37, 40

processed foods, 29, 48

progesterone, 34

pumpkin
Jalapeño, Pumpkin & Corn Pudding, 281
Fall Reset Soup, 160

pumpkin seeds
Miso–Red Curry Black Rice, 120
Seed Cracker Granola, 92
Smoky Pumpkin-Hemp Sprinkles, 79

quinoa, 46, 143
Chicken Satay Meatballs, 155
PB & J Cups, 167
Quinoa Paella with Sausage & Shrimp, 151
Ratatouille Quinoa Bake, 163
Roasted Cauliflower Salad, 146
Seed Cracker Granola, 92
Fall Reset Soup, 160

radicchio
Tricolore Salad, 82
Gnocchi Primavera, 229
Pesto Socca with Antipasti Salad, 318
Seared Tuna Niçoise-ish Salad, 215

radishes
French Lentil & Beet Salad, 315
Ginger-Salmon Burgers, 249
Grilled Skirt Steak & Vermicelli Bowls, 198
Prelude-to-Summer Rolls, 131
Seedy "Avocado Toast" Arepas, 282

raisins
Braised Chickpeas & Broccolini, 323
Carrot Cake Baked Oats, 96
Crispy Polenta Cakes, 272
Roasted Cauliflower Salad, 146

raspberries
Raspberry-Chia Jam, 73
Raspberry Lime Rickey Curd Tart, 111

resistant starches, xii, 3, 41, 51

rhubarb, Strawberry-Rhubarb Polenta Cake, 293

rice
about, 45–46, 116–17
Brussels Sprouts & Wild Rice Salad, 139
Crispy Rice with Spicy Beet Tartare, 125
Gazpacho Rice & Bean Pilaf, 317
Kimchi & Cashew Fried Brown Rice, 133
Low-Sugar Sushi Rice, 121
Minty Green Rice Pilaf, 134

Miso–Red Curry Black Rice, 120
Oven Risotto, 128
Prelude-to-Summer Rolls, 131
Simplest Poke Bowls, 123
substitutions for paleo diet, 52
Moroccan Chicken-Rice Casserole, 119
Mushroom & Wild Rice Soup, 127

rice flour, **brown or white**
Buckwheat Crepes, 149
Ham & Cheese Dutch Baby, 102
Parsnip-Potato Latkes, 225
Raspberry Lime Rickey Curd Tart, 111
Sweet Potato & Cabbage Rosti, 231
Zucchini Skillet Cornbread, 275

rice noodles
Creamy Sesame Noodle Salad, 183
Green Curry Ramen, 181
Grilled Skirt Steak & Vermicelli Bowls, 198
Egg Roll Noodles, 175

ricotta, Pesto Socca with Antipasti Salad, 318

romaine
Tricolore Salad, 82
Grilled Romaine with Parmesan Pangritata, 255

rosemary
French Onion White Bean Dip, 305
Rosemary-Shallot Focaccia-Style Croutons, 241
Spicy Beef Tagine, 220

saliva, 27–28, 31

salmon
Buckwheat Crepes, 149
Ginger-Salmon Burgers, 249
Salmon & Broccoli Noodle Casserole, 188
Simplest Poke Bowls, 123

sausage
Linguine with Chorizo, Clams & Kale, 193
Quinoa Paella with Sausage & Shrimp, 151
Sausage & Greens Minestrone, 312

savory versus sweet, 19–20

seafood
Crab Cake Twice-Baked Potatoes, 223
Creamless Corn & Shrimp Chowder, 277
Linguine with Chorizo, Clams & Kale, 193
Seared Scallops with White Beans, 321

seed sprinkles, 42, 75, 79

sesame seeds
Black Sesame–Buckwheat Banana Bread, 164

Creamy Sesame Noodle Salad, 183
Everything Bagel Granola, 92
Salty Sesame-Sunflower Gomasio, 75

shrimp
Creamless Corn & Shrimp Chowder, 277
Oven Risotto, 128
Quinoa Paella with Sausage & Shrimp, 151

SIBO (small intestinal bacterial overgrowth), ix, 3, 14, 52–53
SIBO Made Simple (Lapine), xiii, 175
skin problems, 12–14
sleep, 32–33
slow carbs, xiii, 3, 14–15, 23, 26–31
smoothies, 24
key strategies to fortify, 30
snacks (snacking), 30
blood sugar–friendly, 31

soba noodles, Ginger-Scallion Chicken Soba Noodle Soup, 196

spinach
Dijon Turkey Meat Loaf with Spinach, 101
Greenhouse Gazpacho, 256
Spanakopita Lasagna, 201
Spinach-Artichoke Dip Mac & Cheese, 173
sprouting grains, 42, 49

squash
Butternut Squash & Leek Stuffing, 259
Cajun Pork Tenderloin with Grits, 279
Lazy-Day Dal, 309
Miso–Red Curry Black Rice, 120
Ratatouille Quinoa Bake, 163
Summer Squash Succotash Enchiladas, 285

stevia, 25

strawberries
Upside-Down Strawberry-Rhubarb Polenta Cake, 293
Fruit & Almond Crisp, 106

strength training, 32
stress management, 34–35
sucrose, 5, 25
sugar
about, 7–15
Added Sugar Cheat Sheet, 20, 22
addiction to, 9–10
measuring carb tolerance, 15–16
sugar reduction, 19–37

sugar snap peas
French Lentil & Beet Salad, 315

Prelude-to-Summer Rolls with Ginger-Walnut Sauce, 131

sunflower seeds
Gnocchi Primavera, 229
Salty Sesame-Sunflower Gomasio, 75
Seed Cracker Granola, 92

sunlight in the morning, 33

sweet peas
Gnocchi Primavera, 229
Ham & Cheese Dutch Baby, 102
Oven Risotto, 128

sweet potatoes, 205
Braised Coconut-Lime Sweet Potatoes & Bok Choy, 226
Brussels Sprouts & Sweet Potato Hash, 212
Chili con Carne Shepherd's Pie, 217
Roasted Sweet Potatoes with Beans & Greens, 311
Spicy Beef Tagine, 220
Sweet Potato & Cabbage Rosti, 231

tahini
Chipotle-Tahini Sauce, 68
Turmeric-Tahini Dressing, 62
Spicy Sesame Dressing, 60

tarragon
Buckwheat Crepes, 149
Grilled Romaine with Parmesan Pangritata, 255
Tarragon-Chive Tartar Sauce, 69

taste buds and sugar, 9–10
testosterone, 14

tomatoes
Cajun Pork Tenderloin with Grits, 279
Chicken Tinga Stew, 288
Cod & Orzo Arrabbiata, 178
Crispy Polenta Cakes, 272
Gazpacho Rice & Bean Pilaf, 317
Greenhouse Gazpacho, 256
Lazy-Day Dal, 309
Quinoa Paella with Sausage & Shrimp, 151
Ratatouille Quinoa Bake, 163
Chicken BLT Panzanella, 243
Smashed Chickpea Shakshuka, 306
Spicy Beef Tagine, 220
Summer Squash Succotash Enchiladas, 285
Summer Tomato-Cashew Dressing, 59

tomatoes, sun-dried
Provençal Chicken Thighs & Slivered Potatoes, 207
Pesto Socca with Antipasti Salad, 318

Rosemary-Shallot Focaccia-Style Croutons, 241

tomato sauce
Low-Fructose BBQ Sauce, 67
Pepperoni Pizza, 262
Summer Squash Succotash Enchiladas, 285

tuna
Basque Tuna Salad Tartines, 257
Seared Tuna Niçoise-ish Salad, 215
Simplest Poke Bowls, 123

turkey
Chili con Carne Shepherd's Pie, 217
Dijon Turkey Meat Loaf with Spinach, 101
Egg Roll Noodles, 175

vinegar, 24, 41–42

walnuts
Banana–Nut Crunch Granola, 91
Carrot Cake Baked Oats, 96
French Lentil & Beet Salad, 315
Ginger-Walnut Sauce, 66
Maple Walnut–Pecan Spice Brittle, 78
Muhammara Roasted Red Pepper Dip, 246
Wellness Project, The (Lapine), 12–13, 65

white beans, 298
All-Day Brothy White Beans, 301
French Onion White Bean Dip, 305
Sausage & Greens Minestrone, 312
Seared Scallops with White Beans, 321

wild rice, 46, 116
Brussels Sprouts & Wild Rice Salad, 139
Mushroom & Wild Rice Soup, 127

yoga, 35

yogurt
Harissa Yogurt, 68
Lemon Poppy Overnight Oats, 95
Savory Yogurt & Granola Bowls, 94
Spanakopita Lasagna, 201

zucchini
Cajun Pork Tenderloin with Grits, 279
Green Curry Ramen, 181
Millet & Zucchini Cakes, 145
Ratatouille Quinoa Bake, 163
Summer Squash Succotash Enchiladas, 285
Zucchini Skillet Cornbread, 275

Index